Working Dogs: An Update for Veterinarians

Editors

MAUREEN A. MCMICHAEL
MELISSA SINGLETARY

VETERINARY CLINICS OF NORTH AMERICA: SMALL ANIMAL PRACTICE

www.vetsmall.theclinics.com

July 2021 • Volume 51 • Number 4

ELSEVIER

1600 John F. Kennedy Boulevard • Suite 1800 • Philadelphia, Pennsylvania, 19103-2899
http://www.vetsmall.theclinics.com

VETERINARY CLINICS OF NORTH AMERICA: SMALL ANIMAL PRACTICE Volume 51, Number 4
July 2021 ISSN 0195-5616, ISBN-13: 978-0-323-79112-0

Editor: Stacy Eastman
Developmental Editor: Axell Purificacion

Photocopying

Single photocopies of single articles may be made for personal use as allowed by national copyright laws. Permission of the Publisher and payment of a fee is required for all other photocopying, including multiple or systematic copying, copying for advertising or promotional purposes, resale, and all forms of document delivery. Special rates are available for educational institutions that wish to make photocopies for non-profit educational classroom use. For information on how to seek permission visit www.elsevier.com/permissions or call: (+44) 1865 843830 (UK)/(+1) 215 239 3804 (USA).

Derivative Works

Subscribers may reproduce tables of contents or prepare lists of articles including abstracts for internal circulation within their institutions. Permission of the Publisher is required for resale or distribution outside the institution. Permission of the Publisher is required for all other derivative works, including compilations and translations (please consult www.elsevier.com/permissions).

Electronic Storage or Usage

Permission of the Publisher is required to store or use electronically any material contained in this periodical, including any article or part of an article (please consult www.elsevier.com/permissions). Except as outlined above, no part of this publication may be reproduced, stored in a retrieval system or transmitted in any form or by any means, electronic, mechanical, photocopying, recording or otherwise, without prior written permission of the Publisher.

Notice

No responsibility is assumed by the Publisher for any injury and/or damage to persons or property as a matter of products liability, negligence or otherwise, or from any use or operation of any methods, products, instructions or ideas contained in the material herein. Because of rapid advances in the medical sciences, in particular, independent verification of diagnoses and drug dosages should be made.

Although all advertising material is expected to conform to ethical (medical) standards, inclusion in this publication does not constitute a guarantee or endorsement of the quality or value of such product or of the claims made of it by its manufacturer.

Veterinary Clinics of North America: Small Animal Practice (ISSN 0195-5616) is published bimonthly by Elsevier Inc., 360 Park Avenue South, New York, NY 10010-1710. Months of issue are January, March, May, July, September, and November. Business and Editorial Offices: 1600 John F. Kennedy Blvd., Ste. 1800, Philadelphia, PA 19103-2899. Customer Service Office: 3251 Riverport Lane, Maryland Heights, MO 63043. Periodicals postage paid at New York, NY and additional mailing offices. Subscription prices are $358.00 per year (domestic individuals), $933.00 per year (domestic institutions), $100.00 per year (domestic students/residents), $451.00 per year (Canadian individuals), $998.00 per year (Canadian institutions), $488.00 per year (international individuals), $998.00 per year (international institutions), $100.00 per year (Canadian students/residents), and $220.00 per year (international students/residents). To receive student/resident rate, orders must be accompanied by name of affiliated institution, date of term, and the *signature* of program/residency coordinator on institution letterhead. Orders will be billed at individual rate until proof of status is received. Foreign air speed delivery is included in all *Clinics* subscription prices. All prices are subject to change without notice. **POSTMASTER:** Send address changes to *Veterinary Clinics of North America: Small Animal Practice*, Elsevier Health Sciences Division, Subscription Customer Service, 3251 Riverport Lane, Maryland Heights, MO 63043. Customer Service (orders, claims, online, change of address): Elsevier Periodicals Customer Service, Elsevier Health Sciences Division Subscription **Customer Service 3251 Riverport Lane Maryland Heights, MO 63043. Tel: 1-800-654-2452 (U.S. and Canada); 314-447-8871 (outside U.S. and Canada). Fax: 314-447-8029. E-mail: journalscustomerservice-usa@elsevier.com (for print support); journalsonlinesupport-usa@elsevier.com (for online support).**

Reprints. For copies of 100 or more of articles in this publication, please contact the Commercial Reprints Department, Elsevier Inc., 360 Park Avenue South, New York, NY 10010-1710. Tel.: 212-633-3874; Fax: 212-633-3820; E-mail: reprints@elsevier.com.

Veterinary Clinics of North America: Small Animal Practice is also published in Japanese by Inter Zoo Publishing Co., Ltd., Aoyama Crystal-Bldg 5F, 3-5-12 Kitaaoyama, Minato-ku, Tokyo 107-0061, Japan.

Veterinary Clinics of North America: Small Animal Practice is covered in *Current Contents/Agriculture, Biology and Environmental Sciences, Science Citation Index, ASCA, MEDLINE/PubMed (Index Medicus), Excerpta Medica,* and *BIOSIS.*

Contributors

EDITORS

MAUREEN A. MCMICHAEL, DVM, MEd
Diplomate, American College of Veterinary Emergency and Critical Care; Professor, Emergency and Critical Care, Department of Clinical Sciences, Auburn University College of Veterinary Medicine, Auburn, Alabama; Inaugural Professor, Carle Illinois College of Medicine, University of Illinois, Champaign, Illinois

MELISSA SINGLETARY, DVM, PhD
Diplomate, American College of Veterinary Preventive Medicine, Assistant Director, Canine Performance Sciences Program, Assistant Professor, Department of Anatomy, Physiology, and Pharmacology, Auburn University College of Veterinary Medicine, Auburn, Alabama

AUTHORS

KARIN BILYARD, DVM, LTC, USAR
Huntley, Illinois

BRIAN D. FARR
Penn Vet Working Dog Center, Clinical Sciences and Advanced Medicine, School of Veterinary Medicine, University of Pennsylvania, Philadelphia, Pennsylvania; Army Medical Department Student Detachment, San Antonio, Texas

PAMELA S. HANEY, MS
Canine Performance Sciences Program, College of Veterinary Medicine, Auburn University, Auburn, Alabama

JACOB JOHNSON, DVM
Diplomate, American College of Veterinary Anesthesia and Analgesia; Associate Professor, Department of Clinical Sciences Auburn, Alabama

STEPHEN JURIGA, DVM
Diplomate, American Veterinary Dental College; Veterinary Dental Center, Aurora, Illinois

LUCIA LAZAROWSKI, PhD
Research Assistant Professor, Department of Anatomy, Physiology and Pharmacology, Research Scientist, Canine Performance Sciences Program, College of Veterinary Medicine, Auburn University, Alabama

ANDREW L. MCGRAW, DVM, MS
Diplomate, American College of Veterinary Internal Medicine (SAIM); Auburn Veterinary Specialists–Gulf Shores, Auburn University Educational Complex, Gulf Shores, Alabama

MAUREEN A. MCMICHAEL, DVM, MEd
Diplomate, American College of Veterinary Emergency and Critical Care; Professor, Emergency and Critical Care, Department of Clinical Sciences, College of Veterinary Medicine, Auburn University, Auburn, Alabama; Inaugural Professor, Carle Illinois College of Medicine, University of Illinois, Champaign, Illinois

ASHLEY MITEK, DVM, MS
Diplomate, American College of Veterinary Anesthesia and Analgesia; College of Veterinary Medicine, Teaching Assistant Professor, University of Illinois, Urbana, Illinois

CYNTHIA M. OTTO
Penn Vet Working Dog Center, Clinical Sciences and Advanced Medicine, School of Veterinary Medicine, University of Pennsylvania, Philadelphia, Pennsylvania

LEE PALMER, DVM, MS, CCRP, EMT-T, NRP, TP-C
Diplomate, American College of Veterinary Emergency and Critical Care; Auburn, Alabama

MEGHAN T. RAMOS
Penn Vet Working Dog Center, Clinical Sciences and Advanced Medicine, School of Veterinary Medicine, University of Pennsylvania, Philadelphia, Pennsylvania

MARCELLA RIDGWAY, VMD, MS
Diplomate, American College of Veterinary Internal Medicine (SAIM); College of Veterinary Medicine, University of Illinois, Urbana, Illinois

BART ROGERS
Canine Performance Sciences, Auburn, Alabama

MELISSA SINGLETARY, DVM, PhD
Diplomate, American College of Veterinary Preventive Medicine, Assistant Director, Canine Performance Sciences Program, Assistant Professor, Department of Anatomy, Physiology, and Pharmacology, College of Veterinary Medicine, Auburn University, Auburn, Alabama

MARTHA SMITH-BLACKMORE, DVM
Visiting Fellow, Animal Law and Policy Program, Harvard Law School, Harvard University, Cambridge, Massachusetts; Forensic Veterinary Investigations, LLC, Boston, Massachusetts; Adjunct Clinical Assistant Professor, Cummings School of Veterinary Medicine, Tufts University, Medford, Massachusetts

TODD M. THOMAS, DVM, MSpVM
Diplomate, American College of Veterinary Surgeons-Small Animal; Auburn Veterinary Specialists–Gulf Shores, Auburn University Educational Complex, Gulf Shores, Alabama

PAUL WAGGONER, PhD
Canine Performance Sciences, Auburn, Alabama

ROBYN R. WILBORN, DVM, MS
Diplomate, American College of Theriogenologists, Associate Professor, Department of Clinical Sciences, College of Veterinary Medicine, Auburn University, Auburn, Alabama

DEBRA L. ZORAN, DVM, PhD, DACVIM (SAIM)
Professor of Small Animal Medicine, Texas A&M Veterinary Emergency Team, Texas A&M Task Force 1 US&R, FEMA Incident Support Team Veterinarian, College of Veterinary Medicine and Biomedical Sciences, Texas A&M University, College Station, Texas, USA

Contents

> The goal of preventive care is to maintain and optimize health by averting preventable problems. Effective preventive care programs for working dogs must incorporate standard procedures applicable to dogs in general with additional elements pertinent to the more specific characteristics of breed, geographic location, living and working conditions, and physical and mental tasks required of the working dog. This article covers the basic essential preventive health guidelines for all working dogs as well as the specific breed, occupational, and regional considerations to be taken into account.

> Working dogs pose unique concerns and challenges to the veterinary practitioner. In this article, the authors review the best practices and clinical pearls for anesthetizing working dogs for both routine and emergent procedures.

> Working dogs serve different functions based on their trained purpose. Due to the nature of their work, they are prone to traumatic dentoalveolar injuries (TDIs). TDIs include tooth wear, fracture, discoloration, and displacement. Undiagnosed or untreated TDIs result in pain, which could lead to poor performance. Veterinarians should educate handlers on potential injuries and perform a thorough oral examination and appropriate diagnostics to identify any oral abnormalities and initiate treatment. The primary goal of treatment is to return dogs to normal function so that they can continue to perform their assigned duty at maximum performance.

> Working dogs are athletes, but have a wide variety of work types and durations that impact their dietary needs. Their basic nutritional needs do not

change: all dogs need a complete and balanced diet, fed in proper proportions to maintain optimal body condition. However, with increasing muscle work and endurance, the amounts of specific nutrients (particularly the macronutrients, protein, fat, and carbohydrates) must be adjusted. This article provides an overview of the key aspects of working canine nutrition and provides the nutritional science behind the recommendations made.

The legal landscape for dogs working in assistance, service, and support roles is complicated and contradictory. Regulations permit access to public places, allow subsets of dogs' emergency transport and treatment, provide elevated protections for K-9s and assistance animals from criminal acts, and make it a crime to fraudulently represent a service animal. Federal and state agencies provide different regulations for dogs to access public places. Identification and verification of the working animal are not standardized. Working dog legislation is a changing landscape that requires veterinarians to be up to date on laws and regulatory guidance.

Canine companions have learned to aid in performing tasks and conducting work for decades. Areas where unique capabilities of working dogs are harnessed are growing. This expansion, alongside efforts to increase domestic purpose-bred stock and awareness of the important role working dogs play in society, is increasing the role veterinarians provide. This article provides a brief overview of 3 key sensory systems in working dogs and highlights considerations for care related to each olfaction, audition, and vision.

Canine sports medicine and rehabilitation recently have evolved to embody the optimization of performance, injury prevention, and mitigation of musculoskeletal degeneration. This article discusses the diverse factors and considerations of working dog wellness and injury prevention and the importance of recognizing normal and abnormal posture and anatomic structure for performance evaluation and early indication of musculoskeletal injury. The importance of a canine physical fitness program is highlighted and the need for a 4-phase recovery plan to determine if a working dog can safely return to work after injury discussed.

Herding and hunting dogs are intense, high-drive dogs that work, and often live, outdoors and in constant or repeated close contact with domestic and wild animals. These dogs are at increased risk for injury and exposure to infectious diseases, toxic substances, and environmental threats. The common practice of feeding or allowing access to raw meat from farm or game animals enhances disease transmission risk. These dogs can be affected by infectious diseases and injurious agents that are rarely encountered in other groups of dogs. In addition, their extreme work ethic may lead to delays in diagnosis.

conditions is paramount in optimizing the delivery of health care. Military personnel rely heavily on the availability of these K-9s, which bring a diverse array of capabilities to myriad operational settings. Anticipating and mitigating common diseases will ensure these dogs continue to serve the needs of US military and allied forces.

Operational K9s encompass a unique population of working dogs that serve as a force multiplier in various civilian law enforcement, force protection, search and rescue, and humanitarian operations. These elite canines do not volunteer to serve, yet they are some of the most faithful and dependable operators in the field. They undoubtedly perform an invaluable service in today's society and are owed a tremendous debt of gratitude for their selfless service, loyalty, and sacrifices. This article describes the unique characteristics and occupational hazards that pertain to the community of Operational K9s.

This article focuses on the areas where harnessing the canine's trainability, mobility, and sociability enables their use for aiding and augmenting humans. This area, which is rapidly expanding, has provided life-changing solutions for persons affected by various impairments and disabilities (eg, visual, hearing, physical, mental).

Herding is done predominantly by breeds developed over centuries to millennia specifically for that purpose. Working-level herding breed dogs are intense, high-drive dogs that will work despite severe illness or pain, thereby masking clues that they are ailing or the nature of their problem. The handler should recognize subtle changes that might signal ill health, and veterinarians should take an active role in training handlers on essential skills. Herding dogs typically work entirely outdoors in rural to wilderness environments with continuous exposure to other domestic animals and wildlife and may be affected by trauma, toxin exposure, infectious diseases, and parasitic infections.

VETERINARY CLINICS OF NORTH AMERICA: SMALL ANIMAL PRACTICE

SERIES OF RELATED INTEREST

Veterinary Clinics of North America: Exotic Animal Practice
https://www.vetexotic.theclinics.com/

THE CLINICS ARE NOW AVAILABLE ONLINE!
Access your subscription at:
www.theclinics.com

Preface

The World of Working Dogs

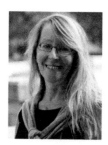 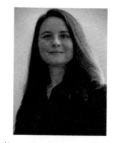

Maureen A. McMichael, DVM, MEd   Melissa Singletary, DVM, PhD

Editors

Ancient artifacts suggest dogs have been helping humans in hunting and herding for thousands of years. The Vikings kept dogs for hunting (Norsk elghund) bear and moose. The Norwegian lundehund hunted puffin, and the Swedish valhund, a close relative of the Welsh corgi, herded cattle. European breeds, the Dutch shepherd, Belgian Malinois, and German shepherd, were originally used for herding sheep and cattle. When World War I broke out, these dogs, recognized for their intelligence, became helpful on the battlefield. In 1916, Germany founded a school to train German shepherds as guide dogs. In 1929, the publicity that resulted from the success of "Buddy" the seeing eye dog led to the expansion of the Seeing Eye in New Jersey. The history of Search and Rescue dogs (S&R) to locate lost people dates back over 300 years to Italy and Switzerland, where St. Bernard dogs were used to find lost people. In the United States, police started using S&R dogs in the 1960s to help track down missing people. To date, dogs have been used to locate (via odor) contraband, narcotics, electronics, explosives, cancer, bed bugs, *Clostridium difficile*, morel mushrooms, pythons, pathogens, and more. Their ability to assist has grown from guide dogs for the visually, hearing, and mobility impaired to medical alert and mental health assistance for posttraumatic stress disorder.

As the importance of working dogs in society grows, there is a need to consolidate critical information on the selection, breeding, training, numerous applications, medical and occupational risks, anatomical nuances, and the complicated legal considerations. This issue is an attempt to amalgamate the experience and knowledge of subject matter experts in the fields of preventative health, anesthesia, dentistry, nutrition, law, sensory systems, sports medicine and rehabilitation, herding and hunting, reproduction, and training in the working dog. It also brings together experts in assistance, military, and operational canines to discuss these unique aspects of working dog care.

Vet Clin Small Anim 51 (2021) xi–xii
https://doi.org/10.1016/j.cvsm.2021.04.016
0195-5616/21/© 2021 Published by Elsevier Inc.

vetsmall.theclinics.com

Working dogs are intelligent, dedicated, and tireless, and we owe it to them to give them the best care available. Our goal is that this issue will add to your working dog toolkit to help you optimize the care and treatment of working dogs in your practice.

The Working Dog

My eyes are your eyes,

To watch and protect you and yours.

My ears are your ears,

To hear and detect evil minds in the dark.

My nose is your nose,

To scent the invader of your domain.

And so you may live,

My life is also yours.

—Author Unknown[1]

Enjoy the issue.

Maureen A. McMichael, DVM, MEd
Department of Clinical Sciences
College of Veterinary Medicine
Auburn University
Auburn, AL 36849, USA

Melissa Singletary, DVM, PhD
Canine Performance Sciences Program
Department of Anatomy, Physiology
and Pharmacology
Auburn University
College of Veterinary Medicine
109 Greene Hall
Auburn, AL 36849, USA

E-mail addresses:
Mam0280@auburn.edu (M.A. McMichael)
mas0028@auburn.edu (M. Singletary)

REFERENCE

1. The Working Dog. Available at: http://www.cpwda.com/poem_the_working_dog. htm. Accessed.

Introduction to Working Dogs

Our canine companions have helped shape the world, as we know it, by serving in roles that enabled humans to advance throughout history. From the earliest domestication where their abilities to effectively and efficiently hunt were harnessed, to present day where their serving of complex roles, improving our safety, security, awareness, productivity, and mobility, is seen. Working dogs have continued to prove themselves an invaluable asset with application and capabilities in areas well beyond their current use. The world of working dogs and working dog health is explored throughout the following 15 articles. Collectively, these articles provide insight into these unique animals, how they are selected, bred, and trained, what makes them good at their job, their various applications, associated occupational risks and medical considerations, and the ever-changing legal landscape related to working dogs.

In the "Considerations in Preventative Health Care" article, Dr Ridgway goes in depth into the essential aspects of prevention that are unique for working dogs as well as specific equipment that veterinarians and handlers should be familiar with. She covers breed disposition to certain diseases, specific injuries more common in working dogs, identification options, immunization protocols, as well as orthopedic soundness and physical exam considerations. Dr Ridgway, a Clinical Professor of Small Animal Internal Medicine and Coordinator of the Working Dog Wellness Program at the University of Illinois College of Veterinary Medicine, is also a search and rescue (S&R) K9 handler. She specializes in the discipline of trailing and further supports K9 first responders through her K9 field first aid training and continuing education presentations related to working dogs, as well as serves as an on-site veterinarian for K9 training seminars.

In the "Anesthetic Considerations in Working Dogs" article, Drs Mitek and Johnson outline the important safety concerns for personnel when working with working dogs as well as the handler presence during anesthesia. They delve into monitoring and essential anesthetic equipment and offer several anesthetic protocols specific to working dogs. Dr Mitek became interested in working dogs during her anesthesiology residency at the University of Illinois, where these patients often present for emergent and elective procedures requiring anesthesia. She is currently a Teaching Assistant Professor at the University of Illinois College of Veterinary Medicine, where she is passionate about advancing the field of working dog veterinary care and teaches students about the best practices in treating these unique patients. She's helped develop the college's working dog policies and has created online and in-person training programs for K9 handlers to help them recognize and treat opioid overdose as well as other life-threatening conditions in their K9s. Dr Johnson is an Associate Professor of Anesthesia and Pain Management at Auburn University. He has served in the US Army Veterinary Corps since 1998 and has been the chief clinical consultant for anesthesia since 2007.

In the "Dentistry for Working Dogs" article, Drs Juriga and Bilyard cover the most common dental injuries and conditions affecting working dogs as well as diagnostic criteria and treatment options. They discuss the importance of handler examinations and veterinarian to handler education since most veterinary physical exams on

Vet Clin Small Anim 51 (2021) xiii–xviii
https://doi.org/10.1016/j.cvsm.2021.04.015
0195-5616/21/© 2021 Published by Elsevier Inc.

security canines do not include an oral exam unless the canine is under general anesthesia. Dr Juriga is the owner of the Veterinary Dental Center, a 3-doctor American Animal Hospital Association–accredited referral dental/oral surgical practice in Aurora, Illinois. He has provided dental and oral surgical services as well as oral health educational seminars for handlers of working dogs since 2005. His goals are to increase awareness of incidence of tooth trauma in working dogs and encourage early identification of tooth injuries through daily handler examinations and annual veterinary examinations. Dr Bilyard was commissioned into the US Army Veterinary Corps in 2007 and served on active duty until 2014. She currently serves as a Lieutenant Colonel in the US Army Veterinary Reserves and is the clinical consultant on working dog oral health within the Department of Defense (DOD). She is pursuing board certification in small animal veterinary dentistry and has provided clinical and emergency care for military and civilian working dogs for over 15 years. Dr Bilyard also manages the Chicagoland Working Dog Veterinary Group, where she and 2 other veterinarians train civilian police and DOD handlers on basic and advanced canine first aid.

In the "Nutrition in Working Dogs" article, Dr Zoran discusses the nutritional considerations of working dogs with an emphasis on security and S&R canines. Dr Zoran, a Professor in the Department of Veterinary Small Animal Clinical Sciences at Texas A&M University, helped found the Texas A&M Veterinary Emergency Team (VET) in 2009. She has been one of the supporting veterinarians for Texas A&M Task Force 1 since 1997, where she provided predeployment and postdeployment canine examinations, first aid training for canine handlers and medics, and programmatic support of the canine program through nutritional and fitness consultations. In her role on the VET and in over 20 deployments, she has been the primary veterinary point of contact with the Urban S&R working dogs in theater and has helped foster advanced training and understanding of working dogs within the Center for Veterinary Medicine. She has also been actively engaged in working dog nutrition and clinical research into hydration and heat tolerance in working dogs, as well as working canine decontamination. In 2019, Dr Zoran was accepted onto the FEMA Incident Support Team as one of 3 veterinary specialists in support of working dogs deployed to large-scale disasters across the United States.

In the "Current Rules and Regulations for Working Dogs" article, the complicated legal logistics are discussed. Drs McMichael and Smith-Blackmore attempt to elucidate the essential aspects that are pertinent to working dogs to provide veterinarians clarification on what may be asked of them. Dr McMichael, a Professor of Emergency and Critical Care at Auburn University, has been dedicated to keeping working dogs healthy since 2001 and has received special recognition from Texas Task Force 1 for her work with their K9s. She has taught K9 first aid and CPR to S&R groups, bomb squads, SWAT teams, emergency medical service (EMS) teams, Arrow Ambulance personnel, and the canine handlers at the Springfield Police Training Institute. She was honored to speak at North American Police Work Dog Association in 2017. She created a Web site to disseminate safety information (www.workingdoghq.com) to help first responders administer emergency first aid for injured K9s in the field. Dr Martha Smith-Blackmore is a veterinarian and Visiting Fellow at Harvard Law School with a focused interest in matters at the intersection of animals and the law. Dr Smith-Blackmore is also an Adjunct Assistant Clinical Professor and a Fellow of the Center for Animals and Public Policy at the Cummings School of Veterinary Medicine in North Grafton, Massachusetts, where she teaches Animal Law & Veterinary Medicine and Veterinary Forensics. Martha also leads Forensic Veterinary Investigations, LLC based in Boston, Massachusetts.

In the "Canine Sensory Systems" article, Drs Singletary and Lazarowski discuss the critical senses of olfaction, audition, and vision in relation to working dogs. The elements of dysfunction in these key sensory systems, significant impacts on performance, and compromising efficacy of these dogs are discussed. Dr Singletary, the Assistant Director of the Auburn University Canine Performance Sciences (AUCPS) program, is also an Assistant Professor of Neuroanatomy at Auburn University College of Veterinary Medicine, Department of Anatomy, Physiology, and Pharmacology. The CPS program is internationally recognized for research and development (R&D) in detection canine sciences. Dr Singletary served as a veterinary officer in the US Army Veterinary Corp, where she supported the military working dog (MWD) mission across multiple locations under her care. She returned to Auburn University to complete a PhD program in biomedical science with a focus in olfactory neuroscience. Dr Lazarowski is a research scientist at the CPS program and Research Assistant Professor in the Department of Anatomy, Physiology, and Pharmacology at the Auburn University College of Veterinary Medicine. She has 13 years of experience in animal olfactory learning and cognition, and 8 years of experience studying olfaction, cognition, and behavior specific to detection dogs. Her research focuses on cognitive and behavioral assessments of detection dog suitability, puppy development, and olfactory learning. She is an affiliate member of the National Institute of Standards and Technology Organization of Scientific Area Committees (OSAC) Dogs and Sensors Subcommittee.

In the "Sports Medicine and Rehabilitation in Working Dogs" article, Drs Otto, Farr, and Ramos discuss performance enhancement, injury prevention, and return to work after injury or illness. They include a discussion of rehabilitation, foundational fitness, behavioral enrichment, and body composition optimization. Dr Otto was involved with the medical care of Urban S&R Dogs as a member of FEMA's Pennsylvania Task Force 1 between 1993 and 2010. She deployed to Hurricane Floyd and 9/11. As a member of the Veterinary Medical Assistance Team, she cared for search dogs during Hurricane Katrina. She has followed the health and behavior of the search dogs of 9/11 for 15 years. In 2012, she founded the Penn Vet Working Dog Center, a research, teaching, and training facility for all types of detection dogs. She has testified before Congress and served on national committees to develop protocols and standards for the care and utilization of working dogs. Dr Farr is an active-duty Army Veterinary Corps Officer and resident in Canine Sports Medicine and Rehabilitation at the Penn Vet Working Dog Center. His primary interest is developing methods suitable for handlers, trainers, and veterinarians to assess and develop working dog physical and mental performance. Dr Ramos is currently a Sports Medicine and Rehabilitation resident at the Penn Vet Working Dog Center. She received her VMD in 2018 from the University of Pennsylvania School of Veterinary Medicine. Following graduation, Dr Ramos began her veterinary specialty internship at Penn Vet while simultaneously pursuing a National Institutes of Health–funded Master in Translational Research through the Institute for Translational Medicine and Therapeutics at the University of Pennsylvania Perelman School of Medicine. Dr Ramos has provided veterinary care and educational seminars focused on preventative medicine, physical fitness, first aid, rehabilitation, and return to work training programs for S&R, law enforcement, single-purpose detection, and medical detection working dogs and their handlers. Dr Ramos is dedicated to advancing the field of canine sports medicine by implementing scientifically valid clinical trials and translational medicine methodologies that not only will benefit elite working dogs but also will impact the canine community at large.

In the "Hunting Dog" article, Dr Ridgway discusses the history and function of hunting dogs. She explores ways that these translate into unique environmental and occupational exposures. There is a thorough discussion of the specific risks associated with hunting, including trauma, infectious diseases, and zoonotic risks. This article is an extensive introduction to understanding the roles and risks of these working dogs. Dr Ridgway also wrote the "Considerations in Preventative Health Care" and the "Herding Dog" articles.

In the "Breeding Management and Production in Working Dogs" article, Dr Wilborn and Ms Haney discuss the optimization strategies involved in managing a colony of high-quality, purpose-bred working dogs to maximize production success. They delve into the capture and organization of population data and discuss appropriate tests and breed-specific health conditions, replacement of breeding stock, and ideal structure of puppy development programs. Dr Wilborn is an Associate Professor at the AU College of Veterinary Medicine and has provided specialty care for the AUCPS breeding program since 2010. Pamela Haney is the Canine Performance R&D Manager for the CPS Program at the Auburn University's College of Veterinary Medicine. She has 10 years' experience contributing to detection dog R&D and has managed the CPS detection dog breeding program for the past 5 years. Pamela Haney has been involved in detection dog research for breeding and selection, early puppy development, nutrition, olfaction, thermoregulation, behavior, physical conditioning, and biomechanics. She has a MS in Exercise Physiology and is currently pursuing a PhD, focusing on Performance Canine Biomechanics, at Auburn University's School of Kinesiology.

In the "Development and Training for Working Dogs" article, Drs Larzarowski, Waggoner, Singletary, and Mr Rogers discuss behavioral suitability, selection, and importance of environmental influence and experience during early development. They highlight critical aspects of puppy development, ideal timing of separation from the dam, and essential factors that affect training and performance later in life. This article introduces Mr Rogers and Dr Waggoner. Bart Rogers is a Chief Canine Instructor of the AUCPS breeding program. He oversees the development and training of candidate detection dogs as well as their selection, evaluation, and placement. Bart has been working with dogs professionally for over 10 years, having trained dogs for various working roles, including explosives detection, wildlife conservation, and service/therapy work. Dr Waggoner is the Co-Director of the CPS Program and Adjunct Associate Professor in the Department of Anatomy, Physiology, and Pharmacology at the Auburn University College of Veterinary Medicine. He is a behavioral scientist with 30 years of experience conducting detection dog–related R&D, test and evaluation, breeding and production, and innovation of operational technology. He is a coinventor of Auburn's patented Vapor Wake detection dog technology. He is a member of the Dogs & Sensors Sub-committee of the National Institutes of Standards and Technology, OSAC, was an original member of the former Scientific Working Group on Dogs and Sensors, and is co-chair of the HR 302 Domestic Detection Dog Production Working Group.

In the "Military Working Dogs" article, Drs McGraw and Thomas discuss the procurement process for how MWDs are sourced, preventative medicine policies, common disease conditions as well as injuries specific to both domestic and deployed MWDs. Dr McGraw is currently medical director at the Auburn Veterinary Specialists–Gulf Shores, Alabama after serving 17 years as a Veterinary Corps Officer in the US Army. He served in 8 separate assignments, 2 of which were combat deployments rendering care to MWDs. He served as principal consultant to the Director of the DOD Military Working Dog Veterinary Service, drafting policy statements on preventive health care for all MWDs. He served as co-editor for the Handbook of Veterinary Care for Military Working Dogs. His career culminated as the Director of the DOD Military Working Dog Veterinary Service, the US Army Veterinary Corps Chief's designated subject matter expert for MWD policy and decision making, and the lone veterinary consultant to the DOD's Joint Service Military Working Dog Committee. Dr Todd Thomas, associate clinical professor at Auburn Veterinary Specialists–Gulf Shores, Alabama, spent 20 years on active duty in the US Army Veterinary Corps. He provided care for a variety of working dogs, including MWDs, Department of Homeland Security canines, Transportation Security Administration canines, and contract working dogs. He was assigned to the DOD Military Working Dog Veterinary Service, LTC Daniel E. Holland Military Working Dog Hospital twice while on active duty, and as an Oak Ridge Institute for Science and Education Knowledge Preservation Program Fellow following retirement in 2016. He was deployed to Afghanistan in 2013 as part of Operation Enduring Freedom. He also spent over 7 years as an instructor in MWD veterinary care at the Army Medical Department Center and School.

In the "Operational Canines" article, Dr Palmer discusses civilian law enforcement, force protection, S&R, and humanitarian operational canines. Specific risks for these canines as well as new laws related to prehospital treatment and transport for these dogs are discussed. Dr Palmer has over 20 years of military, tactical, and operational medicine experience. He has served in the military since 1996 and is currently assigned as the Group Veterinarian for the 20th Special Forces Group, Alabama Army National Guard. Dr Palmer provides training and consultation nationally and internationally in the field of K9 Tactical Casualty Care to military, law enforcement, S&R, and tactical EMS communities. Dr Palmer is a K9 consultant for various military and nonmilitary organizations to include the USAF Pararescue group, US Marshals Service, DHS Federal Protective Services, Domestic Highway Enforcement, and High Intensity Drug Trafficking Areas working group. Dr Palmer is the lead and founder of the K9 Tactical Emergency Casualty Care working group, Medical Education Director for Penn Vet's Working Dog Practitioner program, and active working group member for the Defense Committees on Trauma Canine Combat Casualty Care Committee and K9 TCCC Education and Training Subcommittee.

In the "Assistance, Service, and Therapy Dogs" article, Drs McMichael and Singletary discuss the rapid proliferation of dogs working with individuals with disabilities, impairments, or chronic medical conditions. They also attempt to clarify the confusion about the terminology used to describe these dogs and how to objectively assess the benefits they may provide. An overview of the variety of ways in which these dogs are employed for medical, psychiatric, and social and emotional conditions is given along with some specific examples for use with autism spectrum disorder, diabetes, seizures, and posttraumatic stress disorder. The role of veterinarians in facilitating the successful employment of these working dogs is discussed.

In the "Herding Dog" article, Dr Ridgway discusses the history, breeding, and function of herding dogs. The specific environmental and occupational exposures are discussed as well as the infectious disease and zoonotic risks associated with herding dogs. This article is an extensive introduction to understanding the roles and risks of these working dogs. Dr Ridgway also wrote the "Considerations in Preventative Health Care" and the "Hunting Dog" articles.

We have endeavored to compile current, essential knowledge in one issue to facilitate optimal care and management of these amazing dogs. As best practices, logistical and legal information is constantly changing, and veterinarians need to stay up-to-date. We have provided multiple Web sites throughout the issue to assist in this task in real time. We believe this issue will be an asset to veterinarians and veterinary personnel that treat working dogs in their practices.

Sincerely,

The authors report no conflicts of interest. This document represents current rules and regulations as of the time of this writing. Local, state, and national legislation changes frequently, and veterinarians are advised to remain up-to-date on the changes by accessing real-time data via individual or collective Web sites mentioned in this article.

Maureen A. McMichael, DVM, MEd,
Department of Clinical Sciences
College of Veterinary Medicine
Auburn University
Auburn, AL 36849, USA

Melissa Singletary, DVM, PhD
Department of Anatomy, Physiology
and Pharmacology
Auburn University College of
Veterinary Medicine
109 Greene Hall
Auburn, AL 36849, USA

E-mail addresses:
mam0280@auburn.edu (M.A. McMichael)
mas0028@auburn.edu (M. Singletary)

Preventive Health Care for Working Dogs

Marcella Ridgway, VMD, MS, DACVIM (SAIM)

KEYWORDS

- Dog • Canine • K9 • Working dog • Infectious • Parasites

KEY POINTS

- Careful screening for health problems is essential and includes physical examination at work and rest, targeted imaging, and genetic testing.
- Specific evaluation depending on breed is also important, such as echocardiographic and radiographic assessment for cardiac disease in predisposed breeds, spinal imaging to assess for lumbosacral instability in Labrador retrievers, and pelvic radiographs for hip dysplasia.
- A thorough knowledge of the geographic location in which the dog will work prepares for factors such as temperature and humidity extremes, regionally prevalent infectious diseases, plant or wildlife threats, and variations in terrain to which dogs will be exposed.

INTRODUCTION

The goal of preventive care is to maintain and optimize health by averting preventable problems. Effective preventive care programs for working dogs must incorporate standard procedures applicable to dogs in general with additional elements pertinent to the more specific characteristics of breed, geographic location, living and working conditions, and physical and mental tasks required of the dog. This article applies the definition of working dog as any domestic dog that is operational in a private industry, government, assistance, or sporting context, independently of whether it also performs a role as human companion, as proposed by Carr and colleagues.[1] Breed predispositions to certain diseases have been well characterized for many of the working dog breeds (**Table 1**), and an awareness of and planned monitoring for these conditions are critical in the initial selection and maintenance of healthy working partners. Some conditions to which working dog breeds are prone may be inconsequential or even related to improved capacity for work (eg, Malinois dogs with OCD/spinning behaviors associated with CDH2 gene showing positive correlation with desirable work performance[2]), but problems with special senses (olfaction, vision, and hearing), musculoskeletal soundness, or dysfunction of cardiorespiratory, gastrointestinal,

College of Veterinary Medicine, University of Illinois, Urbana, IL 61802, USA
E-mail address: ridgway@illinois.edu

Vet Clin Small Anim 51 (2021) 745–764
https://doi.org/10.1016/j.cvsm.2021.03.001
0195-5616/21/© 2021 Elsevier Inc. All rights reserved.

Table 1
Breed-associated diseases of the predominant detection, patrol and search-and-rescue dog breeds

Breed	Abnormality	Comments
Belgian Malinois	Orthopedic • Elbow dysplasia • Hip dysplasia Neuromuscular • Lumbosacral stenosis • Epilepsy • SDCA (spongy degeneration with cerebellar ataxia) Eye • Cataracts • Pannus • PRA (especially males) Behavior • Traumatic dental and tail lesions • OCD/spinning • Handler aggression • Hypervigilance Endocrine • Inherited autoimmune thyroiditis GI • GDV Neoplastic • Lymphoma Other • Increased occurrence of heat stroke	SDCA1, SDCA2 genetic tests available Associated with CDH2 gene Associated with SLC6A3, VNTR genes Associated with SLC6A3, VNTR genes 8.4% antithyroid antibody positive Malinois MWD deaths
Dutch shepherd	Orthopedic • Hip dysplasia • Elbow dysplasia Neuromuscular • Masticatory myositis • SDCA (spongy degeneration with cerebellar ataxia) • Polymyositis/Dutch shepherd inflammatory myopathy • Degenerative myelopathy • Epilepsy Behavioral • Spinning Eye[a] • Pannus • Goniodysplasia Skin • Atopy GI • IBD	University of Minnesota Canine Genetics Laboratory test SOD1 genetic test available
German shepherd	Orthopedic • Elbow dysplasia • Hip dysplasia • Panosteitis	26% of cases are GSD SOD1 genetic test available 5× risk, anti-AChR antibody titer 2M antibody test

(continued on next page)

Table 1
(continued)

Breed	Abnormality	Comments
	• Stifle OCD	25% of LE GSD emergency room visits
	• HOD	
	Neuromuscular	5× risk
	• Lumbosacral stenosis	Aspergillosis, leishmaniasis, ehrlichiosis
	• Degenerative myelopathy	
	• Myasthenia gravis	
	• Masticatory myositis	
	• Gracilis contracture	
	• Pectineus hypertrophy	
	Eye	
	• Cataracts	
	• Pannus	
	Behavioral	
	• Aggression	
	• Fearfulness	
	• Separation anxiety	
	Skin	
	• Perianal fistula/furunculosis	
	• Metatarsal fistulae (German dogs)	
	• Atopy	
	• Nailbed diseases	
	• Pyoderma	
	• Lupus	
	GI	
	• EPI	
	• IBD	
	• GDV	
	• Food allergies	
	• Perineal hernia	
	• Megaesophagus	
	Neoplasia	
	• Hemangiosarcoma	
	• Anal sac adenocarcinoma	
	• Colorectal neoplasia	
	• Testicular tumors: seminoma	
	• Lymphoma	
	Cardiac	
	• Congenital heart disease: aortic stenosis	
	• Dilated cardiomyopathy	
	• Fatal ventricular arrhythmia	
	Other	
	• IgA deficiency	
	• Increased infectious disease susceptibility	

(continued on next page)

Table 1
(continued)

Breed	Abnormality	Comments

Golden retriever	Orthopedic
	• Elbow dysplasia
	• Hip dysplasia
	• Shoulder, stifle OCD
	• CCL rupture
	Neuromuscular
	• Laryngeal paralysis
	• Megaesophagus
	• Epilepsy
	• X-linked muscular dystrophy
	• Myasthenia gravis
	Eye
	• Ocular melanoma
	• Retinal dysplasia
	• PRA prcd-PRA, GR-PRA1 tests
	  (Optigen)
	• Cataracts
	• Iris cysts
	Skin
	• Hot spots
	• Pododermatitis
	• Atopy
	• Ichthyosis
	• Nasal depigmentation
	• Otitis externa
	• Seborrhea
	Endocrine
	• Hypothyroidism
	GI
	• GDV
	• Cricopharyngeal achalasia
	• Megaesophagus
	Neoplastic
	• Mast cell tumor
	• Cutaneous, oral melanoma
	• Osteosarcoma
	• Fibrosarcoma
	• Soft tissue sarcoma
	• Lymphoma
	• Hemangiosarcoma
	• Primary brain tumor
	• Histiocytic sarcoma
	Cardiac
	• Congenital heart disease:
	  subaortic stenosis
	Other
	• Lyme nephritis
	• Hemophilia A, B
	• Spectrin deficiency
		DMD, GRMD tests available
		Anti-AChR antibody titer
		Ichthyosis test available
		  (Antagene)
		genetic testing (Cornell,
		  HealthGene)

Labrador retriever	Orthopedic • Elbow dysplasia • Hip dysplasia	Predisposes to lumbosacral stenosis Anti-AChR antibody titer

(continued on next page)

Table 1 *(continued)*		
Breed	**Abnormality**	**Comments**
	• Shoulder, hock OCD • CCL rupture • Transitional vertebrae • Patellar luxation • Ossification of infraspinatus tendon Neuromuscular • Laryngeal paralysis • Epilepsy • Distal polyneuropathy • Labrador myopathy • Myasthenia gravis • Exercise-induced collapse (30% carriers, 3% affected) • Centronuclear myopathy Eye • Ocular melanoma • Retinal dysplasia • PRA • Cataracts • Entropion, ectropion Skin • Hot spots • Pododermatitis • Atopy • Drug-associated pemphigus foliaceous • Seborrhea • Nasal depigmentation • Hereditary nasal hyperkeratosis Endocrine • Hyperadrenocorticism (Cushing) • Diabetes mellitus • Hypothyroidism GI • GDV • IBD • Perianal fistulae • Chronic hepatitis Neoplastic • Mast cell tumor • Digital SCC • Nasal tumor • Lymphoma • Histiocytic sarcoma Cardiac • Congenital heart disease: tricuspid dysplasia, pulmonic stenosis • Arrhythmias: reentrant tachycardia, AV block Other • Lyme nephritis	EIC test (University of Minnesota Veterinary Diagnostic Laboratory) CNM test (Alfort Laboratory, Animal Genetics) RD/OSD test (Optigen) prcd-PRA test (Optigen) HNPK genetic test (Animal Genetics)

(continued on next page)

Table 1 (continued)		
Breed	**Abnormality**	**Comments**
Bloodhound	Orthopedic disease • Hip dysplasia • Elbow dysplasia • Shoulder OCD Neuromuscular • Degenerative myelopathy Eye • Ectropion, entropion • Retinal dysplasia • Cataracts • Cherry eye • Pannus Endocrine • Thyroiditis GI • GDV Cardiac • Congenital heart disease: VSD, aortic stenosis	26% affected 15% affected SOD1 genetic test available PRA (University of Missouri, Animal Health Trust)
English springer spaniel	Orthopedic • Hip dysplasia • Elbow dysplasia • Patellar luxation Neuromuscular • Epilepsy • Rage syndrome • Fucosidosis • GM-1 gangliosidosis • myasthenia gravis • Congenital hypomyelinization Eye • PRA • Retinal dysplasia • Cataracts • Pectinate ligament dysplasia • Persistent pupillary membranes • Glaucoma: primary and secondary • Ectropion, entropion Skin • Allergic dermatitis • Otitis • Seborrhea • Pemphigus foliaceus • Sebaceous adenitis • Lichenoid-psoriasiform dermatosis	Test available (PennGen, AHT) Anti-AChR antibody titer PFK deficiency test available Genetic test (Animal Genetics)

(continued on next page)

Table 1 (continued)		
Breed	**Abnormality**	**Comments**
	Endocrine • Hypothyroidism GI • Chronic hepatitis Cardiac • Congenital heart disease • DCM Other • RBC abnormalities: PFK deficiency, IMHA • Malignant hyperthermia	
German shorthaired pointer	Orthopedic • CCL • Shoulder OCD • Hip dysplasia • Elbow dysplasia • Panosteitis Neuromuscular • Hemivertebrae • Myasthenia gravis • GM-2 gangliosidosis • Epilepsy • Acral mutilation syndrome Eye • Cone degeneration (day blindness) • Entropion • Distichiasis • Cataracts • Persistent pupillary membrane • Retinal dysplasia Skin • Atopy • Food allergy • Cutaneous lupus erythematosus • Epidermolysis bullosa • Seasonal flank alopecia Endocrine • Hypothyroidism • Hypoadrenocorticism GI • Malocclusion: brachygnathism • GDV Neoplastic • Mast cell tumor Cardiac • Subaortic stenosis Other • Cryptorchidism • XX sex reversal • Factor VIII, IX, XII deficiency • von Willebrand disease type II	34.5% affected Anti-AChR antibody titer AMS genetic test (Animal Genetics) CD genetic test (Optigen) Tests available (VetGen, Cornell, and so forth) vWD testing (VetGen)

(continued on next page)

Table 1
(continued)

Breed	Abnormality	Comments
Border collie	Orthopedic • Shoulder, stifle OCD • Hip dysplasia • Patellar luxation Neuromuscular • Congenital and adult-onset deafness • Border collie collapse • Epilepsy • Neuronal ceroid lipofuscinosis • Steroid-responsive meningitis-arteritis • Neuroaxonal dystrophy • Achilles tendon rupture • Gastrocnemius musculotendinopathy Eye • Collie eye anomaly/choroidal hypoplasia • Cataracts • Primary lens luxation • PRA • Retinal dysplasia • Persistent pupillary membranes • Pannus • Glaucoma Endocrine • Diabetes mellitus • Hypothyroidism GI • Cobalamin (vitamin B_{12}) malabsorption • Portosystemic shunt Cardiac • Congenital heart disease: patent ductus arteriosus Other • Trapped neutrophil syndrome • ABCB1 mutation • Malignant hyperthermia	Genetic test (Optigen, AHT) CEA/CH (Optigen) No genetic test for BC PRA BCG genetic test (Animal Genetics) Marker test (U New South Wales) MDR1 test (Washington State University) Genetic test (Animal Genetics)

Abbreviations: AChR, acetylcholine receptor; AV, atrioventricular; CCL, cranial cruciate ligament; GDV, gastric dilatation-volvulus; GI, gastrointestinal; HOD, hypertrophic osteodystrophy; IBD, inflammatory bowel disease; MWD, military working dogs; OCD, obsessive-compulsive disorder; SCC, squamous cell carcinoma; VSD, ventricular septal defect; vWD, von Willebrand disease.

neurologic, or other systems can obviously have a significant deleterious effect on a dog's ability to perform. The relative degree to which specific disorders affect the dog's working performance varies by the individual activities required of the dog and the drive of the dog. Here drive is defined as "the propensity of a dog to exhibit a particular pattern of behaviors when faced with particular stimuli."[3]

Careful screening for health problems includes (1) careful and thorough physical examination, preferably at work as well as at rest and performed on a regular schedule (more frequently in young dogs and dogs whose work imposes a high risk for injury), (2) targeted radiographic or other imaging evaluation (eg, echocardiographic and radiographic assessment for cardiac disease in predisposed breeds, spinal imaging to assess for lumbosacral instability in Labrador retrievers, pelvic radiographs for hip dysplasia), and (3) genetic testing to screen for those breed-related problems for which such testing is available (genetic mutation or markers associated with the condition have been identified). Geographic location in which the dog will work introduces factors such as temperature and humidity extremes, regionally prevalent infectious diseases, plant or wildlife threats, and variations in terrain to which dogs will be exposed.

PHYSICAL EXAMINATION

To ensure ongoing suitability for work as well as early detection and intervention to optimize health outcomes, working dogs benefit from undergoing twice-annual physical examination and routine laboratory testing (complete blood count [CBC], serum chemistry, urinalysis, fecal testing for parasites, annual heartworm/tick-borne disease screening) to establish a baseline for the dog and to screen for subclinical problems. In this regard, the veterinarian plays a critical role in not only safeguarding the health of the dog but also ensuring the quality of the dog's work, which has important human health and safety implications.

Veterinarians caring for working dogs should make a point of instructing the dogs' handlers in performing a thorough physical examination of their dogs. Handlers should examine their canine partners routinely and before and after deployment to augment scheduled veterinary visits and ensure optimal monitoring so that problems can be identified and addressed promptly.

Working dogs are often energetic, high-drive individuals and may be difficult to restrain for a thorough physical examination. However, a comprehensive examination is imperative to ensure suitability for performing their jobs and to reliably detect problems to which these dogs may be more prone because of the services they are providing, with significant ramifications if a working dog is unable to perform at peak. Conscientious use of sedation (discussed elsewhere in this issue) when needed facilitates thorough evaluation as well as personnel safety. Owners/handlers of these dogs are generally very knowledgeable about effectively handling them and can partner with veterinary personnel in planning and implementing their management in the clinic setting. For potentially dangerous dogs (eg, high-drive law enforcement and military working dogs), communication between the veterinarian and the handler in advance of the visit is recommended for planning care to proceed smoothly.

Basic parameters of body temperature, pulse, and respiratory rate (TPR) can vary dramatically in a given dog depending on level of arousal, ambient conditions under which the dog is transported and examined, and current state of physical conditioning (eg, well-conditioned athletic dogs may have a lower-than-expected heart rate at rest). Owner/handlers should be advised to record the dogs' TPR at rest, when working, and when recovering from work to establish a baseline to which the veterinarian can refer when the dog is presented for a routine wellness examination or because of illness or injury.

These records are especially helpful if the dog needs to receive care from a different provider when away from the home location or when the dog has to be examined during active work periods: some dogs reach body temperatures of 42.4°C (108.3°F) without apparent consequence during work periods, but knowledge of this unusual normal would be important to distinguish genuine problems normally indicated by increased body temperatures (see the article "Operational K9s" in this issue).

Some aspects of the physical examination warrant particular attention. Teeth should be carefully evaluated: even subtle dental problems can compromise the performance of dogs doing bite work, retrieving (can affect the dog's pleasure in a toy reward as well as formal retrieving in hunting, obedience), or pulling with the mouth (water sports, water rescue, human assistance activities). In addition, dogs using their teeth in these ways may be prone to oral or dental injury (see elsewhere in this issue). Vision is important for many activities, especially jumping, getting on or off equipment or structures, retrieving, or negotiating difficult terrain. Some working breeds are predisposed to eye disease (see **Table 1**), and dogs may sustain injury to the eye by impalement (equipment, building material, plant material), blunt force trauma or falling (retinal detachment), ocular foreign body (ash, building debris, plant material), or bite/scratch from another animal in the course of their work. An initial ophthalmic examination to evaluate fitness for work is indicated and evaluation by a board-certified veterinary ophthalmologist and Canine Eye Registration Foundation or Companion Animal Eye Registry certification is desired for breeds with hereditary eye disease as a criterion for their work suitability.

Verification of orthopedic soundness is critical for dogs in occupations that require extreme athleticism and endurance. A complete orthopedic examination, including gait evaluation and examination while awake and while sedated, should be included in the initial determination of suitability for work and whenever performance is reportedly impaired. Handlers know their dogs and should be believed when they report a decline in a dog's performance, although the problem may be below the threshold for detection by a veterinary professional: that fact should be admitted to the handler. The handler is usually correct. Serial orthopedic examinations plus or minus imaging) over time may help to elucidate problems not initially detectable. Several the working breeds are predisposed to orthopedic disease (see **Table 1**), and initial assessment and targeted testing should be performed as a baseline and for monitoring for occurrence or progression. In addition, dogs may sustain an orthopedic injury in the course of their work, and having a baseline for comparison can be helpful in defining acquired abnormalities. Feet and toenails should be carefully inspected. Active dogs may snag and partially avulse toenails, which may be inapparent without palpation/manipulation of each nail. Footpad or interdigital injuries are common from intense activities on roadways, equipment, building structures, and natural terrain. Work on hot surfaces can cause heat injury. Plant foreign bodies may affect feet, especially interdigital tissues, in dogs working outdoors. Handlers benefit from instruction in routine examination of the feet and first aid for minor foot injuries.

DISEASE SCREENING
General

Comprehensive health assessment including a thorough physical examination and routine clinicopathologic screening (CBC, serum chemistry profile, and urinalysis) should be completed at least every 6 months in actively working dogs. Veterinarians should consider breed differences in hematologic and biochemical reference ranges when interpreting laboratory test results.[4–12] Dogs should undergo routine infectious disease screening appropriate for the area, recognizing that their work may put them at increased risk of exposure to environmental reservoirs of infection and invertebrate vectors. Dogs that travel widely may need additional screening to address diseases present in the other regions in which they work. Owners/handlers should be advised to maintain updated logs of travel locations and dates and to have this information readily available for veterinarians. In traveling, dogs may contract diseases not common in their home environments, with resulting delay in diagnosis by primary veterinarians who do not typically see those cases or know about the dogs' potential exposure to geographically restricted diseases such as pythiosis, coccidioidomycosis and other systemic fungal diseases, hepatozoonosis, leishmaniasis, and trypanosomiasis. Because of regional differences in infectious disease prevalence and other health threats (eg, venomous snakes, feral hogs, frequent trapping or baiting), it is prudent for owners/handlers to contact veterinarians in nonlocal work areas for information on the particular canine health hazards of that region. This approach also allows them to establish relationships with veterinarians to provide urgent or emergent veterinary care while away from home. It is important for veterinarians to be aware that many working dogs, especially law enforcement and military dogs, are imported from other countries, which may have different endemic infectious diseases. If diseases present in the country of origin are not considered, diagnosis may be delayed or missed, which may adversely affect outcomes for the veterinary patient and additionally permit introduction of a foreign disease into a nonaffected country.

Screening for Breed-associated Disease

Awareness of the breed-associated health problems of dogs in various occupational roles as well as consideration of the physical and mental demands of a particular occupation are important for veterinarians assessing suitability to work and monitoring for occurrence or progression of disease conditions. Many breeds require screening for abnormal structure (hip dysplasia, elbow dysplasia) or functional abnormalities, which can be performed as an initial examination for selection of qualified prospects. For some abnormalities, there are genetic tests available that allow identification of dogs likely to develop the condition even before clinical abnormalities are present. **Table 1** summarizes breed-associated diseases in working dogs that can impair working ability. Ultimately, the degree to which abnormalities disqualify a dog from working depends on the severity of the abnormality, the type of work to be done, the dog's drive or determination, and the degree to which an individual dog excels at the work or possesses other desirable traits to a degree to offset the disadvantage presented by the abnormality.

IDENTIFICATION

Working dogs should be individually identified by a permanent identification method. The nature of their activities may preclude external identification tags or collars because of the risk of these being detached as the dog moves through difficult terrain or close quarters, or, worse, causing the dog to become snagged on vegetation, equipment, or other structures and subsequently injured or unable to return to the handler (**Figs. 1 and 2**). In addition, the inherent value of the dogs dictates permanent identification that cannot be removed and can provide proof of ownership should the dog be lost or stolen. Tattoos provide a permanent visible identification mark and are usually placed on the dog's ventral abdomen or thigh: tattooing of the inside of ears is less desirable because ears can be accidently torn or intentionally amputated, foiling identification. Tattoos remain the most readable when applied when the dog is mature/no longer growing. They may blur or fade over time, requiring refreshing, and can be intentionally altered to disguise a dog's identity. Tattoos must be registered to provide traceability and the owner/handler must be conscientious about updating contact information (telephone numbers, address, email). Individuals finding a tattooed dog may not know to look for a tattoo, may not see a tattoo obscured by the animal's position or haircoat, may not realize that tattoos can be

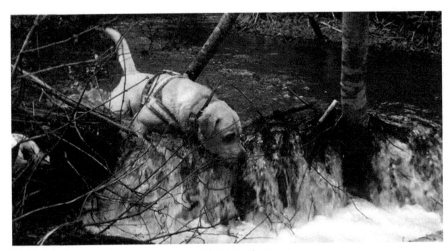

Fig. 1. Working search-and-rescue (SAR) dog wearing vest.

registered, or may not know what registry to contact. This problem can be addressed by combining a tattoo with a tag worn by the dog indicating the registering agency (eg, National Dog Registry, AKC Reunite, BeKind PetFind, Canadian Kennel Club) and how to contact them. Microchip implants offer several advantages

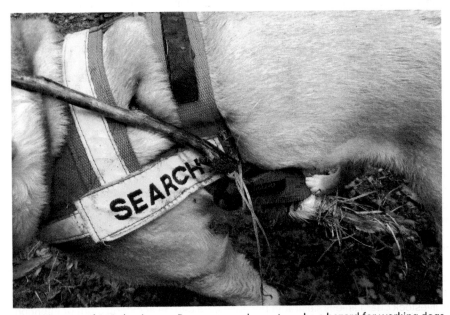

Fig. 2. Close up of SAR dog in vest. Dog-worn equipment can be a hazard for working dogs. This SAR dog's vest became entangled in vegetation despite the vest being a proper snug fit. The attentive handler was able to identify the situation and extricate the dog. Some handlers opt to work their dogs without any collars, harnesses, or vests to avoid the risk of entanglement or strangulation but, in so doing so, assume other risks: dogs without readily visible identification as being owned or working may be perceived as a threat and captured or harmed (shot) and are absent a solid handle to catch, restrain, or use to lift or assist the dog out of a difficult position. (Photos by Mike Ritcey, SFD K-9 of BC. Used by permission.)

compared with tattoos. Once implanted, a microchip is expected to last for the lifetime of the dog. Each microchip is programmed with a unique, unalterable code and manufacturer identification: like tattoos, microchips must be registered to provide full traceability but, because microchip codes are cross-referenced to the veterinary hospital or other agency placing the microchip, there may be some level of traceability even if the owner/handler fails to register the chip or update contact information. Unlike tattoos, found dogs are routinely screened for microchips. Although microchips provide no visible evidence that a dog is permanently identified, they can be paired with a tag identifying the registering agency and/or a tattoo to alert finders to the fact that the dog is owned. It is always helpful to the finder for the dog to be identified as well by some visible identification with the owner's contact information (identification tags, personalized collars) so that a dog can be directly and immediately reunited without needing to contact a registry. A rabies vaccination license tag provides traceability through the licensing body as well as verification of immunization status in the case of a human being injured by the dog. For dogs that have already been tattooed or implanted with a microchip, careful recording and cross-referencing of identification information is warranted because fraudulent representation of the animal by sellers does occur.

IMMUNIZATION

Working dogs may be less likely to experience exposure to other dogs in boarding kennels, dog parks, or grooming facilities often implicated in infectious disease transmission in pet dogs. However, many have repeated exposure to dogs from other environments at group training events or competitions (where equipment or training/performing surfaces as well as kenneling and toileting areas may be shared) or deployment of K-9 teams from multiple agencies (eg, search-and-rescue [SAR] or law enforcement operations, hunting camps), and may be kenneled in a home environment with multiple dogs that originate from different sources, with different dogs coming and going for breeding, training, or deployment purposes. They often travel widely, sometimes internationally (eg, SAR dogs, competition sport dogs). Law enforcement, SAR, and hunting dogs may work in environments that put them in varying and unpredictable risks of exposure to diseases with environmental or wildlife reservoirs. In addition to possibly enhanced risk of exposure from working environments, illness in these dogs has more extensive ramifications because it may prevent the dog from effectively performing vital work in drug or explosive detection, protection, search, or service dog functions. Therefore, comprehensive immunoprophylaxis is warranted to protect their health and sustain their ability to work.

Working dogs should receive all core vaccinations: murine leukemia virus or recombinant canine distemper virus, adenovirus-2, parvovirus with or without parainfluenza virus, and rabies virus vaccines. Rabies virus carries public health significance in addition to health implications for the dog, and maintaining current rabies immunoprophylaxis is of heightened importance for all dogs performing bite work and for dogs such as livestock guardian dogs and hunting dogs with greater likelihood of interacting with domestic or wild animals that may be infected. Vaccination records from other countries are difficult to authenticate and are sometimes falsified to reduce incurred costs or expedite transfer to a new owner; imported dogs should be vaccinated as though they are vaccine naive, even if there is accompanying documentation of vaccination. Recognition that rabies vaccination status may be inaccurate is of particular significance because dogs are commonly imported from countries with higher rabies prevalence than the destination country.

When determining appropriate noncore vaccines, the veterinarian should consider that working dogs typically travel more widely and more frequently than pet dogs and, in those nonhome locations, are more likely to have greater exposure and direct interactions in new environments as they engage in training events, competitions, or deployment for their work. Consequently, vaccines considered core or noncore based on regional disease prevalence may be considered core for these dogs: Leptospira vaccines should be considered core for working dogs. Leptospirosis is a potentially severe to fatal disease in dogs and is zoonotic, posing health risks to handlers as well as other dogs. Pathogenic Leptospira bacteria are widely distributed in urban, suburban, rural, and wilderness areas, maintained in the environment by domestic and nondomestic animal hosts and persisting in moist soil, plant litter, and water, especially stagnant pools. Therefore, dogs working in almost any environment risk exposure and should be protected by immunization. There is minimal cross-protection across Leptospira serovars so administration of a 4-serovar (not a 2-serovar) vaccine is advised. Leptospira vaccines have been anecdotally associated with an increased incidence of adverse vaccine reactions, but controlled investigation with currently available products shows no greater likelihood of adverse reactions than other canine vaccines.[13,14] Current products confer good immunity of at least 1 year's duration so annual (rather than every 6 months) revaccination is recommended.[14] Working dogs may travel internationally, which may dictate additional immunization considerations: the specific Leptospira serovars implicated in clinical disease vary across different regions of the world and vaccines are available for some of these other serovars.

Because canine infectious respiratory disease complex (CIRDC), or kennel cough, is highly contagious and can significantly interfere with work and training, Bordetella vaccination is recommended for all dogs that will be boarded, exposed to nonworking dogs in the course of work (TSA, service dogs), or congregated with dogs from other sources for training or work. Whether intranasal vaccines interfere with olfaction is uncertain: until this can be determined, intranasal vaccines should be avoided in working detection dogs unless they can be held off duty for the week following vaccination because of the potential for extreme ramifications of impaired detection (see the article on olfaction in this issue). Canine influenza virus (CIV) is a highly contagious agent contributing to CIRDC but disease is uncommon and associated with intermittent outbreaks that tend to be limited to particular geographic locations when they occur. CIV vaccines (especially H3N2) may be advised for dogs traveling widely and/or congregating with dogs from diverse sources at training and competitions. CIV circulates widely in South Korea and China and should be considered in dogs traveling to or from those areas, although a serologic study of military working dogs in Korea showed a 0% seropositivity.[15] CIV has not been a prevalent or significant pathogen in dogs in Europe.[16–18] Dogs maintained in closed populations without exposure to noncohort dogs do not require Bordetella, canine parainfluenza, or canine influenza vaccines, although vaccination on initial intake may be advisable.

Borrelia burgdorferi vaccines are indicated for dogs living or traveling to Lyme disease–endemic areas, especially dogs (eg, SAR, herding, guardian, and hunting dogs) that work in wooded and other natural areas and therefore are at higher risk of exposure to tick vectors. Borrelia vaccination should always be adjunctive to and not in place of rigorous tick control (tick preventives/acaricides, prompt removal of ticks, management of the home yard environment).

Other noncore vaccines include canine enteric coronavirus (CCV) vaccine and Crotalus atrox vaccine. CCV vaccination is not recommended because infections are asymptomatic to mild and self-limiting, generally restricted to puppies 6 weeks of age or younger, and vaccination may not be effective. *C atrox* (rattlesnake) vaccine contains components of western diamondback rattlesnake venom and is intended to stimulate neutralizing antibodies, which can reduce morbidity and mortality in dogs bitten by western diamondback and perhaps some other species of rattlesnakes. There is limited evidence showing some benefit in mice,[19] but efficacy in dogs has not been assessed. A study of outcomes of rattlesnake bites in dogs showed no difference between vaccinated and unvaccinated dogs.[20] Vaccination may be associated with adverse reactions to the toxoid and, concerningly, may sensitize dogs to the venom so that envenomated vaccinated dogs may experience an anaphylactic response to the venom.[21] Although some agencies do vaccinate dogs at risk of frequent rattlesnake encounters, the complete lack of data on safety and efficacy of the rattlesnake vaccine precludes its recommendation. Vaccinated dogs must still receive emergency veterinary care following a rattlesnake bite.

PARASITE CONTROL

All dogs should receive consistent and comprehensive parasite management appropriate to their region. Working dogs often require more intensive parasite management because they travel widely, potentially encountering parasites not endemic in their home environments, and because they may have greater exposure to parasites and vectors in their work environments. Many preventive products, including combination products covering flea-tick, heartworm, and/or intestinal parasites, are available commercially and can be selected based on the preferences of the owner/handler for optimizing compliance. Products with repellant properties are advantageous for dogs that are frequently outdoors. External parasite control must also include treatment of all cohort dogs and other host animals in the household or kennel as well as environmental management to eliminate potential flea or tick reservoirs. Dogs that work in natural areas may need a multiple-pronged approach to control ticks: a systemic acaricide with a tick collar (Seresto) or flea-tick spray applied before deployment with careful examination and tick removal after outdoor sessions.

Conscientious heartworm preventive administration and routine testing are imperative for working dogs, who may be deployed in areas where heartworms have developed resistance to preventive drugs.[22–25] Some handlers of hunting and other scent detection dogs report anecdotally that administration of heartworm preventives adversely affects olfaction. Although these products have not been specifically evaluated for their effect on scenting ability, some other types of medications have been shown to adversely affect olfaction and, because some preventives are associated with neurologic signs in dogs, it is possible that commonly used preventives may affect neurologic functioning of the olfactory system. However, the benefit of heartworm prevention outweighs a transient reduction in detection ability. Until studies elucidating the effect, if any, of preventive medication on scenting ability are completed, precautions of taking treated detection dogs out of service for 3 to 5 days after administration or, if multiple detection dogs are available, staggering administration dates to ensure availability of dogs not recently treated for detection tasks may be considered.

SPECIAL PREVENTIVE CONSIDERATIONS
Prophylactic Gastropexy

Many of the working dog breeds are predisposed to gastric dilatation-volvulus (GDV), which usually affects larger deep-chested dogs and is immediately life threatening. Bloodhounds are the second most frequently affected breed after Great Danes, but

German shepherd dogs, Belgian Malinois, Labrador retrievers, and springer spaniels are also at increased risk. Other documented risk factors include increasing age, deep-chested conformation (thorax depth to width ratio >1.6), a relative with GDV, and once-daily feeding regimen.[26–30] GDV is a significant cause of mortality in law enforcement and military working dogs[31–33] and may occur at any time of day (when panting during training or deployment may contribute to initial gastric distension and veterinary care may not be readily accessible) or night (when dogs may be unattended and therefore not identified and presented for veterinary care). Dogs that survive GDV are prone to recurrence of GDV. Gastropexy, in which the stomach is secured in position by a surgical attachment to the body wall, prevents recurrence and reduces mortality in the face of recurrence; prophylactic gastropexy, performed before any GDV occurrence, provides significant protection, reducing incidence of GDV (to 0% in some studies) and severity if it occurs (stomach can still dilate but not torse).[34–40] Prophylactic gastropexy can be performed laparoscopically, reducing recovery time for the procedure, or be paired with ovariohysterectomy in female dogs. Prophylactic gastropexy should be performed for all working dogs of an at-risk breed or body type.

Physical Conditioning

Physical conditioning should be considered a vital component of preventive care. Development and maintenance of balanced muscle strength and appropriate strength and function of tendons and ligaments are critical for maximizing ability and preventing injury in these dogs, from which extreme athleticism and endurance are often required. Musculoskeletal health and appropriate warm-up activities are also important for tolerance of temperature extremes and prevention of heat stroke: by promoting proper muscle metabolism and blood flow, muscle functions more efficiently, generating less heat with exercise, and reaction times improve (see the article, "Sports Medicine and Rehabilitation," in this issue).

Proper Use of Equipment

Owners/handlers are generally knowledgeable about types of dog gear and equipment and the situations for which these are used but are often much less familiar with the associated potential health risks. It is fairly typical for choke collars to be left on dogs around the clock rather than appropriately only while the dog is actively being handled. Although any collar can pose a choking/hanging risk, the full-slip choke collars are the most dangerous because there is no limit to the extent that they constrict and, because they usually compose chain links with rings on the ends, they readily snag and can be difficult for the handler to loosen to disengage the dog. Handlers should be implored to not leave choke collars on between handling sessions and to use them carefully during handling to prevent injury to delicate underlying structures (hyoid apparatus, larynx and laryngeal nerves, jugular vein, vagus nerve, carotid artery, trachea). Pendant-style identification tags and rabies vaccination tags can be caught in wire fencing or grates or otherwise get snagged: risk of injury because of this is greatest if the tags are on a full-slip choke collar. Muzzles can contribute to development of heat stroke when dogs cannot open the mouth and extend the tongue to adequately breathe and dissipate heat. Improperly fitted muzzles can cause injury to underlying tissues, and generally only properly fitted basket muzzles should be used. Harnesses are divided into 2 categories: restrictive and nonrestrictive. Restrictive harnesses are those designed with a chest strap that crosses the plane of the shoulder and may predispose to biceps brachii tendon injury. Both types of harness have been shown to result in a shortening of the dog's stride[41–43] and may cause irritation of underlying structure by rubbing or if something gets caught between the harness and the dog's skin, which is more likely with harnesses constructed of fabric or that have a soft lining. Jute and heavy canvass used to make toys or bite equipment are abrasive and contribute to tooth wear. Tennis balls, commonly used as a play reward for working dogs, have a very abrasive outer surface and likewise can promote dental attrition (see the article, "Working Dog Dentistry," in this issue, for further recommendations).

Lumbosacral Stenosis Monitoring

Lumbosacral stenosis (LSS) is a common disorder in large dogs, and breeds used across several working disciplines are predisposed, including German shepherd dogs (most commonly affected breed) and Labrador retrievers. Genetic factors, congenital abnormalities, and repetitive use or abnormal motion contribute to the condition of lumbosacral (LS) instability, intervertebral disc degeneration, soft tissue proliferation, and cartilage and bone changes leading to stenosis of the spinal canal and progressive compression of the cauda equina and blood supply to nerve tissue. Labrador retrievers may be predisposed because of an increased occurrence of transitional vertebrae in the breed. The average age at presentation across all dogs is 7 years, but clinical signs may be subtle early in the course of the disease: pain and impaired performance may affect working dogs far earlier than pet dog owners might observe problems, but diagnosis at this stage may be missed because of mild to absent clinical findings, lack of suspicion, and overlap with signs of other problems, including muscle strain: these active dogs are asked to perform very athletic tasks, which may in turn predispose them to lumbosacral stenosis through repetitive extreme activities. It is therefore important for veterinarians to maintain a high index of suspicion for this condition in working dogs and to pursue evaluation for LSS in response to handler observation of changes in the dog's working ability or comfort level when other causes are not identified. Ideally, preliminary screening for LS instability or predisposing abnormalities (transitional vertebrae) should be made part of a preliminary fitness for work evaluation, but this significantly escalates the cost of preliminary examinations because accurate assessment for LSS requires advanced imaging studies (computed tomography or MRI).

SUMMARY

Veterinarians providing care for working dogs carry a great deal of responsibility for assessing fitness for work in working dog candidates and in sustaining the health of working dogs in the face the tremendous physical and mental demands placed on these dogs and their increased risk of injury and disease exposure. Comprehensive preventive care is vital for working dogs to maintain peak performance, which can be a matter of life and death for the people these dogs serve as well as the dogs themselves, and to prolong their working lives, understanding the significant investment that these skilled dogs represent. Veterinarians must be especially astute in assessing these dogs. Health problems may be subtle but still significantly impair performance. The dogs often show minimal signs because of a high pain threshold and tremendous eagerness to work. In recognizing breed-related problems, tailoring preventive care plans to meet each dog's needs, and addressing the specific risks and demands of the specialized tasks these dogs perform, veterinarians play a key role not only in the health and welfare of working dogs and their handlers but also in myriad aspects of community health and national and international security served by these dog-handler teams.

DISCLOSURE

The author declares no conflicts of interest.

REFERENCES

1. Cobb M, Branson N, McGreevy P, et al. The advent of canine performance science: offering a sustainable future for working dogs. Behav Process. 2015;110: 96–104.
2. Cao X, Irwin DM, Liu Y, et al. Balancing selection on CDH2 may be related to the behavioral features of the Belgian Malinois. PLoS One 2014;9(10):e110075.
3. SWGDOG 2011 Scientific working group on dog and orthogonal detector guidelines. Available at: https://ifri.fiu.edu/research/detector-dogs/swgdog/.
4. Harper EJ, Hackett RM, Wilkinson J, et al. Age-related variations in hematologic and plasma biochemical test results in Beagles and Labrador Retrievers. J Am Vet Med Assoc 2003;223(10):1436–42.
5. Matwichuk CL, Taylor S, Shmon CL, et al. Changes in rectal temperature and hematologic, biochemical, blood gas, and acid-base values in healthy Labrador Retrievers before and after strenuous exercise. Am J Vet Res 1999;60(1):88–92.
6. Sharkey L, Gjevre K, Hegstad-Davies R, et al. Breed-associated variability in serum biochemical analytes in four large-breed dogs. Vet Clin Pathol 2009; 38(3):375–80.
7. Greenfield CL, Messick JB, Solter PF, et al. Results of hematologic analyses and prevalence of physiologic leukopenia in Belgian Tervuren. J Am Vet Med Assoc 2000;216(6):866–71.
8. Ruggerone B, Giraldi M, Paltrinieri S, et al. Hematologic and biochemical reference intervals in Shetland Sheepdogs. Vet Clin Pathol 2018;47(4):617–24.
9. Bourgès-Abella NH, Gury TD, Geffré A, et al. Reference intervals, intraindividual and interindividual variability, and reference change values for hematologic variables in laboratory beagles. J Am Assoc Lab Anim Sci 2015;54(1):17–24.
10. Chang YM, Hadox E, Szladovits B, et al. Serum biochemical phenotypes in the domestic dog. PLoS One 2016;11(2):e0149650.
11. Miglio A, Gavazza A, Siepi D, et al. Hematological and biochemical reference intervals for 5 adult hunting dog breeds using a blood donor database. Animals (Basel) 2020;10(7):1212.
12. Lawrence J, Chang YM, Szladovits B, et al. Breed-specific hematological phenotypes in the dog: a natural resource for the genetic dissection of hematological parameters in a mammalian species. PLoS One 2013;8(11):e81288.
13. Moore GE, Guptill LF, Ward MP, et al. Adverse events diagnosed within three days of vaccine administration in dogs. J Am Vet Med Assoc 2005;227:1102–8.
14. Klaasen H, Adler B. Recent advances in canine leptospirosis: focus on vaccine development. Vet Med (Auckl) 2015;6:245–60.
15. Kim H, Yang D, Seo B, et al. Serosurvey of rabies virus, canine distemper virus, parvovirus, and influenza virus in military working dogs in Korea. J Vet Med Sci 2018;80(9):1424–30.
16. Schulz B, Klinkenberg C, Fux R, et al. Prevalence of canine influenza virus A (H3N8) in dogs in Germany. Vet J 2014;202(1):184–5.
17. Hiebl A, Auer A, Bagrinovschi G, et al. Detection of selected viral pathogens in dogs with canine infectious respiratory disease in Austria. J Small Anim Pract 2019;60(10):594–600.

18. Mitchell JA, Cardwell JM, Leach H, et al. European surveillance of emerging pathogens associated with canine infectious respiratory disease. Vet Microbiol 2017;212:31–8.
19. Cates CC, Valore EV, Couto MA, et al. Comparison of the protective effect of a commercially available western diamondback rattlesnake toxoid vaccine for dogs against envenomation of mice with western diamondback rattlesnake (Crotalus atrox), northern Pacific rattlesnake (Crotalus oreganus oreganus), and southern Pacific rattlesnake (Crotalus oreganus helleri) venom. Am J Vet Res 2015;76(3):272–9.
20. Leonard MJ, Bresee C, Cruikshank A. Effects of the canine rattlesnake vaccine in moderate to severe cases of canine crotalid envenomation. Vet Med (Auckl) 2014;5:153–8.
21. Petras KE, Wells RJ, Pronko J. Suspected anaphylaxis and lack of clinical protection associated with envenomation in two dogs previously vaccinated with Crotalus atrox toxoid. Toxicon 2018;142:30–3.
22. Bourguinat C, Lee A, Lizunda R, et al. Macrocyclic lactone resistance in Dirofilaria immitis: failure of heartworm preventives and investigation of genetic markers for resistance. Vet Parasitol 2015;210:167–78.
23. Bourguinat C, Keller K, Xia J, et al. Genetic profiles of ten Dirofilaria immitis isolates susceptible or resistant to macrocyclic lactone heartworm preventives. Parasit Vectors 2017;10(Suppl 2):504.
24. McTier TL, Six RH, Pullins A, et al. Efficacy of oral moxidectin against susceptible and resistant isolates of Dirofilaria immitis in dogs. Parasit Vectors 2017;10(Suppl 2):482.
25. McTier TL, Pullins A, Inskeep GA, et al. Microfilarial reduction following ProHeart® 6 and ProHeart® SR-12 treatment in dogs experimentally inoculated with a resistant isolate of Dirofilaria immitis. Parasit Vectors 2017;10(Suppl 2):485.
26. Glickman LT, Glickman NW, Pérez CM, et al. Analysis of risk factors for gastric dilatation and dilatation-volvulus in dogs. J Am Vet Med Assoc 1994;204(9):1465–71.
27. Glickman LT, Glickman NW, Schellenberg DB, et al. Incidence of and breed-related risk factors for gastric dilatation-volvulus in dogs. J Am Vet Med Assoc 2000;216(1):40–5.
28. Glickman LT, Glickman NW, Schellenberg DB, et al. Non-dietary risk factors for gastric dilatation-volvulus in large and giant breed dogs. J Am Vet Med Assoc 2000;217(10):1492–9.
29. Raghavan M, Glickman N, McCabe G, et al. Diet-related risk factors for gastric dilatation-volvulus in dogs of high-risk breeds. J Am Anim Hosp Assoc 2004;40(3):192–203.
30. Pipan M, Brown DC, Battaglia CL, et al. An Internet-based survey of risk factors for surgical gastric dilatation-volvulus in dogs. J Am Vet Med Assoc 2012;240(12):1456–62.
31. Moore GE, Burkman KD, Carter MN, et al. Causes of death or reasons for euthanasia in military working dogs: 927 cases (1993-1996). J Am Vet Med Assoc 2001;219(2):209–14.
32. Evans RI, Herbold JR, Bradshaw BS, et al. Causes for discharge of military working dogs from service: 268 cases (2000-2004). J Am Vet Med Assoc 2007;231(8):1215–20.
33. Miller L, Pacheco GJ, Janak JC, et al. Causes of death in military working dogs during operation iraqi freedom and operation enduring freedom, 2001-2013. Mil Med 2018;183(9–10):e467–74.

34. Ward MP, Patronek GJ, Glickman LT. Benefits of prophylactic gastropexy for dogs at risk of gastric dilatation-volvulus. Prev Vet Med 2003;60(4):319–29.
35. Allen P, Paul A. Gastropexy for prevention of gastric dilatation-volvulus in dogs: history and techniques. Top Companion Anim Med 2014;29(3):77–80.
36. Gazzola KM, Nelson LL. The relationship between gastrointestinal motility and gastric dilatation-volvulus in dogs. Top Companion Anim Med 2014;29(3):64–6.
37. Ullmann B, Seehaus N, Hungerbühler S, et al. Gastric dilatation volvulus: a retrospective study of 203 dogs with ventral midline gastropexy. J Small Anim Pract 2016;57(1):18–22.
38. Loy Son NK, Singh A, Amsellem P, et al. Long-term outcome and complications following prophylactic laparoscopic-assisted gastropexy in dogs. Vet Surg 2016; 45(S1):O77–83.
39. Coleman KA, Boscan P, Ferguson L, et al. Evaluation of gastric motility in nine dogs before and after prophylactic laparoscopic gastropexy: a pilot study. Aust Vet J 2019;97(7):225–30.
40. Benitez ME, Schmiedt CW, Radlinsky MG, et al. Efficacy of incisional gastropexy for prevention of GDV in dogs. J Am Anim Hosp Assoc 2013;49(3):185–9.
41. Carr BJ, Zink C, Dreese K. Harnesses for agility dogs. In: Clean run magazine. 2017.
42. Carr BJ, Dresse K, Zink MC. The effects of five commercially available harnesses on canine gait. Proc ACVS Surg Summit 2016.
43. Lafuente MP, Provis L, Schmalz EA. Effects of restrictive and non-restrictive harnesses on shoulder extension in dogs at walk and trot. Vet Rec 2019;184(2):64.

Anesthetic Considerations for Working Dogs

Ashley Mitek, DVM, MS[a],*, Jacob Johnson, DVM[b]

KEYWORDS

- K9 • Canine • Law enforcement K9 • Sedation • Analgesia

KEY POINTS

- Working dogs can cause serious bodily injury, and practitioners should prioritize human safety when working with these patients.
- When possible, every effort should be made to thoroughly plan a working dog's anesthetic event to maximize efficiency and safety and to prevent miscommunication.
- The K9 handler plays an important role in the working dog's care. It is essential for the veterinary team to effectively communicate and include the handler in the K9's care.

INTRODUCTION

Working dogs pose unique anesthesia and pain management considerations compared with the typical pet canine presenting to a practitioner. As more agencies use the talents of working dogs for various responsibilities, veterinarians will more frequently be asked to provide elective and emergency anesthesia and pain management to these patients. Because of their value to society, cost to obtain, and lengthy training, it is imperative that anesthesia and pain management be provided that meets the highest standard of care and gives the patient the best opportunity to return to work.

Working dogs are used for numerous tasks, including, but not limited to, scent detection (for example, narcotics, explosive, arson, search and rescue, cadaver, and currency detection), apprehension/protection, assistance animals, and service animals. Many working dogs in the United States used by police agencies are dual purpose, meaning they do bite work in addition to detection. The list of possible tasks a working dog may perform is constantly growing. New research suggests that canines may be able to identify COVID-19 in human respiratory secretions.[1]

There are no conflicts of interest or disclosures to report.
[a] College of Veterinary Medicine, University of Illinois, 1008 West Hazelwood Drive, Urbana, IL 61821, USA; [b] Department of Clinical Sciences, 1010 Wire Road, Auburn, AL 36849, USA
* Corresponding author.
E-mail address: Ashleymitek@gmail.com

Veterinarians should identify the type of work the dog performs, their current level of training, and their relationship with the handler, before creating anesthesia and pain management plans. An all-inclusive review of every type or breed of working dog and their unique concerns under anesthesia is beyond the scope of this review. Dual-purpose law enforcement canines (LEK9s; narcotic detection and protection/apprehension) are the focus of this article because they are most frequently seen by veterinarians and pose unique challenges.

SAFETY CONCERNS AND RECOMMENDATIONS
Veterinary Personnel and Handler Safety

The most important concern surrounding LEK9s is human safety. Many of these dogs have been trained to bite with excessive force and can cause serious bodily injury. LEK9s presenting for routine screening examination immediately after importation or purchase (which may require sedation or anesthesia, especially if the examination includes orthopedic examination and radiographs) may not be fully trained and can pose additional risks to veterinary personnel.

Undoubtedly a veterinary practice is a new environment to most LEK9s, inciting anxiety in these patients for many reasons, including new smells, sounds, people, and other animals. In addition, the LEK9 may be in pain when presented, which may make the patient more prone to reactive behavior.

At the author's institution (A.M.), all LEK9s are required to have a basket muzzle placed before entering the facility, and their handler is expected to accompany them at all times, when possible, including during induction and recovery. Cloth muzzles are not recommended on an LEK9 because they do not allow the patient to ventilate (pant) appropriately when excited or hot, which may result in adverse outcomes. Only experienced personnel should work with the hospitalized LEK9.

Most handlers are comfortable restraining their LEK9. However, the veterinarian supervising care should discuss this with the handler before treating the patient. In some instances, new handlers are not comfortable restraining their LEK9, which can lead to severe injury to the veterinary team and/or handler if not clarified before restraint. Alternatively, handlers are often aware of how the LEK9 prefers to be restrained, or how the patient has responded in the past. Communicating with the handler regarding these issues can be invaluable to the safe and efficient treatment of the patient. If this is the first time a handler has been with an LEK9 during sedation, induction, and recovery, the authors strongly encourage the veterinarian to educate the handler about these events so they can actively participate and be prepared to be part of the patient's anesthetic team. Most handlers readily accept this responsibility.

Veterinarians are aware that allowing the "owner" of a patient to assist with restraint may put them in uncertain legal liability territory if the patient bites the owner or staff member. The authors encourage veterinarians to review their liability coverage and regulations when these questions arise. In the authors' experience, having the handler present often leads to a better overall experience for the LEK9, the veterinary staff, and the handler, as many LEK9s have important bonds with their handler and readily respond to their commands.

Safety Recommendations for Entering/Exiting a Facility

In addition to considering the safety of both the handler and the veterinary personnel, it is important to consider the safety and comfort of other patients and clients in the hospital. If possible, LEK9s should enter the facility from a separate entrance than other patients. Entering the facility from a separate entrance prevents unnecessary exposure to other patients in the facility (waiting room) and decreases the chances of an interaction between the LEK9 and another client or animal. LEK9s should immediately be placed into an examination room upon entering the facility.

Specific safety concerns pertaining to prehospital sedation, in-hospital premedication, induction, and recovery are covered in later discussion.

Stressed LEK9s, particularly at recovery, can in rare circumstances injure themselves. The anesthetic recovery section in later discussion covers mitigating these risks.

GENERAL ANESTHESIA CONSIDERATIONS OF THE LAW ENFORCEMENT CANINES

All canine patients, including working dogs, should have an individualized treatment plan. Every patient may have different anesthetic and procedural concerns, preexisting conditions, breed considerations, responses to anesthetic drugs, work expectations, personalities, and pain tolerances, in addition to many other factors.

In later discussion, the authors have listed common considerations the veterinary team should evaluate before performing anesthesia on an LEK9.

Planning and Timing

The anesthesia of an LEK9 can be an ideal time to plan and conduct routine surveillance examinations as previously discussed. Readers are directed to the LEK9 Anesthesia Checklist in **Box 1**. Using a checklist can help prevent miscommunications, optimize patient care, and curate a collaborative team approach.[2]

LEK9 patients often benefit from being the first case of the day. Being the first case of the day may allow the patient to have a more limited exposure to other animals and give them the best chance of recovering before personnel may need to leave for the day. Because LEK9s are often discharged as soon as they are stable, an early surgery time best positions staff to identify any postoperative complications before discharge.

Before any drug administration, discussions with the handler regarding their expectations as well as requirements for the dog to return to duty should occur. The effects of anesthetic drugs on canine performance, especially olfaction, is unknown, and an extended convalescent period after an anesthetic procedure is recommended (see Melissa Singletary and Lucia Lazarowski's article, "Canine Special Senses: Considerations in Olfaction, Vision, and Audition," in this issue). If the dog is required to return to duty within 24 hours of anesthesia, special consideration toward using drugs that are reversible or rapidly eliminated is advisable.

Breed Concerns

Many, but not all, LEK9s are large-breed dogs, typically averaging 25 to 35 kg. Several of the commonly used breeds are predisposed to gastric dilatation and volvulus. The veterinarian should discuss gastropexy with the owner/handler of any LEK9 that is undergoing anesthesia. Many government agencies now mandate or strongly recommend LEK9s have a prophylactic gastropexy before commencing their service. When appropriate, it can be beneficial to have 1 anesthetic event that encompasses several procedures, minimizing the number of trips the patient must make to the hospital.

Many large-breed dogs used for law enforcement are predisposed to or have preexisting orthopedic conditions. In addition, they may have undiagnosed dental disease or fractures from bite work (see Stephen Juriga and Karin Bilyard's article, "Working Dog Dentistry," in this issue) When anesthesia is planned, it is the ideal time to perform a complete oral and orthopedic examination and take dental, hip,

---

Box 1
Anesthesia checklist for law enforcement K9s

Prehospital:
☐ Schedule and coordinate all procedures throughout the hospital, if needed.
  ☐ LEK9s often benefit from being the first case of the day.
☐ Communicate with the LEK9's handler regarding the perianesthetic plan and their role in the procedures.
  ☐ Ask the handler if the patient needs any of the following performed so it can be scheduled in advance:
    ☐ Vaccination
    ☐ Oral examination/radiographs
    ☐ Orthopedic examination/radiographs
    ☐ Complete blood count, chemistry, urinalysis, or other diagnostics
    ☐ Gastropexy
    ☐ Toe nail trim
    ☐ If warranted, discuss and plan a postoperative analgesic plan that may include epidural or other locoregional anesthetics.
☐ Ensure patient wears a basket muzzle before entering the building.

Perianesthetic:
☐ Premedicate patient
☐ Perform physical examination
☐ Remove all collars, especially pronged and choke collars
☐ Place IV catheter
  ☐ Consider placing IV in hindlimb if possible to maintain distance from patient's face at induction and recovery
  ☐ Collect blood as necessary:
    ☐ PCV/TP
    ☐ BUN
    ☐ Glucose
    ☐ Additional blood samples can be saved for CBC and chemistry, if warranted
    ☐ Consider performing urinalysis, if warranted

Recovery:
☐ When possible, have handler available
☐ Have a recovery area set up in a quiet space
☐ Place basket muzzle before extubation (can insert a photograph of ET tube coming out of basket muzzle)
☐ Additional induction agent/analgesic and/or sedative readily available for poor recovery/emergence delirium (example: dexmedetomidine 0.5 μg/kg IV)

---

spine, stifle, and elbow surveillance radiographs. Nail clipping and, if needed, auricular examination can be done during recovery as long as the dog is muzzled. Veterinarians should coordinate in advance with necessary personnel to insure these multiple procedures are done efficiently to minimize anesthesia time.

Some LEK9s have previously diagnosed osteoarthritis but can continue to work and maintain a good quality of life. The anesthetic team should be vigilant of the affected joints and ensure that the patient is well padded and positioned, and carefully moved while anesthetized in order to prevent further injury and pain at recovery.

Preanesthetic Physical Examination

Every attempt should be made to complete a thorough physical examination of an LEK9 when the patient can be safely examined, with minimal stress. However, many LEK9s will not tolerate this, and/or it poses significant risks to the veterinary care team. At the author's institution (A.M.), LEK9s are routinely premedicated before examination, because it poses minimal risk to a young healthy dog. The risks (usually minimal) of sedating a patient before physical examination should be communicated to the handler.

Preanesthetic Bloodwork

It is often not possible to draw blood from an LEK9 before premedication. In ASA (American Society of Anesthesiologists) I and II patients, preprocedural bloodwork has not been shown to change patient outcome.[3] However, the authors recommend that blood be collected during intravenous (IV) catheter placement before anesthetic induction if abnormalities are detected on the history or physical examination. At a minimum, a blood glucose, packed cell volume/total protein (PCV/TP), and blood urea nitrogen (BUN) should be checked because abnormal results can change the anesthetic plan and/or procedure and spur additional necessary diagnostics.

Fasting

Considerable debate exists around fasting recommendations in canines. The 2020 American Animal Hospital Association Anesthesia Guidelines recommends that a healthy canine be fasted for 4 to 6 hours before anesthesia.[4] If the patient has a history, or is at considerable risk of regurgitation, the anesthesia plan should be amended to facilitate rapid and continuous control of the airway.

Selection of Pharmacologic Agents

There is no perfect anesthetic agent for all LEK9s, but the ideal drug profile is rapidly acting and easily reversible. Ketamine and tiletamine/zolazepam (Telazol) can be used in working dogs and may provide some benefits in certain situations but should be used knowing that they cannot be reversed. Benzodiazepines should be used with caution in healthy LEK9s because of their propensity to induce paradoxic excitement and behavioral changes. Although LEK9s are often stoic, analgesics, such as opioids, should never be withheld from the patient when warranted. Acepromazine is not reversible, is long acting, and may cause unexpected side effects in working dog breeds. If cardiac arrest occurs in a dog that was medicated with acepromazine, epinephrine reversal will occur, which is characterized by a drop in blood pressure after administration of epinephrine while alpha-blockers are on board.

Anosmia/Hyposmia

Several drugs, and general anesthesia, are known to induce anosmia, a loss of the sense of smell, in people in very rare circumstances[5–7] (see Melissa Singletary and Lucia Lazarowski's article, "Canine Special Senses: Considerations in Olfaction, Vision, and Audition," in this issue). The authors are unaware of these disorders occurring in dogs as a result of general anesthesia or sedation, although it has been shown to occur with antibiotics.[8] Although the authors are unaware of any case reports of LEK9s losing their sense of smell after anesthesia or sedative events, interested readers are directed to a more comprehensive veterinary reviews on the topic[9] and to see Melissa Singletary and Lucia Lazarowski's article, "Canine Special Senses: Considerations in Olfaction, Vision, and Audition," in this issue. Because there are case reports of humans permanently losing their sense of smell after lidocaine application to the nasal epithelium, the authors recommend that no local anesthetics be applied intranasally in LEK9s.[10]

Vaccination Although Anesthetized

There is considerable debate surrounding whether to vaccinate patients while anesthetized. Although rare, patients may be at risk of developing life-threatening anaphylaxis, which can prove fatal under anesthesia. It may be challenging to safely vaccinate an LEK9, and the authors recommend that in some instances, vaccination can be safely performed while anesthetized as long as the patient is monitored for any signs of anaphylaxis. Anaphylaxis can be difficult to detect during anesthesia, and classic signs in dogs would be tachycardia and hypotension. The risks of performing vaccination while anesthetized should be communicated with the handler.

Sedation Versus General Anesthesia

Many veterinarians think that "sedation" is less risky than "general anesthesia." Evidence shows that there is no difference in mortality between the two, and clinically differentiating these 2 states may prove challenging.[3]

Both sedation and general anesthesia may compromise homeostasis and impair the body's normal compensatory mechanisms. Although general anesthesia may produce a more profound loss of consciousness and insult to important body systems that control ventilation, oxygenation, and cardiovascular stability, patients are often more appropriately and intensely monitored while "anesthetized," which is key in identifying adverse changes before they become life threatening.

Furthermore, LEK9s often require a deeper sedative plane and larger doses of sedative drugs for safe handling. These facts may lead to LEK9s being "anesthetized" when the practitioner was intent on only having the patient "sedated."

Semantics aside, when a procedure on an LEK9 is expected to last greater than 20 to 30 minutes, the authors recommend that the patient be intubated and anesthetized, with complete monitoring. The Monitoring section discussed next provides additional recommendations.

MONITORING

LEK9s should be monitored during sedative and anesthetic events. The American College of Veterinary Anesthesia and Analgesia recommends the following[11]:

- An experienced individual be solely dedicated to monitoring the patient
- This individual should monitor the following parameters at least every 5 minutes and document this information on the patient's anesthetic record:
  o Heart rate
  o Respiratory rate
  o Temperature
  o Mucus membrane color
  o Anesthetic depth
- The following equipment should be used to monitor the patient:
  o Capnograph
  o Electrocardiograph
  o Blood pressure cuff
  o Pulse oximetry monitor
  o Thermometer

The importance of having an experienced anesthetist that is completely focused on monitoring the patient with the recommendations above may help prevent many adverse events.

Because LEK9s are typically well-conditioned athletes, their physiologic parameters may be different under anesthesia. Depending on their level of activity and excitement before sedation, they may have an elevated body temperature, but in the absence of other signs of heat-related injury, this does not require intervention. Their heart rate is generally lower and second-degree atrioventricular block is not uncommon. Intervention is not necessary unless either bradycardia or heart block is affecting the cardiac output. Under anesthesia, a drop in cardiac output would be demonstrated by hypotension and decreased end-tidal carbon dioxide ($ETCO_2$) concentrations on capnography. If ventilation is constant, then a drop in $ETCO_2$ represents decreased carbon dioxide return to the lungs (hypoperfusion) or machine error. Transient apnea and lower respiratory rates are more common than in comparably sized pet dogs, but this does not require intervention unless severely hypercapnic ($ETCO_2 > 60$) for a prolonged duration (eg, ~5–10 minutes).

RECORDKEEPING

A patient's past anesthetic records may be helpful in predicting future issues. For this reason, any LEK9 that is sedated or anesthetized should have a complete record of the medications used, any issues such as hypotensive events, and any negative effects of specific medications used. A copy should be given to the handler. These documents can be helpful when deciding on an anesthetic plan for an LEK9. Thorough recordkeeping is also vital for liability reasons. Many LEK9s are insured for significant values.

ANESTHETIC PLANNING CONSIDERATIONS FOR ELECTIVE PROCEDURES

There are numerous anesthetic drug combinations that can be effective in LEK9s, and each patient's unique history, type of work, comorbid conditions, and previous anesthesia experiences should be taken into account to create an individualized treatment plan. In the later sections, the authors outline several anesthesia/analgesia plans that may be effective.

At-Home Premedication

The anesthetic plan can be initiated at home, if necessary. Handlers can give a sedative by mouth before arriving at the clinic if the patient has a history that would demonstrate this as a benefit. Drugs, such as oral trazodone and gabapentin, may have varying sedative effects. In general, these oral agents are not always reliable, but some patients may benefit from anxiolysis or sedation before arrival at the hospital. Transmucosal detomodine[12] or dexmedetomidine[13] can also be administered before arrival at the clinic to facilitate more reliable sedation if needed. Consideration should be given to how these medications will interact with the other drugs to be used for sedation and anesthesia.

In-Hospital Premedication

Once in the hospital, the most effective and reliable way to sedate an LEK9 is with intramuscular (IM) administration of drugs. After a muzzle is in place, the handler can often restrain the patient so that the veterinary team member can quickly inject sedating agents in the hindlimb or epaxial region. The authors recommend an 18- to 20-g luer-lock needle and less than 2 mL of injectate to facilitate rapid drug administration. Luer-lock needles are ideal because they may prevent the needle from separating from the syringe if a patient moves during injection. Although aspiration is often recommended before IM injection, for safety reasons, IM injection can under extenuating circumstances be performed without aspiration in LEK9s.

After IM injection, noise should be kept to a minimum to facilitate a smooth and rapid transition to a sedative state. Depending on the medications administered, least 20 minutes should be allowed for the desired sedative effect to occur. The muzzle should not be removed when an LEK9 appears sedate. Serious injury has occurred in veterinary personnel when the patient appeared to be sedate and the muzzle was removed, only to have the LEK9 startle and bite. Muzzles should remain on the patient until the point of intubation.

Sample IM premedication (or sedation only) protocols for a healthy LEK9
10 µg/kg dexmedetomidine + 0.1 mg/kg hydromorphone
OR
10 µg/kg dexmedetomidine + 0.4 mg/kg butorphanol

Note the following cautions.

The combination of dexmedetomidine + opioid can be a favorable and reliable combination for most LEK9s. Dexmedetomidine can be paired with several different types of opioids, but the authors recommend a full mu-agonist be included in painful procedures. If available, methadone may cause less vomiting and nausea in comparison to hydromorphone and morphine.

In LEK9s that are exceptionally aggressive, or who have proven challenging to sedate in the past, ketamine or tiletamine/zolazepam at 1 to 5 mg/kg IM can be included in the above protocols. At the higher end of the dose range, these combinations are likely to induce general anesthesia. The patient should be closely monitored, and equipment should be available for intubation should the patient lose airway control. The addition of a dissociative may also improve the quality of the patient's recovery.

Although rare, some LEK9s may fail to become sedate after initial premedication. If this occurs, confirmation that the appropriate amount of time elapsed after IM drug administration and that the correct medications and doses were selected should commence. Patients may fail to become sedate for many reasons, but most commonly in LEK9s, it is because the full dose was not injected IM because of poor patient compliance/user error, or because the patient is exceptionally anxious. After the appropriate amount of time has elapsed from the time of premedication administration, and the patient shows no signs of becoming sedate, the full dose of the premedication combination that was selected should be given. If the patient has only become mildly sedated, and it is not yet safe to place an IV catheter, the premedication should be repeated at one-half of the dose.

Once the patient is sedated, the handler can assist in lifting the patient onto a gurney and transporting to the anesthetic preparation area/or alternate space where induction will take place. During this transport period, personnel can begin to take vital signs, perform a physical examination, and place an IV catheter. If the procedure allows, it may be beneficial to place the IV in a hindlimb to help personnel maintain further distance from the LEK9's face during induction and recovery.

Induction

LEK9s should be preoxygenated with a basket muzzle on for approximately 5 minutes before administration of the induction agent.[14] During this time, an IV catheter can be placed, a blood sample is taken, vital signs are assessed, and monitoring equipment are readied for a seamless induction and transition to general anesthesia.

There are numerous rapid-acting IV induction agents available to practitioners. Propofol, alfaxalone, tiletamine/zolazepam, and ketamine/midazolam are all appropriate induction agents in the healthy LEK9. Rapid-acting hypnotics (propofol and alfaxalone) are preferred, as they are less likely to persist during the recovery period. Perhaps the 2 most common differences between induction of a pet canine and an LEK9 is (1) it is helpful to have the handler remain with the LEK9 through premedication and induction because the patient may startle or premedications may wear off, and (2) it is important to achieve an appropriate plane of anesthesia before removing the muzzle, attempting to open the LEK9s mouth and intubating them. The basket muzzle should stay in place until the patient's eyes have rolled ventrally and they have a minimal or no palpebral reflex, at which point intubation can be attempted.

Maintenance

Inhalant and injectable agents can be used to provide multimodal anesthesia and analgesia. There is no 1 maintenance protocol that is best. A combination of an inhalant agent, such as isoflurane or sevoflurane, in combination with premedications discussed above should provide an appropriate plane of anesthesia for most procedures when titrated appropriately.

Recovery

LEK9s may pose a serious safety concern to their handler and veterinary personnel at recovery. Practitioners can promote a smooth and safe recovery by doing the following:

- Basket muzzle should be placed before recovery.
    - The endotracheal tube can easily be placed through one of the openings to allow the patient to wear the muzzle while recovering.
- Individualized anesthetic drug plan should be chosen, assuring it provides appropriate level and duration of anesthesia.
    - Anxiolysis
    - Analgesia
        - Note: It can be challenging to differentiate postoperative pain from dysphoria. It is imperative that all LEK9s receive appropriate analgesics.
    - A rapid transition from general anesthesia to regaining consciousness should be prevented because it may increase the risk of dysphoria.
- Communication between the handler and the veterinary care team on the plan for recovery should include the following:
    - Location
        - The recovery room should be quiet to minimize overly stimulating the patient.
        - The patient should be placed in the run/cage before recovery. Attachment of a length of gauze or string to the endotracheal tube facilitates extubation at a distance from the patient.
    - Timing
    - Monitoring
    - Personnel that should be present:
        - The role of the handler in recovery should be discussed before induction. Most handlers will sit with their LEK9 (near the head) in the recovery cage or room. This can be very helpful to the veterinary care team if the patient wakes up dysphoric.

- If the handler chooses to leave the building during the maintenance phase of anesthesia, anesthesia personnel should have the handler's cell phone number in order to notify them when recovery will occur.
  - Organizing any needed equipment:
    - Supplemental oxygen
    - Heat support
    - Monitoring devices
      - A pulse oximeter can be placed on the hind limb toe web as a noninvasive way to measure heart rate and saturation in recovery.
  - Additional injectable drugs should be prepared and easily accessible in recovery for controlling pain and/or dysphoria at extubation. As an example, the authors recommend having the below available:
    - 0.5 to 2 μg/kg of dexmedetomidine, which can be administered IV to control a dysphoric recovery.
    - Propofol or alfaxalone IV to effect sedating the patient can also be beneficial (continue to monitor the patient's oxygenation and ventilation).
    - A rapid-acting analgesic, such as hydromorphone at 0.1 mg/kg, can be administered to control pain.
  - Only experienced veterinary personnel should directly handle the LEK9.

A low-volume fluid line can be attached to the IV catheter (preferably in a hind limb) to allow veterinary personnel to administer any medications from a safe distance, if needed. This low-volume fluid line can be set up before recovery, so that if the patient does wake up dysphoric, the veterinary team is not struggling to place a needle into a moving IV catheter hub, which may lead to inadvertent human injection, and failure to administer sedating agents to the LEK9.

There is no evidence in healthy canines to support the commonly taught principle that the endotracheal tube should be removed only when the patient swallows many times. In the authors' experience, extubating any canine patient, especially an LEK9, after they are conscious enough to swallow several times can lead to an increased incidence of poor recovery and injury to personnel. In young healthy LEK9s who have no history of regurgitation, or an increased procedural risk of regurgitation, it may be of benefit to remove the endotracheal tube when the patient begins to show signs of waking (eg, moving head, eyes opening, attempting to vocalize) but before the patient is able to swallow.

Dexmedetomidine is often administered to LEK9s as part of a balanced anesthetic protocol, but the doses can exceed the typical dose administered to pet canines and more align with the manufacturer's recommendation. It can be beneficial at recovery to have clinically relevant plasma concentrations of dexmedetomidine still present from the premedication, which can facilitate a slower and smoother recovery.

However, if the patient does not regain consciousness within a reasonable amount of time (approximately 20–30 minutes) after inhalants or other agents are discontinued, practitioners can consider administering incremental doses of atipamezole IM and monitor response to therapy. Administration of the recommended dose of atipamezole may lead to a sudden and violent recovery and should be used with caution.

Alpha-2 agonists like dexmedetomidine make it difficult for patients to concentrate urine. Frequently, LEK9s will need to void a large volume of urine shortly after recovery. If possible, the patient's bladder should be expressed before recovery. When it is safe for them to walk, the veterinary team should encourage the handler to allow the LEK9 to urinate outside. Handlers should also be informed that the LEK9 may need to urinate more frequently for the next 24 hours.

Postoperative Analgesics

Preemptive analgesia should be included in any anesthetic drug protocol for patients who may experience a painful procedure. It is the first step in preventing postoperative pain that can lead to a poor recovery and chronic pain syndromes.

Various analgesic agents are available that act on the different pain pathways (transduction, transmission, modulation, and the perception). Readers are encouraged to review pain management guidelines and recommendations that have been previously published for canines.[15] When possible, a multimodal analgesic plan should be created for the individual and procedural needs of each patient. A few unique concerns of analgesia in LEK9s are listed as follows:

- LEK9s are often "stoic," and the detection of pain may be challenging. It is imperative that analgesic agents not be withheld when warranted.
- Many LEK9s are high energy and may not do well when hospitalized. Every effort should be made to discharge them as soon as possible, assuming their pain can be controlled at home.
- Long-acting locoregional anesthetics may be beneficial by decreasing the need for systemic analgesia leading to a shorter hospital stay. Consideration should be given to how regional anesthesia may affect ambulation postoperatively. Prolonged loss of motor control may lead to stress in high-energy working dogs and delay the ability to discharge the patient.
- Handlers should be educated by the veterinary team to recognize pain in their LEK9, and breakthrough pain should be treated promptly.

Postoperative Nausea and Vomiting

Postoperative nausea and vomiting (PONV) is a common, and an often underdiagnosed, sequelae of anesthesia and should be treated promptly. It is recognized through signs of nausea, such as licking the lips, hypersalivation, or anorexia. Maropitant and ondansetron are 2 effective agents in preventing and controlling PONV.

ANESTHETIC PROTOCOL CONSIDERATIONS FOR EMERGENCY PROCEDURES

LEK9s are often presented for emergency conditions. The 2 most common reasons are gastric dilatation volvulus and a traumatic injury while in the line of duty (eg, stabbing or gunshot wound). As previously discussed, safety is paramount, especially because these LEK9s may present in extreme pain. The handler, if available, should place a basket muzzle before the patient enters the facility. If possible, the handler should be included in the patient's care team, remain with the patient until intubation, and be available to assist at recovery. Handlers often readily accept this role and have a unique bond with their LEK9. Many handlers are capable and well trained in handling stressful situations, but it is imperative that the veterinary team effectively communicates with them during this period. If pain is suspected, the patient should be administered a full mu-agonist IV or IM on arrival as part of the overall stabilization process. Uncontrolled pain can lead to fatal arrhythmias and other systemic demise, in addition to making an LEK9 more challenging to examine and treat.

Analgesics for Emergency Cases (Premedication)
Methadone 0.3 mg/kg IM or IV
Morphine 0.5 to 1 mg/kg IM or slow IV
Fentanyl 5 µg/kg loading dose and then 5 µg/kg/h IV (or titrated to effect)
Hydromorphone 0.1 mg/kg IV or IM

The LEK9 should be optimally resuscitated to the extent possible before being anesthetized. One sample protocol for an LEK9 undergoing emergency anesthesia is discussed below.

Premedication

Premedication should include midazolam, 0.5 mg/kg, and hydromorphone, 0.2 mg/kg IV. If the canine cannot be intubated within 60 seconds, propofol is given incrementally at 1 mg/kg until intubation can be achieved. Although dexmedetomidine is a good selection for healthy patients, it should be avoided in compromised patients because of its significant cardiovascular effects.

Induction

A slow, small bolus of propofol to effect is often appropriate when the patient has been premedicated. In unstable patients, the amount of induction agent needed is lowered and insult to the cardiovascular system is mitigated, by administering additional full mu-agonists, such as fentanyl, hydromorphone, and methadone IV as a coinduction agent. Alternatively, lidocaine, administered at 2 mg/kg IV, can be used as a coinduction agent.

Maintenance

Every effort should be made to use inhalant-sparing techniques by using additional analgesic and anesthetic agents that induce minimal cardiovascular depression. These agents include using a fentanyl and/or lidocaine constant rate infusion (CRI) that is titratable.

CRI for emergency anesthesia:
Fentanyl CRI: 5 to 40 μg/kg/h (with a 5-μg/kg loading dose)
Hydromorphone CRI: 20 to 50 μg/kg/h (with a 50-μg/kg loading dose)
Morphine CRI: 0.1 to 0.25 mg/kg/h (with 0.25-mg/kg loading dose, slow)
Lidocaine CRI: 3 to 6 mg/kg/h (with a 2-mg/kg loading dose)

Monitoring

In addition to baseline monitoring (see above), emergency cases may also benefit from the placement of an arterial catheter to monitor blood pressure invasively and evaluation of serial blood gases, during both anesthesia and early recovery. However, leaving an arterial catheter in place after extubation may create serious complications if the dog is difficult to restrain.

In addition to the stable patient recovery and hospitalization recommendations, emergency patients that need to be hospitalized may benefit from the use of low-flow lines and auxiliary ports to allow for hands-off administration of postoperative medications. Telemetry and other monitoring devices that allow the patient to be assessed without arousing or stressing them may also be beneficial. Accommodations should be made to allow the handler to stay with the patient whenever possible.

SUMMARY

LEK9s present unique challenges to the veterinary anesthesia team when presented for routine or emergency anesthesia. With careful planning, vigilance, and a healthy respect for the safety risks in working with LEK9s, the anesthesia team can provide these patients with the best chance of a positive anesthetic experience.

CLINICS CARE POINTS

- Before any drug administration, the veterinarian should communicate with the handler about their involvement before, during, and after the procedure. If the patient must return to duty within 24 hours, special consideration to using drugs that are reversible or rapidly eliminated is advisable.

- Ketamine and tiletamine/zolazepam (Telazol) can be used in working dogs and may provide some benefits in certain situations, but should be used knowing that they cannot be reversed.

- Benzodiazepines should be used with caution in healthy law enforcement canines because of their propensity to induce paradoxic excitement and behavioral changes.

- Because law enforcement canines are typically well-conditioned athletes, their physiologic parameters may be different under anesthesia. Their heart rate is generally lower, and second-degree atrioventricular block is not uncommon.

- In preparation for recovery, a length of gauze or string can be attached to the endotracheal tube to allow extubation at a distance from the patient.

- At recovery, low-volume fluid line can be attached to the intravenous catheter (preferably in a hind limb) to allow veterinary personnel to administer any medications from a safe distance, if needed.

- Consideration should be given to how regional anesthesia may affect ambulation postoperatively. Prolonged loss of motor control may lead to stress in high-energy working dogs and delay the ability to discharge the patient.

REFERENCES

1. Jendrny P, Schulz C, Twele F, et al. Scent dog identification of samples from COVID-19 patients – a pilot study. BMC Infect Dis 2020;20:536 [article: 536].
2. Pucher PH, Aggarwal R, Almond MH, et al. Surgical care checklists to optimize patient care following postoperative complications. Am J Surg 2015;210(3):517–25.
3. Brodbelt Dave. Perioperative mortality in small animal anaesthesia. Vet J 2009;182(2):152–61.
4. Grubb T, Sager J, Gaynor JS, et al. 2020 AAHA Anesthesia and Monitoring Guidelines for dogs and cats. J Am Anim Hosp Assoc 2020;56(2):59–82.
5. Mayell A, Natusch D. Anosmia–a potential complication of intranasal ketamine. Anaesthesia 2009;64(4):457–8.
6. Dhanani NM, Jiang Y. Anosmia and hypogeusia as a complication of general anesthesia. J Clin Anesth 2012;24(3):231–3.
7. Elterman KG, Mallampati SR, Kaye AD, et al. Postoperative alterations in taste and smell. Anesth Pain Med 2014;4:e18527.
8. Jenkins EK, Lee-Fowler TM, Angle TC, et al. Effects of oral administration of metronidazole and doxycycline on olfactory capabilities of explosives detection dogs. Am J Vet Res 2016;77:906–12.
9. Jenkins EK, DeChant MT, Perry EB. When the nose doesn't know: canine olfactory function associated with health, management, and potential links to microbiota. Front Vet Sci 2018;5:56.
10. Salvinelli F, Casale M, F Hardy J, et al. Permanent anosmia after topical nasal anaesthesia with lidocaine 4%. Br J Anaesth 2005;95:838–9.
11. American College of Veterinary Anesthesia & Analgesia Monitoring Guidelines. Available at: https://acvaa.org/wp-content/uploads/2019/05/Small-Animal-Monitoring-Guidlines.pdf. Accessed November 5, 2020.

12. Hopfensperger MJ, Messenger KM, Papich MG, et al. The use of oral transmucosal detomidine hydrochloride gel to facilitate handling in dogs. J Vet Behav 2013;8(3):114–23.

13. Cohen AE, Bennett SL. Oral transmucosal administration of dexmedetomidine for sedation in 4 dogs. Can Vet J 2015;56(11):1144–8.

14. McNally EM, Robertson SA, Luisito SP. Comparison of time to desaturation between preoxygenated and nonpreoxygenated dogs following sedation with acepromazine maleate and morphine and induction of anesthesia with propofol. Am J Vet Res 2009;70(11):1333–8.

15. Epstein M, Rodan I, Griffenhagen G, et al. 2015 AAHA/AAFP pain management guidelines for dogs and cats. J Feline Med Surg 2015;17(2):251–72.

Working Dog Dentistry

Stephen Juriga, DVM[a],*, Karin Bilyard, DVM, LTC, USAR[b]

KEYWORDS

- Canine • Tooth injury • Tooth fracture • Tooth wear • Tooth luxation • Oral trauma

KEY POINTS

- Normal anatomy and function of the canine oral cavity
- Considerations for working dog management, workflow, and hospital safety
- Recognition of common oral conditions and traumatic dentoalveolar injuries
- Treatment or referral of the dog within the context of their function
- Discussion of strategies for maintaining oral health and preventing traumatic injuries

Working dogs are categorized into subgroups by the American Kennel Club (AKC) groupings.[1] The AKC breed groups are sporting, herding, nonsporting, working, terrier, toy, and hound. The working group includes breeds that traditionally are used for guarding, pulling, and other physically demanding tasks. Working dogs also have been described by their career certification to include law enforcement dogs, military service dogs, detection dogs, assistance dogs, and canine athletes.[2]

Working dogs develop periodontal disease at similar prevalence to companion dogs. Untreated periodontal disease has local and systemic effects. Local effects include pain, gingival recession, bone loss, periodontal abscess, rhinitis, retrobulbar cellulitis, oronasal fistula, and potential tooth loss.[3] Systemic effects of chronic inflammatory mediators and bacteremia have been shown to result in histopathologic changes in the liver, kidneys, and heart tissue.[4,5]

Oral health in working dogs is essential because the oral cavity, teeth, and nasal cavities are juxtaposed. The olfactory system is used for scent detection so maintenance of oral health is vital to many working dogs' ability to perform their assigned task. Moreover, oral pain associated with trauma or infection can affect a working dog's advancement in training, minimize performance potential, and negatively affect a dog's overall health.

Depending on their defined performance or task(s), working dogs are more prone to oral trauma, specifically traumatic dentoalveolar injuries (TDIs), which include tooth wear, fracture, discoloration and displacement. TDI has a prevalence of 26.2% in

[a] Veterinary Dental Center, 345 Sullivan Road, Aurora, IL 60506, USA; [b] U.S. Army Public Health Activity-Fort Knox, 18N663 Carriage Way Lane, Huntley, IL 60142, USA
* Corresponding author.
E-mail address: stephenjuriga@yahoo.com

Vet Clin Small Anim 51 (2021) 779–802
https://doi.org/10.1016/j.cvsm.2021.04.002
0195-5616/21/© 2021 Elsevier Inc. All rights reserved.
vetsmall.theclinics.com

the general population of dogs.[6] The most common TDIs are tooth fractures with pulp exposure,[6,7] a source of pain and infection. Law enforcement (police and military) dogs are more prone to tooth trauma due to their guard or police work, training, housing, and play.[8,9]

This article focuses on working dogs used by local law enforcement and government agencies. These types of working dogs are certified to perform single or multi-purpose tasks to include patrol, tracking, narcotics, explosives, and search and rescue. Moreover, due to the higher prevalence of TDIs, the traumatic injuries common in these working dogs are discussed and illustrated.

TOOTH ANATOMY

An accurate assessment of a dog's dentition is dependent on a veterinarian's familiarity with normal tooth anatomy (**Fig. 1**). The tooth is composed of an enamel covering, a dentinal wall beneath, and a centrally located pulp. The crown of the tooth (visible part of the tooth) is covered by enamel. Enamel is a hard, calcified tissue that is 0.1 mm to 0.6 mm[10] in dogs. Tooth enamel is formed prior to eruption and cannot repair itself from abrasive wear, fracture, or decay.

Dentin is a hard tissue that lies beneath the enamel. It is the structurally strong wall of the tooth and extends the entire vertical length of the tooth. Dentin is produced throughout the life of the tooth by a cell known as an odontoblast and is composed

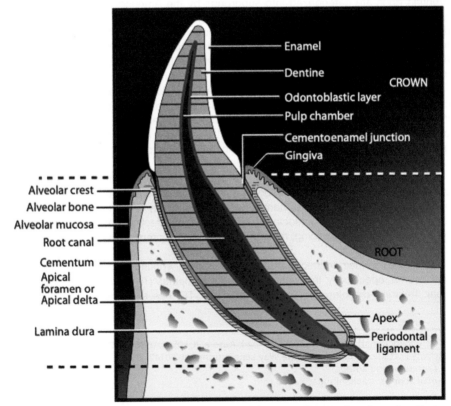

Fig. 1. Tooth anatomy. *Courtesy of* Image created by Janet Sinn-Hanlon, iLearning Center, University of Illinois Veterinary Medicine.

of microscopic tubules. Primary dentin is formed prior and during eruption. Secondary dentin is produced continuously over the lifetime of the tooth, resulting in a thickening of the tooth wall and gradual reduction in pulp chamber size. Tertiary or reparative dentin is formed as a reaction to wear, fracture, or caries.[11] This reparative tissue appears as a central brown spot on the tooth surface. When dentin loses its covering, enamel of the crown or cementum of the root, the dentin tubules may serve as a pathway for bacteria to enter the pulp depending on the age of the patient and depth of the exposure.

Pulp chamber or root canal is in the center of the tooth and contains nerves, blood vessels, and connective tissue. The pulp is the living tissue that nourishes the odontoblasts, strengthening a tooth over time, and has the nerve fibers that sense heat or cold. Initially, the pulp canal is large and the dentinal wall is thin. As the tooth matures, the odontoblasts produce secondary dentin, resulting in the tooth wall thickening, the root lengthening, and closure of the apex (**Fig. 2**).

PERIODONTAL ANATOMY

The periodontium describes the tissue that supports and surrounds the tooth (see **Fig. 1**). It includes the gingiva, alveolar bone, cementum, and periodontal ligament. The gingiva surrounds the teeth and protects both the bone and periodontal ligament. Loss of this tissue by trauma, accumulation of tartar, or gingivitis may result in a periodontal pocket, gum recession, infection of the bone, or tooth loss. The alveolar bone is the bony process (socket) that encases individual teeth of the mandible and maxilla. The alveolar bone acts as the foundation of attachment and anchors the teeth to the jaw. Cementum is a hard connective tissue that covers the root and serves as point of attachment of the periodontal ligament. The periodontal ligament is composed of collagen fibers in a specific orientation that attach the tooth to the alveolar bone. The periodontal ligament fibers suspend the tooth within the alveolus and provides a shock absorber effect to prevent fracture of teeth during forceful occlusal action and allows a dog to sense pressure.

TOOTH TYPES AND FUNCTION

The dog has 6 incisor teeth of the maxilla and mandible. Each has a single root and the function is for grasping and tearing hide as well as grooming. Distal to the incisors is a single canine tooth in each quadrant. Canine teeth have a long, conical crown that

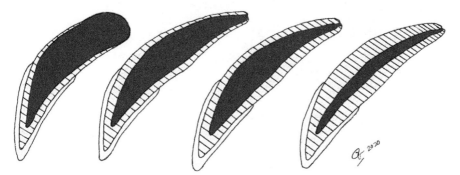

Fig. 2. Illustration of tooth maturation at 7 months of age (*left*), 12 months, 2 years, 4 years of age (*right*). (*Courtesy of* Jo Banyard, DVM, DAVDC.)

curves distally and tapers to a point. Their function is for grabbing, holding, and killing prey as well as protection and defense. The canine tooth length, rostral location in the oral cavity, and function make them prone to trauma or fracture.[7] There are 4 premolar teeth of the maxilla and mandible, which are located distal to the canine teeth. Their pyramidal crowns interdigitate with the premolars of the maxilla and mandible and they should appear in a saw-toothed or interdigitated orientation when viewed from the side. Premolar function is to hold prey and shear meat from larger prey. The molars are located behind the premolars and their function is to grind food. Dogs have 4 carnassial teeth: 2 maxillary fourth premolars and 2 mandibular first molars; their function is to cut meat.[11] Working dogs that perform apprehension or protection are trained to bite with their full mouth. Therefore, the maintenance of tooth structure and oral health includes the maxillary incisors/canines/premolars and mandibular incisors/canines/premolars and first molar teeth.

WORKING DOG CONSIDERATIONS FOR HOSPITAL SAFETY

Prior to rendering services, it is recommended to have a protocol or standard operating procedure for the examination and treatment of working dogs in place. Temperament and behavioral considerations in the management of working dogs are extremely important with regard to veterinary staff, handler, and dog safety. The handler is a valuable asset in reducing fear, anxiety, and stress of the dog in the veterinary clinic setting. It is important to discuss with the handler the dog's temperament and behavior prior to any physical examination. Training veterinary staff to recognize fearful or aggressive canine body language and how to safely restrain with handler assistance increases overall safety.

All working dogs must be on leash, accompanied by the handler, wearing a properly fitted and secured basket muzzle,[12] until the dog's temperament is evaluated (**Fig. 3**). If possible, the working dog team should enter the building through a quiet entrance

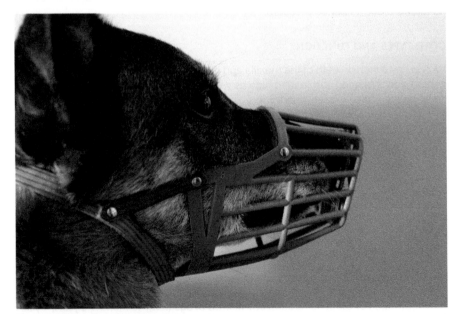

Fig. 3. Working dog with a basket muzzle.

and directly into a large examination room to decrease social interaction with other dogs and people. If possible, the handler should be present at all times during the examination, admission, recovery, and discharge.

Clinical history should include a dog's certification (job), husbandry (in home or kennel), handling tips for the examination, and typical behavior in the clinic setting. Often, the handler can discuss what has worked well for restraint or positioning guidance to minimize fear or aggression. Staff always should ask the handler if it is okay to approach the dog and communicate to the handler the procedures and restraint required. It usually is easier to restrain and control working dogs on a raised table and, if needed, ask the handler permission prior to lifting the dog. If the examination is performed on the ground, staff should never sit or kneel but always should squat and be prepared to quickly step back if a dog becomes aggressive.

Once the overall physical examination is performed, if the working dog is cooperative and the handler agrees, the basket muzzle can be removed to perform a thorough oral examination (**Fig. 4**). If the working dog is not cooperative and the handler is comfortable touching the dog's mouth, then the handler should maneuver the mouth for a brief examination by the veterinarian. Many times, the handler can lift the lips for a buccal observation (from rostral to caudal) in order to document occlusion, calculus, gingival inflammation, missing teeth, and worn or fractured teeth (**Figs. 5** and **6**). If the veterinarian or handler is unable to perform an oral examination due to fearful behavior, anxiety, or aggression, then the dog needs sedation or general anesthesia for the safety of the dog and the veterinary staff (see article on Anesthesia of Working Dogs).[12] In addition, previsit anxiolytics can be administered and prescribed for future visits. Careful consideration of a dog's handling capabilities is important when determining best treatment because follow-up care can be difficult to provide in the uncooperative dog.

For sedation or general anesthesia, safety and handler involvement of working dog management are instrumental. Working dogs that are not cooperative should wear a basket muzzle until an induction agent is administered. Once the procedure is

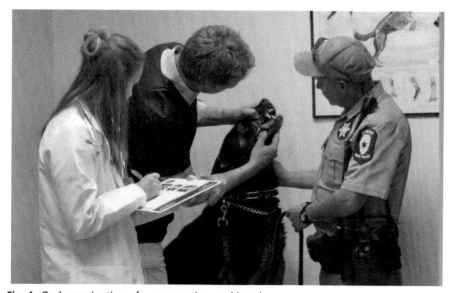

Fig. 4. Oral examination of a cooperative working dog.

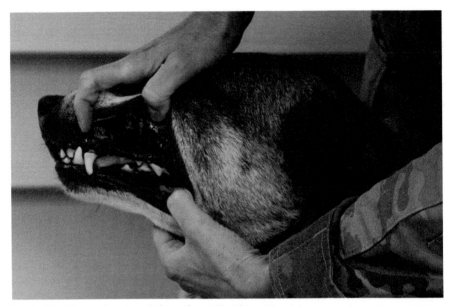

Fig. 5. .Handler performing daily oral examination.

complete, prior to recovery/extubation, an intravenous microdosage of a sedative agent generally is indicated to provide a slow, predictable recovery. The veterinary staff should safely move the working dog to a preselected recovery area with the handler present. As soon as the dog is extubated, the handler should place a basket muzzle back on the dog. Working dogs generally do not like being crated in unfamiliar locations away from their handler, so minimal time spent in the hospital or kennel is recommended.

Examination findings are to be recorded in the patient's medical record, preferably using a standardized dental examination chart, and are used to generate an initial

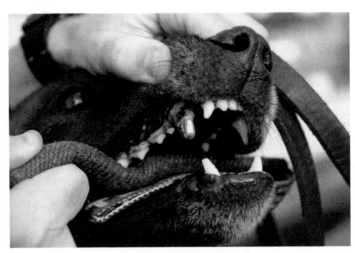

Fig. 6. Handler-assisted oral examination utilizing a reward object.

treatment plan. Because working dog handlers are very involved in their dog's care and motivated to assist,[13] the chart and photographs (**Fig. 7**) should be shared with the handler to serve as a reference for daily handler directed oral examinations.

CLINICAL SIGNS

Clinical signs of oral disease in companion dogs often are vague or subtle. They may include halitosis, gingivitis, drooling, reluctance to chew or play with toys, sneezing, pawing at the mouth, or dropping food from the mouth. A working dog's temperament, training, and performance, however, can lead to more specific, observable signs. Handlers may report a failure to advance in training, decoy bite avoidance, shallow bite, early reward release, oral bleeding, reluctance to eat, nasal discharge, unilateral facial swelling, or weight loss.

Few fractured or nonvital teeth are associated with clinical signs of oral pain, visible swelling, or drainage. Many infected teeth establish drainage into the oral cavity along the periodontal ligament of the tooth or an intraoral fistulous tract, which may not be visualized easily. The maxillary canine teeth extend into the nasal cavity and are more likely to abscess and drain into the nasal cavity than present with facial swelling due to the increased thickness of the buccal alveolar bone. Some diseased teeth result in a fenestration through the buccal bone near the root tip and visually cause swelling or drainage through skin. This occurs most commonly with a fracture of the maxillary fourth premolar or first molar, which drains through the skin of the face rostral and ventral to the eye.

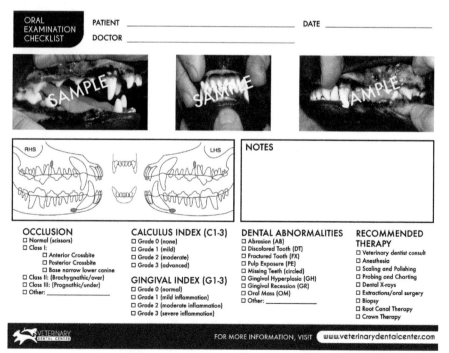

Fig. 7. Example of an oral examination chart with patient reference photos taken on the date of the examination.

TRAUMATIC DENTOALVEOLAR INJURIES

TDIs include injuries to the tooth (crown or root) and/or tooth-supporting structures (periodontal ligament or alveolar bone) sustained as a direct result of a traumatic force.[6] These include tooth wear, fracture, discoloration, or displacement, and treatment is dependent on the extent of trauma. These injuries affect 26.2% of dogs[6] and 70% of dogs with concurrent maxillofacial fractures.[14] The most common TDIs are tooth fractures with pulp exposure,[9] a source of pain and infection.

TDIs occur due to interactions with other animals, vehicular accidents, blunt force trauma, falls, or chewing activities. Working dogs tend to have a higher prevalence of tooth fractures due to their training, behavior, and abrasive and aggressive nature of their work.[8] Working dogs can develop TDIs from injuries in training (bite sleeve or aggressive pulling on a reward), housing or environmental (bowls, fence, crate, or car enclosure), abnormal behavior (interactions with their housing or spinning), or during performance (protection, defense, or apprehension).[12] The consequences of these injuries include pain, infection, tooth loss, bacteremia, and osteomyelitis and can contribute to systemic disease.[15] Ultimately, traumatized teeth have a direct effect on a working dog's function.

There are several systems used to classify TDI. The American Veterinary Dental College (AVDC) has published a classification system that defines tooth fractures (**Fig. 8**). These include enamel infarction, enamel fracture, enamel/dentin fracture, enamel/dentin/pulp fracture, crown/root fractures that do not involve the pulp, and crown/root fractures that involve the pulp and root fractures. This system also uses the terms, uncomplicated and complicated, to infer whether the pulp is not exposed or exposed respectively. This classification, however, does not include luxation injuries (concussion, subluxation, luxation, and avulsion) or alveolar fractures. Soukup and colleagues[6] recommend a universal classification system modified from human traumatology, which includes dental fractures, luxation injuries, and alveolar fractures (**Fig. 9**).

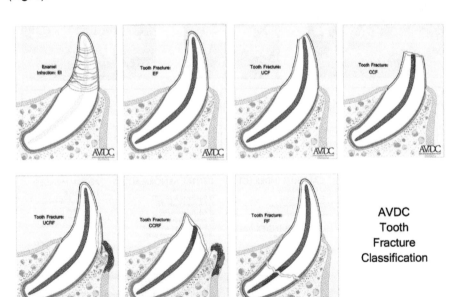

AVDC
Tooth
Fracture
Classification

Fig. 8. Classification adopted by the AVDC.

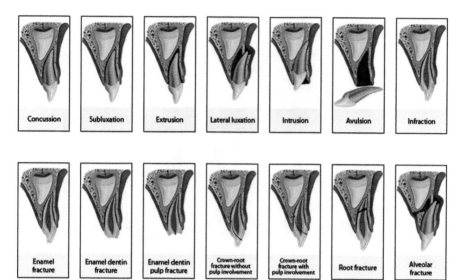

Fig. 9. Classification system for TDIs. (Source modified and reprinted with permission from Andreasen J.O., Lauridsen E., Gerds T.A. (2012) Dental Trauma guide: a source of evidence based guidelines for dental trauma. Dent Traumatol. 28: 345-350.)

TOOTH WEAR (ATTRITION OR ABRASION)

Tooth wear is the physiologic process from mastication that results in the loss of enamel and/or dentin and may result in pulp exposure. Two types of tooth wear are attrition and abrasion. Attrition is the result of tooth-on-tooth contact or malocclusion of teeth. Abrasion is the loss of enamel and dentin due to contact with a nondental object, such as a dog's housing or enclosure, bones, antlers, other hard objects, or even softer abrasive objects like tennis balls.

Tooth wear results in loss of enamel exposing dentin. If wear is gradual, the odontoblasts produces tertiary or reparative dentin to protect the pulp. Tertiary dentin often appears as a central brown spot on the occlusal surface (**Fig. 10**). If the tooth wear progresses faster than the odontoblasts can form dentin, however, the pulp can become exposed (**Fig. 11**).

Working dogs are prone to tooth wear due to excessive chewing of bowls, kennel structures such as cage doors, or excessive grooming.[12] Bowl or bucket chewing results in general crown wear, whereas cage or cage door chewing results in loss of tooth structure on the distal aspect of the canine teeth (**Fig. 12**). This abrasive wear pattern on the distal tooth surface of canine teeth weakens the tooth and results in a higher incidence of crown fracture. Excessive or chronic self-grooming result in loss of tooth structure of the maxillary and mandibular incisor teeth.

Evaluation of teeth with abrasive or attrition tooth wear is accomplished by examining the worn surface with a dental explorer for pulp exposure and utilizing radiographic imaging (dental radiographs or computed tomography [CT]). Abnormal radiographic findings include periapical lucency (**Fig. 13**), condensing osteitis (excessive bone mineralization around the apex), and root resorption or pulp canal asymmetry compared with the contralateral tooth or adjacent teeth. Treatment of teeth affected by tooth wear includes behavioral/housing/training modification and crown therapy.

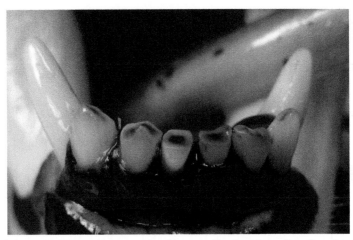

Fig. 10. Photograph illustrating centralized brown discoloration of tertiary dentin formation secondary to tooth wear.

TOOTH FRACTURE

Tooth fractures are common in dogs. A study of 63 dogs anesthetized for reasons other than oral disease revealed 27% of patients had dental crown fractures.[16] Tooth fractures with pulp exposure mostly affected canine teeth with a reported frequency of 35.5% to 57.1%.[6,16] Fractured teeth are painful and result in pulp necrosis. Strategic teeth (canine, maxillary fourth premolar, and mandibular first molar) were the fractures sustained most commonly that exposed the pulp. These teeth are termed, *strategic*, due to their importance in daily function of prehension, defense and mastication.[6]

Trauma to the tooth can be classified by the tooth structure that is damaged (see **Fig. 8**), such as enamel, dentin, or root as well as whether there is pulp exposure (enamel/dentin/pulp) or fractures without pulpal exposure (enamel/dentin). An injury exposing pulp is described as complicated whereas an injury that does not expose the pulp is described as uncomplicated.

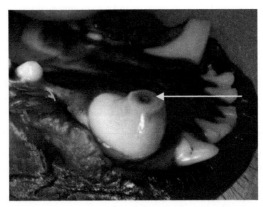

Fig. 11. Clinical image of pulp exposure (*arrow*) secondary to abrasive tooth wear.

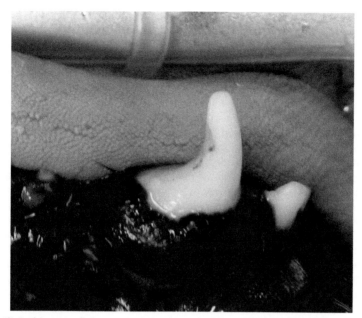

Fig. 12. Clinical image of abrasion on the distal surface of the canine teeth.

Enamel fractures can be hard to visualize because enamel is very thin. The incisors and premolars are the teeth affected most commonly. Because dentin is not exposed, these injuries do not cause pain or compromise the pulp. Treatment of an enamel fracture includes removal of sharp enamel and monitoring the tooth for discoloration.

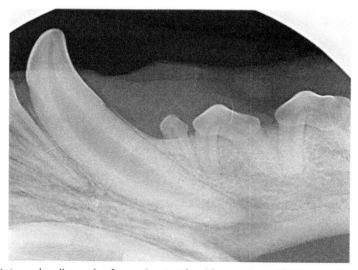

Fig. 13. Intraoral radiograph of a canine tooth with a periapical lucency consistent with pulpal necrosis and periodontitis.

Enamel/dentin fractures (uncomplicated) describe fractures confined to enamel and dentin (**Fig. 14**). Dentin is composed of tubules that extend from the pulp to the enamel. These fractures result in pain and may allow bacteria to access or insult the pulp. The depth of an enamel/dentin fracture has a direct effect on the likelihood of pulp exposure.[17] Treatment of an enamel/dentin fracture involves sealing of all the exposed dentin tubules as soon as possible. The tooth should be monitored for discoloration and radiographed annually for a widened root canal and periapical disease. A near pulp exposure appears as a central pink hue of the tooth fracture (**Fig. 15**). This pinkish hue is visible when 0.5 mm of dentin overlays the pulp. Many of these teeth develop pulpal death and should be treated as an enamel/dentin/pulp fracture with either root canal therapy or extraction.

Fractures that involve enamel/dentin/pulp (**Figs. 16** and **17**) result in pain, pulp inflammation, and pulp death over weeks to months.[15] Working dog function (apprehension and defense) leads to a higher incidence of canine tooth fracture. The canine tooth's rostral location in the oral cavity and the high crown height–to–base diameter ratio both contribute to the higher incidence of fracture.[7] The canine teeth penetrate into objects during training and performance (bite sleeves or suspect apprehension). The forces transmitted to the teeth are unpredictable in magnitude and direction, which ultimately results in a higher incidence of canine tooth fractures.[18] Abrasive wear occurs on the distal aspect of the canine teeth due to behavior directed at their enclosure: cage, crate, or transport vehicle.[12] This loss of tooth structure weakens the crown and contributes to canine tooth fracture.

Evaluation of a tooth fracture is accomplished by examining the crown defect with a dental explorer and utilizing radiographic imaging (dental radiographs or CT). Abnormal radiographic findings include widening of the periodontal ligament at the apex, periapical lucency, condensing osteitis (excessive bone mineralization around the apex), root resorption (**Fig. 18**), or pulp canal asymmetry compared with the contralateral tooth or adjacent teeth.

A fractured tooth with pulp exposure requires either root canal therapy or extraction. If left untreated, these teeth develop pulp necrosis and death.[19] Root canal therapy is the preferred therapy for functionally or strategically important teeth and is discussed later.

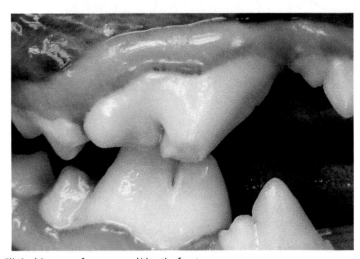

Fig. 14. Clinical image of an enamel/dentin fracture.

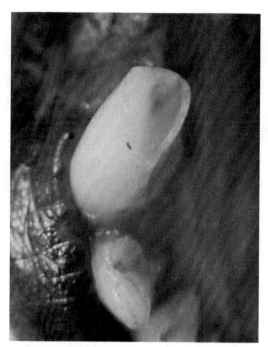

Fig. 15. Clinical image of an enamel/dentin fracture with a centralized pink hue consistent with a near pulp exposure.

TOOTH DISCOLORATION

Discolored teeth occur from concussive or blunt trauma without the loss of crown structure can result in reversible or irreversible inflammation to the pulp. Reversible pulpitis usually is caused by minor trauma, and the tooth survives the insult. The teeth

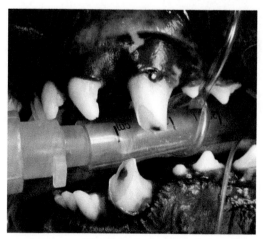

Fig. 16. Clinical image of an enamel/dentin/pulp fracture of the left maxillary and mandibular canine teeth.

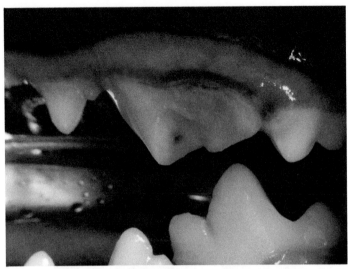

Fig. 17. Clinical image of an enamel/dentin/pulp fracture of the left maxillary fourth premolar.

may appear pink for a week but then return to normal color. Irreversible pulpitis is a result of severe pulp inflammation and subsequent pulp necrosis. These teeth initially appear pink and then over weeks turn purple or gray (**Fig. 19**). One study revealed that 92% of teeth with crown discoloration were nonvital.[20] In animals, these teeth initially are painful and prone to infection. A tooth that has sustained trauma without fracture and appears discolored should be considered nonvital. Dental radiography or CT imaging is used to assess the discolored tooth for root fracture, root resorption, periapical lucency or wide pulp cavity compared with the contralateral tooth (**Fig. 20**). These

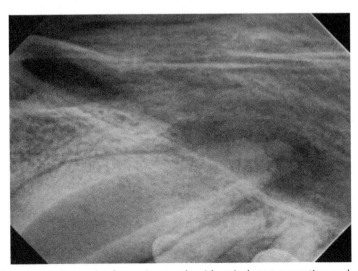

Fig. 18. Intraoral radiograph of a canine tooth with apical root resorption and periapical lucency consistent with pulpal necrosis and periodontitis.

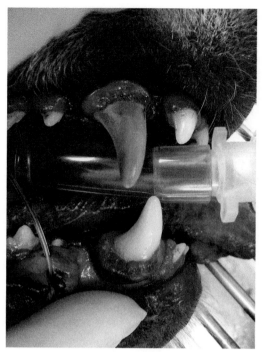

Fig. 19. Pinkish-purple discoloration of a maxillary canine tooth consistent with concussive injury.

teeth should receive root canal treatment or extraction similar to a tooth with direct pulp exposure.

TOOTH DISPLACEMENT

Luxation injuries result in trauma to the periodontal ligament, cementum, alveolar bone, and neurovascular supply to the tooth. These injuries fall into 6 categories,[14,21,22] which can be listed in increasing severity: concussion, subluxation, lateral luxation, extrusive luxation, intrusive luxation, and avulsion (see **Fig. 9**).

Concussion is injury to a tooth that does not result in displacement but leads to some degree of pulpitis. Subluxation describes an injury to the supporting tissues (periodontal ligament) with mobility (bleeding around the tooth) without clinical or radiographic displacement of the tooth. Concussive and subluxation injuries should be evaluated radiographically to rule out root fracture and monitored for pink/blue/gray discoloration. Discoloration occurs from pulpal hemorrhage and if it persists has a direct correlation to pulp viability (see **Fig. 19**).

In lateral luxation the tooth appears tilted labial (outward), lingual or palatal (inward), or mesial/distal (**Fig. 21**). Extrusive luxation is an injury in which the tooth is displaced in a coronal direction and appears longer than its contralateral tooth. Teeth that have sustained lateral or extrusive luxation injury are mobile, may or may not have gingival laceration(s), and radiographically have widened periapical space.[15]

Intrusive luxation is a condition in which a tooth is displaced deeper (apical) within alveolar bone. The most common tooth affected is the canine, resulting in displacement into the nasal cavity. Avulsion describes a tooth that has been completely

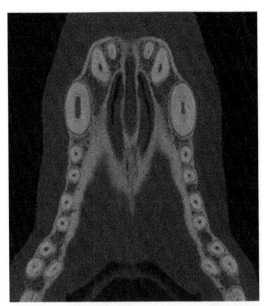

Fig. 20. Cone beam CT image of a nonvital left maxillary canine tooth. Note the larger pulp canal of the left canine tooth (*arrow*) compared with the contralateral canine.

displaced out of the alveolus (**Fig. 22**). If the handler witnessed the injury, immediate reimplantation of the tooth is recommended.

Tooth luxation has been reported to be more common in young patients (<3 years of age), due to the result of a traumatic force being transferred from the tooth to a more flexible tissue (periodontal ligament and alveolar bone) resulting in tooth luxation rather

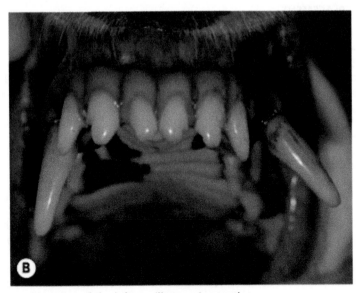

Fig. 21. Lateral luxation of the left maxillary canine tooth.

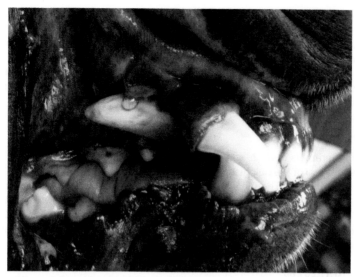

Fig. 22. Avulsion of the right maxillary canine tooth.

that crown fracture.[6] The incidence of tooth displacement has not been studied in working dogs but is likely more common than the general dog population due to the bite forces and variable angle(s) of attack on the bite sleeve in training.

Diagnosis and evaluation of displacement require sedation or anesthesia. Tooth mobility and radiographic evaluation is performed.[19] Treatment may include anatomic repositioning, stabilization and root canal therapy if the neurovascular supply to the tooth has been compromised.[15] Concussive and subluxation injuries are treated with analgesics, soft diet, and restricted bite training for 2 weeks. Lateral luxation and extrusive luxation are treated by tooth repositioning, repair of gingival lacerations if present, splinting, and root canal therapy. Intrusive luxation requires extraction therapy as orthodontic extrusion is not possible in dogs. Lateral, extrusive, and intrusive luxation injuries all result in pulp necrosis and without treatment the teeth are prone to root resorption and/or infection.[21,22] Treatment of an avulsed tooth depends on the age of the patient, extraoral time, and whether extraoral storage media (milk, saliva, and saline) was utilized,[15] and immediate referral to a veterinary dentist is recommended. All teeth with displacement injuries need to be re-evaluated with follow-up radiographs in 6 months to 12 months.

TREATMENT CONSIDERATIONS

The goal of treatment of working dogs always should be the retention of functionally important teeth if at all possible. Referral to an AVDC board-certified veterinary dentist (see www.avdc.org) always is recommended for tooth trauma, maxillofacial trauma, difficult extractions, endodontic treatment, or restoration of teeth with composites or metal crowns. Veterinary dentists have experience handling working dogs, have advanced imaging modalities (intraoral dental radiography and CT or cone beam tonometry) as well as treatment strategies (root canal, metal crown therapy, and intraoral splinting) to retain or restore function.

When discussing treatment recommendations, it is important to communicate the amount of time likely to be lost from work while the dog is recovering. Some programs might have to delay treatment in order to keep shifts covered, training sustained, or after inspection and certification. Most working dogs are trained and rewarded with a toy (usually a rubber chew toy, ball, or rope tug). All dogs that receive oral surgery or preparation for crown therapy must be restricted from training and chewing behavior during healing or until the crown is placed. Odor detection dogs also have limitations in regard to work unless the handler is able to use verbal praise or soft treats for their reward.

ROOT CANAL THERAPY

Root canal therapy is performed to preserve tooth structure and tooth function. It involves the removal of the pulp tissue by shaping and cleaning the canal with a series of files and disinfectants. The clean and disinfected root canal then is obturated (filled) with root canal sealer and an inert material to seal the apex and walls of the tooth (**Fig. 23**). The crown of the tooth is sealed from the oral cavity by a composite restorative material followed by radiographs in 6 months to 12 months and every year thereafter to confirm success.

EXTRACTION THERAPY

Extraction therapy is the recommended treatment of a fractured tooth with endodontic disease that does not receive root canal therapy. The decision to extract a tooth in a working dog is dependent on the tooth affected, function of the working dog (patrol, tracking, or narcotics), severity of the fracture (at or below the gingiva or root involvement), and radiographic evaluation (periapical disease or internal or external root

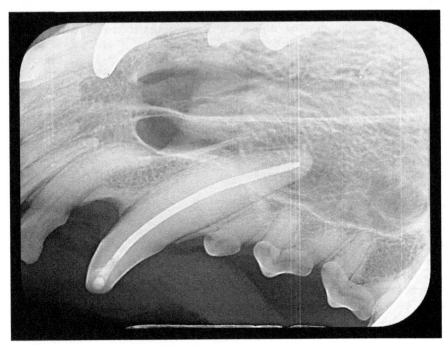

Fig. 23. Intraoral radiograph of the left maxillary canine tooth after receiving root canal therapy.

resorption). A majority of extractions performed in working dogs are surgical extractions. These patients receive a mucoperiosteal flap, some degree of bone removal, tooth sectioning of multirooted teeth, complete root removal, and primary closure. A soft diet and restriction of reward objects are recommended for 2 weeks. If the dog is a cage/enclosure chewer, a breathable basket muzzle can be worn to prevent unsupervised oral trauma to the oral surgery site. Moreover, there should be consideration of bone healing time in the extraction of the mandibular canine and first molar teeth.

Prosthodontic Crown

Crown therapy is indicated to restore lost tooth structure, protect the teeth from further damage as well as to allow the patient to return to normal function.[23,24] Due to the high bite forces generated by working dogs, crown therapy is highly recommended for teeth that have received root canal therapy (**Fig. 24**). Moreover, canine teeth that have developed abrasive wear on the distal tooth surface from cage chewing are more prone to fracture and benefit from three-quarters or full crown therapy (**Fig. 25**).

Crown therapy requires 2 anesthetic episodes. The first may be performed with the root canal procedure in which the tooth is shaped and impressions are taken. The impression, full mouth study models, and bite registration are sent to a dental laboratory for crown fabrication. The next anesthetic procedure is performed in the following weeks for crown fitting and cementation. This results in a period of time in which the dog cannot work or train, and the handler must be counseled on how to prevent further tooth injury.

Working dogs require crown materials with strength and maximum protection. A full-cast metal crown is the preferred material and many are fabricated with titanium for strength and biocompatibility.[24,25] The use of crown lengthening techniques, tooth height, axial grooves, convergence angles, and resin-based cements all contribute to retention and success.[7,23,25] Finally, crown therapy does not completely eliminate future tooth fractures for aggressive chewers or cage-chewing behavior. Consultation with a behavioral specialist should be considered for these patients.

PREVENTION AND STRATEGIES FOR MAINTAINING ORAL HEALTH

Veterinarians, handlers, trainers, and program managers need to work together to maintain oral health and prevent oral trauma. The overall health and maintenance of a working dog requires a team approach through education.

From an early age, all potential working dogs should receive routine oral examination on veterinary visits and by their caregiver in order to acclimate the puppy to manipulation of their oral cavity. Similar to frequent grooming, desensitization, and early socialization skills, puppies need to be accustomed to handlers and veterinarians performing oral examinations. Once the team enrolls in a training program, it is vital that the handler builds rapport with their canine and that a daily oral examination becomes part of the grooming routine.

Veterinarians play an integral role in oral disease prevention, recognition, and treatment and should use visual tools (models, illustrations, or photos) of tooth injuries to educate handlers on normal and abnormal tooth structure.[15] Handler education resources (*Oral Examination Reference Guide* and *Self-Study Guide*) can be found at https://workingdoghq.com/k9-handler-resources/.

All working dogs should receive an annual oral examination by their veterinarian. Many veterinarians find an oral examination of an awake working dog to be

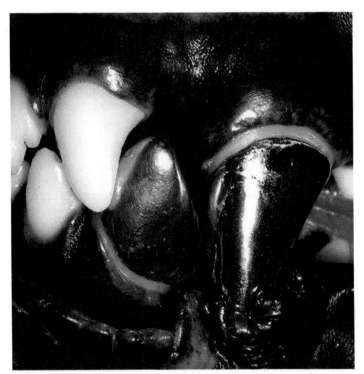

Fig. 24. Full metal crown of the left maxillary and mandibular canine teeth post–root canal therapy for crown fractures.

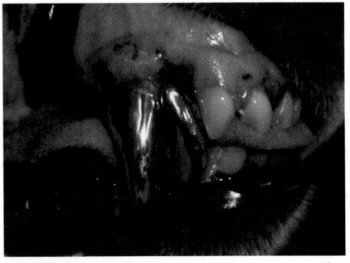

Fig. 25. .Metal crown therapy for abrasive tooth wear of the distal crown of canine teeth secondary to cage chewing.

challenging, which is why an examination under anesthesia that includes cleaning, probing, and dental radiography is so important. Canine programs should require and budget for routine oral examinations under anesthesia so that oral disease can be identified and treated early, thereby prolonging the working ability of the team.

Daily oral hygiene should be a goal for all working dogs. The Veterinary Oral Health Council (www.vohc.org) has a list of products with clinical evidence for use. These include but are not limited to toothbrush, dental diets, chew treats, toothpaste, oral gel, and water additive.

Considerations for working dog husbandry and management in order to prevent tooth trauma are based on the authors' experiences. In the authors' opinion, the majority of oral trauma observed in working dogs generally is linked to their environment, behavior, or a training or duty incident.

Working dogs are selected based on their intense drive and athletic capabilities. These traits often lead to less than desirable behavioral patterns, such as separation anxiety, obsessive-compulsive disorder, and destructive tendencies. Tooth trauma can occur on crates, flooring, and kennel bars and inside the duty vehicle. Many cage chewers need their enclosure fitted with plexiglass or a design without bars. Dogs that are agitated in the vehicle can wear a basket muzzle or be housed in an enclosed kennel. Excessive self-grooming due to dermatology, gastrointestinal, or behavioral conditions can cause incisor tooth wear. This can be prevented by properly diagnosing and treating underlying medical conditions.

Selection of appropriate reward and play objects are essential because repetitive tugging or chewing on hard objects can cause abrasive wear or fractures. rubber chew toys, hard rubber toys, and rope tugs are safe options but working dogs should not be allowed to have free access to these items due to their inherent nature to chew. Hard bones, plastic, sticks, and rocks should be avoided.

Tooth injuries commonly are reported during training sessions. These can be prevented by selection of a properly designed bite sleeve and decoy protective clothing. Equally important is the communication between the handler and decoy on the dog's bite work behavior or style. The decoy should be certified to present themselves for a full bite/grip and appropriately absorb the dog with each catch. Once on the wrap, many dogs with abrasive tooth wear can fracture a tooth if the decoy inappropriately falls, jams, or swings the canine. All training sessions and duty shifts should conclude with a brief oral examination to immediately identify any oral abnormalities.

Prevention and strategies for maintaining oral health in working dogs are lifetime processes. A working dog uses its oral cavity as a tool in order to perform trained tasks. A progressive oral health program must be incorporated and performed by the handler, trainer, program, and veterinarian.

SUMMARY

Maintaining oral health in working dogs is an integral part of their care. Untreated tooth or oral pain can affect the ability to perform their assigned duty at optimal performance. Due to their high drive and stringent training, working dogs hide pain and continue to perform their tasks while concurrently suffering from oral pain. Tooth trauma is painful, inhibits performance, and requires treatment. Veterinarians play an important role in the diagnosis and education of handlers on the common oral conditions affecting working dogs. Veterinarian and handler-assisted oral examinations should be performed at every visit; otherwise, an annual sedated or anesthetized examination is recommended. This article illustrates the causes, consequences, and treatment of tooth wear, fractures, discoloration, and displacement. Veterinarians must identify, record, treat, or refer to a veterinary boarded dentist for appropriate treatment. Handlers, trainers, and managers must perform oral exams, identify, and advocate for immediate evaluation and treatment. It is a team effort to recognize the importance of oral health in working dogs. Resolution of these conditions improve patient comfort and maintain optimal performance. Preventive strategies in training and housing also are important considerations in the prevention of TDIs in the working dog.

CONFLICT OF INTEREST STATEMENT

The authors declare that the research was conducted in the absence of any commercial or financial relationships that could be construed as a potential conflict of interest.

DISCLOSURE

The authors have nothing to disclose.

CLINICS CARE POINTS

- Veterinarians play an important role in the diagnosis and education of handlers on common oral conditions that affect working dogs.
- Depending on their defined performance, working dogs are more prone to oral trauma, which include tooth wear, tooth fracture, tooth discoloration, and tooth displacement.
- Handler-assisted examinations should be performed at every visit, or annual sedated or anesthetized examinations are recommended.
- Veterinary board certified dentists with working dog experience can help design treatment strategies in order to retain and restore oral function.

Working dog dentistry pearls and pitfalls

Pearls
Veterinarians play an important role in the diagnosis and education of handlers on common oral conditions that affect working dogs.
Staff training and hospital protocols need to be implemented prior to examination or treatment of working dogs.
Encourage handlers to train their working dogs to allow voluntary oral examinations.
Handler-assisted examinations should be performed at every visit, or annual sedated or anesthetized examinations are recommended.
Veterinary board certified dentists with working dog experience can help design treatment strategies in order to retain and restore oral function.

Pitfalls
Working dogs have a higher prevalence of tooth trauma due to their guard or police work, training, housing, and play.
Handlers that are unable to perform oral examinations on their working dog after training sessions and duty shifts must recognize that their working dog is more likely to have tooth trauma that goes undiagnosed and untreated.
Few working dogs exhibit clinical signs of oral pain due to their high drive and training.
Delayed diagnosis of oral pain associated with tooth trauma or infection can affect a working dogs advancement in training, performance, and negatively affect the dog's overall health.

REFERENCES

1. American Kennel Club. The complete dog book. 19th edition. New York: Wiley; 1998.
2. Otto CM, Cobb M, Wilsson E, editors. Working dogs: form and function. 2nd edition. Lausanne: Frontiers Media SA; 2020.
3. Stepanik K. Clinical signs associated with periodontal disease. In: Lobprise HB, Dodd JR, editors. Wigg's veterinary dentistry. 2nd edition. Hoboken (NJ): Wiley & sons; 2019. p. 81–108.
4. Debowes LJ, Mosier D, Logan E, et al. Association of periodontal and histologic lesions in multiple organs from 45 dogs. J Vet Dent 1996;13:57–60.
5. Pavlica Z, Petelin M, Juntes P, et al. Periodontal disease burden and pathological changes in organ from dogs. J Vet Dent 2008;25:97–105.
6. Soukup JW, Hetzel S, Paul A. Classification and epidemiology of traumatic dentoalveolar injuries in dogs and cats: 959 injuries in 660 patient visits (2004-2012). J Vet Dent 2015;32(1):6–14.
7. Soukup JW, Collins C, Ploeg HL. The influence of crown height to diameter ratio on the force to fracture of canine teeth in dogs. J Vet Dent 2015;32:155–63.
8. Le Brech C, Hamel L, LeNihouannen JC, et al. Epidemiological study of canine teeth fractures in military dogs. J Vet Dent 1997;14:51–5.
9. Capík I, Ledeck V, Evãík A. Tooth fracture evaluation and endodontic treatment in Dogs. Acta Vet 2000;69:115–22.
10. Crossley DA. Tooth enamel thickness in the mature dentition of domesticated dogs and cats- preliminary study. J Vet Dent 1995;12(3):111–3.
11. Lemmons M, Beebe D. Oral anatomy and physiology. In: Lobprise HB, Dodd JR, editors. Wigg's veterinary dentistry. 2nd edition. Hoboken (NJ): Wiley & sons; 2019. p. 1–24.
12. Army Technical Bulletin Medical 298: Veterinary care and management of the military working dog. May 09, 2019.
13. Burghardt WF. Behavioral considerations in the management of working dogs. Vet Clin Small Anim 2003;33:417–46.
14. Soukup JW, Mulherin BI, Synder CJ. Prevalence and nature of dentoalveolar injuries among patients with maxillofacial fractures. J Small Anim Pract 2013; 54:9–14.
15. Soukup J. Traumatic dentoalveolar injuries. In: Lobprise HB, Dodd JR, editors. Wigg's veterinary dentistry. 2nd edition. Hoboken (NJ): Wiley & sons; 2019. p. 109–30.
16. Golden AL, Stoller N, Harvey CE. A survey of oral and dental disease in dogs anesthetized in a veterinary hospital. J Am Anim Hosp Assoc 1982;18:891–9.
17. Fouad A, Levin LG. Pulpal reactions to caries and dental procedures. In: Hargreaves KM, editor. Cohen's pathways to the pulp. 11th edition. St Louis (MO): Mosby; 2011. p. 573–98.
18. van Valkenburgh B. Incidence of tooth breakage among large, predatory mammals. Am Nat 1988;131:291–302.
19. Trope M, Barnett F, Signurdsson, et al. The role of endodontics after dental traumatic injuries. In: Hargreaves KM, editor. Cohen's pathways to the pulp. 11th edition. St Louis (MO): Mosby; 2011. p. 758–92.
20. Hale FA. Localized intrinsic staining of teeth due to pulpitis and pulp necrosis in dogs. J Vet Dent 2001;18:14–20.
21. Ulbricht RD, Marretta SM, Klippert LS. Mandibular canine tooth luxation injury in a dog. J Vet Dent 2004;21:77–83.

22. Startup S. Wire-composite splint for luxation of the maxillary canine tooth. J Vet Dent 2010;27:198–202.

23. Lisa F, Reiter AM. Assessment of 68 prosthodontic crowns in 41 pet and working dogs (2000-2012). J Vet Dent 2015;32:148–54.

24. Coffman C, Visser C, Soukup J, et al. In: Lobprise HB, Dodd JR, editors. Wigg's veterinary dentistry. 2nd edition. Hoboken (NJ): Wiley & sons; 2019. p. 387–410.

25. Mestrinho LA, Gordo I, Gawor J, et al. Retrospective study of 18 titanium alloy crowns produced by computer aided design and manufacturing in dogs. Front Vet Sci 2019;6:97.

Nutrition of Working Dogs

Feeding for Optimal Performance and Health

Debra L. Zoran, DVM, PhD, DACVIM (SAIM)*

KEYWORDS

- Canine nutrition • Performance dogs • Performance diet

KEY POINTS

- Nutrition plays an important role in optimizing working canine performance.
- Individual nutrients are key to supporting and sustaining the athletic aspects of their working career.
- The veterinarian should consider the nutritional needs of each canine individually in light of their unique mission or athletic purpose.

INTRODUCTION AND OVERVIEW

Working dogs are an essential part of today's society, providing critical roles as partners to police, security officers, first responders, and individuals, using their athleticism, strength, special senses, and trainability to perform a specific task. Working canines are dogs with very specific training doing intensive jobs, and the roles they serve vary not only in type of effort but also in the degree of athleticism and special training the work requires. There are many variables that come into play determining optimal performance as a working canine: genetics, conformation, and behavior are innate, but environmental inputs, such as nutrition, fitness, and health care, also play key roles. The focus of this article is to review the role of nutrition and key nutrients in optimizing working canine performance and their ability to sustain that capability to complete their mission.

The focus of this review is on the nutritional needs of protection and detection canines, a group of working dogs with a distinct requirement for athleticism and the potential to be involved in difficult or continuous work over multiple days or weeks. Protection canines fall into the category of working police, patrol, livestock, guard, and security dogs that serve to alert, deter, or assist in defense of self, humans, or the animals they protect when threatened or when there is a perceived threat.[1–4] Many protection canines are members of state and federal law enforcement agencies

Texas A&M Veterinary Emergency Team, Texas A&M Task Force 1 US&R, FEMA Incident Support Team Veterinarian, College of Veterinary Medicine and Biomedical Sciences, Texas A&M University, College Station, TX 77843-4474, USA
* Corresponding author.
E-mail address: dzoran@cvm.tamu.edu

Vet Clin Small Anim 51 (2021) 803–819
https://doi.org/10.1016/j.cvsm.2021.04.014
0195-5616/21/© 2021 Elsevier Inc. All rights reserved.

and may also be dual function trained as both a protection and a detection canine. Detection canines are specifically trained to alert to the presence of a scent or odor of any number of illicit, dangerous, human, ecological, medical, or biological substances.[4] See Chapter 14: Operational Canines.

The type of work that a protection canine in a police or security unit is likely to perform is most closely aligned to a sprint athlete, as they typically run short distances to apprehend and grapple with a target, using both power and strength to complete that task. Protection canines that are dual trained in detection are also working to detect illicit or specific substances (eg, drugs or weapons) and often do this work at a walk in relatively controlled environments, such as searching in schools or airports. However, some protection canines work in very broad, environmentally difficult areas, such as those patrolling the border, will work in high heat, and may be required to apprehend suspects over a large search area. Thus, the workload can be quite variable depending on their mission tasking; however, most protection canines are not routinely engaged in moderate- or high-intensity work activities over a long distance or prolonged time (eg, they are not endurance athletes). As a result, the baseline nutritional and energy needs for most protection canines are not dissimilar to those calculated for an active pet dog. However, these canines must maintain a very high level of muscle strength and balance and must also be in optimal (ideal) body condition for sprinting and athletic performance, both of which may require adjustments (up or down) in the dietary levels of protein or fat.[5] Conversely, detection canines are a group of working dogs that have been selected and trained for specific characteristics: high drive, fearlessness on very unstable surfaces, trainability, stable personality (not aggressive or fearful), and their willingness to detect specific odors for reward.[6] There are a variety of health-related, training, and physiologic aspects to optimal detection canine effectiveness[7]; however, the nutritional needs of these specific categories of working canines only recently have been the focus of research studies.[8–10] Most previous work on the nutrition of the canine athlete concentrated heavily on endurance dogs (sled dogs) and sprinters (racing greyhounds), and there is a considerable database of knowledge about the physiology, metabolism, and the nutritional needs of sprint and endurance canines.[9–12] However, most working police, odor detection, or search and rescue (S&R/SAR) canines do not fall into these functional categories of work, and in fact, working detection dogs and particularly S&R canine activities are typically a blended athletic endeavor, requiring nutritional recommendations to be adapted to their specific and individual work. For example, in disaster response, S&R canines are best described as performing low- to moderate-intensity, intermediate- to long-duration work in a work environment that requires balance, core strength, and athleticism in addition to moderate endurance.[9,10] As a result of this incredible variability of work, the nutrition and energy requirements for an S&R canine may vary significantly depending on the intensity and length of the deployment, and on the differences in the work environment (ie, heat, cold, humidity) and terrain. The broad outlines defining work requirements for protection and detection canines reveal the reasons that the diet, energy needs, and nutrient profile must be tailored to the individual canine working conditions, but also illustrate the challenges associated with making that determination.

ENERGY NEEDS OF WORKING CANINES: DURATION AND INTENSITY

The daily energy and nutrient requirements for dogs are established by the National Research Council (NRC).[13] Energy for muscle activity and movement, as well as basic body functions, is obtained from adenosine triphosphate (ATP) created by the cellular metabolism of protein, fat, and carbohydrates. To better understand energy needs of dogs, the contributions of different parts of the diet to the energy equation, and some of the common energy calculation guidelines, it is important to first review some basics. One gram of protein, fat, or carbohydrate will generate a specific amount of energy that can be used when formulating diets and is important in understanding energy requirements. This number is traditionally given on the label of a food as metabolizable energy (ME). The ME of a nutrient is the amount of energy available to the dog after taking into account losses from digestion (nutrients in foods are not 100% digested), urine losses, and losses in exhalation of gases. These numbers are generally given a value of 4 kcal/g for protein and carbohydrate, and 9 kcal/g for fat based on the Atwater equation (a calculation used in human nutrition).[13] However, because manufactured pet food contains relatively less digestible ingredients than whole foods, the equation has been modified (literally the modified Atwater equation). Using this equation, the available energy from protein and carbohydrate in dog food is 3.5 kcal/g, and the energy from fat is 8.5 kcal/g.[13] Thus, energy density for whole foods compared with commercially processed foods in dogs is different and should be considered, particularly when assessing the energy content of a diet that is a mixture of whole and processed food (a common situation in some working canine diets). The concentrations of protein and carbohydrate are energetically important but contribute less to ME than fat, and thus, fat levels should be adjusted to maintain appropriate caloric intake as work or training requirements increase or decrease in their dogs. Many factors have a significant impact on calorie needs and include changes in workload or work environment, seasonal (heat or cold), and environmental changes (working in rough or hilly terrain), medical conditions that impact metabolism, such as hypothyroidism, or the reduction in energy needs that will occur following an ovariohysterectomy or neuter.[7,10,14–17] In addition, working canines also typically have greater muscle mass (thus greater muscle volume and mitochondrial density) and less fat mass than pet dogs, which also influence protein and energy needs.[7,10,18–21]

The energy needs of working canines, which by definition are performing as athletes and have much different energy requirements, do not fall easily or adequately into the traditional equations. As such, a large body of research has been collected studying the energy utilization of exercising dogs using indirect calorimetry.[7,10,13,15] Indirect calorimetry is a procedure that determines energy utilization by measuring the maximum volume of oxygen used or Vo_2 max. The Vo_2 max is a reflection of the maximum energy generated by oxygen utilization from muscle generation of ATP within muscle cell mitochondria.[7,13]

To understand the energy requirements of the canine athlete, it is important to recognize the differences in canine muscle composition that influence the energy preferences and needs for sustaining maximum muscle work with different types of work. First, canine muscle has higher concentrations of type I (low-myosin ATPase) and type IIa (aerobic) muscle fibers than other species.[18–20] These types of muscle fiber in dogs permit higher rates of aerobic (low-intensity, longer duration) metabolism during muscle work, especially from fatty acid sources.[22–25] In addition, unlike in humans, who use carbohydrate loading to increase stamina, in dogs, exhaustion does not correlate with glycogen depletion. Dogs in moderately intense, long-term work are able to continue to generate energy from fat oxidation, thought to be due to their high-aerobic activity in skeletal muscle.[7,10,26,27] In multiple studies in dogs investigating energy intensity and duration of activity to determine energy utilization (using Vo_2 max), dogs will use fat for energy (aerobic metabolism) when at 40% or less of their maximum aerobic effort, will use a combination of both carbohydrates (from protein oxidation) and fat for exercise between 40% and 70% of their maximum aerobic capacity, and when exercising at greater than 70% of their maximum aerobic capacity (eg, sprinting), will use glucose for energy (anaerobic metabolism of glycogen).[7,10,12] The oxidation of fatty acids in dogs begins rapidly after the onset of activity, peaking at 30 minutes of sustained activity, and is maintained when exercising at 30% to 50% of Vo_2 max.[7] A fit working dog that is exercising at 30% to 50% Vo_2 max is using fatty acids for energy and can maintain this level of activity for many hours with minimal fatigue.[14,24–27] Carbohydrate oxidation becomes a major source of energy for long-term exercise at greater than 50% of Vo max as long as glycogen is present, which dogs derive from muscle stores in the short term, but in the longer term derive carbohydrate-based energy from protein oxidation and gluconeogenesis.[12,22,27,28] In multiple studies of endurance canines, the dogs perform equally well with diets containing no carbohydrate, versus those with increasing carbohydrate content, as long as the protein content was high enough to maintain muscle mass, and fat content was increased to match energy demands.[26,27] These studies all point to the adaptation of dogs to perform aerobic work using fat and protein, and sparing muscle glycogen during endurance work.[25]

In contrast to the energy needs of endurance dogs, most, if not all, protection and detection working canines will be involved in either short sprinting work (as protection/police canines) or moderate-intensity, longer-term activities (detection, S&R, hunting, field trial, high-activity service dogs). The energy needs for this type of work, and the nutrient proportions used in their diets, must be adjusted to meet each canine's intended purpose. This is well illustrated in a study evaluating the maintenance energy requirements (MER) of 20 detection canines (odor, explosive, and human remains detection) under typical work conditions (short searches, detection areas in urban or confined areas).[5] The researchers found that the energy needs in this population of working dogs was essentially the same as the NRC recommendations for active, adult canines ($2 \times$ resting energy requirement [RER] or 132 kcal $\times$ BW$^{0.75}$).[5] There are no studies assessing the energy needs of S&R canines working in disaster field conditions, over multiple hours in a day, or over multiple days of work. However, these conditions are similar in many aspects to the duration and type of work required of hunting dogs: moderate-intensity, sustained intermediate-duration work. Studies of hunting dogs completed to assess energy needs in a variety of working conditions (extreme heat, high humidity, extreme cold, terrain differences, and so forth) reveal that energy demands are much higher during their work/training periods ($5–8\times$ MER), but do not reach the levels of energy needed by endurance sled dogs, even in extremely cold weather conditions.[10,16,17,29] The differences observed in energy needs of working dogs in these diverse conditions illustrate 2 important points: (1) energy needs for working dogs at rest (not in active training or deployed) are not significantly different from other dogs, and (2) during training (which may be intense and year-around) or when actively engaged in performing work of moderate intensity (field search) and long duration (hours to days), dogs may require significant increases in energy intake ($5–10\times$ MER) to sustain their muscle function and capacity to maintain work.

As has been noted previously, there are numerous studies using field and treadmill exercise demonstrating the increasing energy needs of greyhounds, foxhounds, and Alaskan sled dogs during extended exercise periods.[11,12] These data points provide important insight into the energy needs for each specific types of activity, but at the same time, these studies do not take into account the impact on energy needs created by changes in the working environment that occur in field work conditions of wilderness and disaster S&R canines. Some of the most important variables that will impact energy use during work are environmental temperatures (high heat, cold, or humidity), variability in the terrain (significant inclines can double or triple energy use), thermal regulation requirements (panting), and surface irregularities (sand vs snow, and so forth) that impact workload for many working dog activities. Thus, even with general guidelines for energy requirements based on activity type and duration (which are the critical starting point), the needs of a working protection or detection canine cannot be generalized. A combination of careful attention of the handler to their dog's ideal or competitive body weight, making assessments of increased energy needs based on working conditions, maintaining the dog in ideal body condition (3 or 4 out of 9) (**Fig. 1**), and monitoring muscle condition (**Fig. 2**) to provide awareness

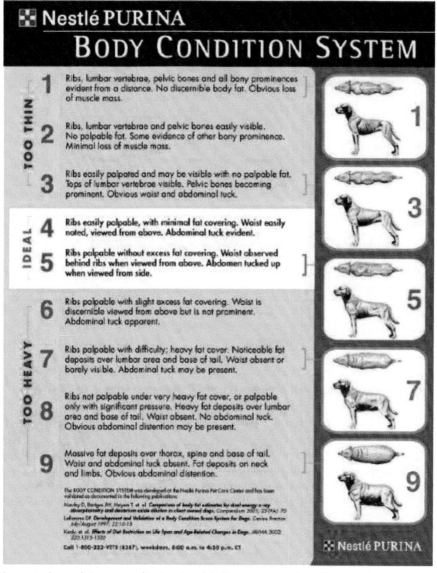

Fig. 1. Body condition scores (Purina 9 scale). (From petnutritionalliance.org).

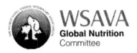

Muscle Condition Score

Muscle condition score is assessed by visualization and palpation of the spine, scapulae, skull, and wings of the ilia. Muscle loss is typically first noted in the epaxial muscles on each side of the spine; muscle loss at other sites can be more variable. Muscle condition score is graded as normal, mild loss, moderate loss, or severe loss. Note that animals can have significant muscle loss if they are overweight (body condition score > 5). Conversely, animals can have a low body condition score (< 4) but have minimal muscle loss. Therefore, assessing both body condition score and muscle condition score on every animal at every visit is important. Palpation is especially important when muscle loss is mild and in animals that are overweight. An example of each score is shown below.

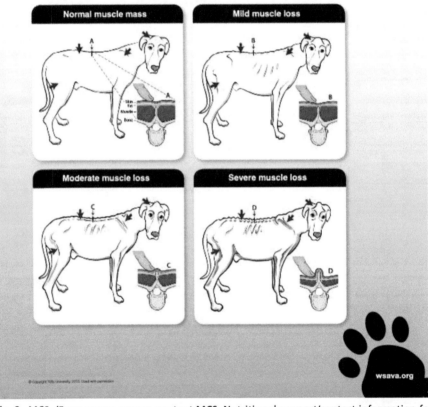

Fig. 2. MCS. (From wsava.org.wp-content MCS. Nutritional support/contact information for Veterinary Nutritionists: www.acvn.org/directory/. The Web site for the American College of Veterinary Nutritionists has a Web directory of board-certified nutrition specialists and their contact information for people needing to find a nutrition person to consult on commercial or a homemade diets.)

of muscle mass norms for their dog, is required to assist handlers and support personnel in assuring that appropriate adjustments can occur.

Calculation of the RER is the first and most important equation in the process of developing a calorie target. RER is an estimate of the minimal energy needs of dogs to support basal metabolism and simple activity.[13] There have been several different approaches to calculating RER (**Table 1**), but for ease of use in a clinical setting, the linear equation $[(BW_{kg}) \times 30] + 70$ is the most serviceable starting point. The MER equation is used to account for increased activity or physiologic needs (increased work/activity, lactation, reproduction, and so forth) and is calculated by multiplying RER by a factor (typically $1.5-2\times$)[13] (see **Table 1**). However, a working dog under moderate-intensity, long work hours, or extreme conditions (high heat, extreme cold, difficult terrain), may require 3 to $8\times$ more energy than this baseline.[7,10,14] An example of the challenge in determining an appropriate intake was illustrated by the extreme conditions that dogs experienced working the Oso, Washington mudslide.[17] The working conditions disaster required dogs to search on an inclined grade in heavy mud conditions (6–12 in deep) where the environmental conditions were challenging because of rain and temperatures in the 30°F to 40°F range. The dogs were all being fed their standard rations (energy levels at $2-3\times$ MER) at the outset. However, it was quickly realized that all of the dogs were losing weight and muscle mass despite

Table 1
Energy calculation equations for resting energy requirement and maintenance energy requirement[29]

Energy Value	Calculation Examples
Resting energy requirement (*RER*): the energy required in a normal, intact animal at rest	$RER = 70(BW_{kg})^{0.75}$ RER (linear) = $30(BW_{kg}) + 70$ (only if BW between 2 and 45 kg) On average, RER = 70 kcal/d/kg body weight
Maintenance energy requirement (*MER*): the energy required in a normal, intact, adult animal for moderate activity in a thermoneutral environment	$MER = 140(BW_{kg})^{0.75}$ MER = 1.5–2.0 (RER) for modestly active companion dogs For moderate work intensity over a long time, MER must be increased to 2 to $8\times$ (RER) or higher based on conditions Neutered dogs may require up to 25% fewer calories to maintain an ideal body condition
MER of racing greyhounds (sprinting)	$150-160(BW_{kg})^{0.75}$ or RER × 2.2–2.5 Increase needs likely due to increased muscle mass
MER of hunting dogs (intermediate endurance)	$155-280(BW_{kg})^{0.75}$ or RER × 4 Needs adjusted to training vs multiday events over long distance
MER of sled dogs (long distance exercise)	$228-1052(BW_{kg})^{0.75}$ or RER × 15 The greatest energy needs occur in the coldest temperatures and with mountainous or difficult terrain conditions
MER of working dogs (intermediate work)	$150-350(BW_{kg})^{0.75}$ or RER × 2–5 Needs adjusted to environmental conditions, work intensity, and duration of work (deployment) over days

increasing their intake. The dogs' condition was not stabilized until caregivers provided higher protein/energy food and increased their intake to 8 to 10× RER.[17] This example illustrates that not only do energy needs vary by the individual and the type of work they do, but also the specific circumstances of the mission. The need for careful determination of energy needs and real-time adjustment is critical to the dog's ability to complete the mission, as well as maintaining their ability to detect odor and reducing risk of injury.

One of the most widely recognized tools for physical assessment of a dog relative to the need for adjusting their dietary energy levels is monitoring their body condition score (see **Fig. 1**).[30] Body condition scoring is a well-known and relatively simple, but reliable and repeatable tool to assess the fat mass of an individual.[30] Working canines must be able to work under a variety of conditions and be able to sustain this effort for hours or days. This requires not only physical fitness but also a healthy body weight, ideal or thin body condition (4/9), and excellent muscle condition. Dogs working in high-heat, high-humidity conditions are less heat tolerant and less able to sustain work if they are carrying excess body fat or are poorly conditioned.[31,32] Increased body fat also increases adipokines that change the balance of hormones controlling appetite, metabolism, muscle utilization of glucose, and inflammatory cytokines that are detrimental to optimal athletic performance and promote increased risk of injury.[33,34] All canine handlers should obtain and record regular body weights, using the same scale, on their canine partners and learn to assess body condition as 2 methods of determining whether they are appropriately meeting (or exceeding) the energy needs of their working canine.

A less well-known, and less well-studied, but potentially helpful tool for handlers and veterinarians to use in the assessment of muscle mass of the working canine is the muscle condition score (MCS) (**Fig. 2**). MCS is a relatively new tool, and because of the variability of canine breeds, sizes, and conformation, has met with some difficulty in general use and validation. Recently, MCS was compared with muscle ultrasound measurements for determination of muscle mass loss in dogs, and although mild changes were not detectable by MCS, moderate or significant muscle loss detection was comparable.[35] Muscle mass is not a true measure of muscle fitness or function, but it is an indication of muscle loss or lack of muscle tone that may be due to nutritional, fitness-related issues, or injury-caused atrophy that if identified can be corrected and optimize both health and performance. Nevertheless, the use of MCS as a part of regular assessment (like body condition score or body weight) by the handler and the veterinary support personnel can provide another more objective measure of the nutritional and physical status of this working canine athlete.

NUTRIENTS FOR PERFORMANCE: PROTEIN, FAT, CARBOHYDRATES, AND WATER
Protein

Dietary protein is important for maintenance of nitrogen balance, providing the essential amino acids required for health, normal immune function, muscle function, and repair through support of the essential proteins of body chemistry (albumin, total protein, and other acute phase proteins) important in immune function.[36] According to the NRC, dogs require only 20 g/1000 kcal of diet (or about 10% protein in a typical dry food) to maintain their basic nitrogen balance.[36] However, in working canines, there is an increased need for dietary protein for maintenance of increased muscle mass and function, but also as an energy substrate during moderate, sustained exercise. The need for increased protein in endurance activities (eg, sled dogs) has been well documented, both in field and in experimental treadmill conditions.[12] There is general agreement that endurance activities in dogs require a minimum of 26% protein ME (from either animal source or mixed animal/plant based sources) to prevent muscle catabolism and protect protein functions at the cellular level.[9,12] The ideal amount of protein for optimal performance in endurance canines has not been firmly established, but studies show the most consistent performance and ability to sustain work are achieved when they are fed protein at 28% to 32% ME.[9,10,37,38] Conversely, in dogs engaged in sprinting activities (eg, greyhounds), there is less direct evidence for a performance benefit of a high-protein concentration in the diet.[22] This effect is likely a result of the high-intensity but extremely short-term anaerobic activity for which stored glycogen is the primary energy source. Furthermore, in 1 study, a lower dietary protein concentration (18% protein ME) and higher carbohydrate to serve as an energy source resulted in a better sprinting performance in the greyhounds than those fed high- (>35% protein ME) protein, low-carbohydrate diets typical of greyhound rations.[22]

The protein requirements for optimal performance in canines working at moderate-intensity levels for intermediate durations of time (eg, protection or detection canines) have not been extensively evaluated. Wakshlag and Schmalberg[9] and others recommend a minimum of 22% to 24% protein ME for working S&R canines to provide the necessary protein for cellular functions, muscle energy use, and maintenance of muscle mass. In a treadmill exercise study of intermediate- or moderate-intensity work comparing the physiologic response of dogs fed diets with either high protein/high fat (27:57), high protein/low fat (27:32), or low protein/high fat (18:57), researchers found important benefits on cellular metabolism in the dogs fed the high-protein diets (low or high fat), but conversely, dogs fed the lower-protein, higher-fat diets had a slightly better thermal recovery (not statistically significant) following work in high-temperature environments.[39] At this time with the information available, the baseline recommendations for dietary protein of working canines are providing protein at 22% to 24% ME.[9,10] However, protein may need to be increased to 25% to 28% ME (or higher) for maintenance of muscle, or when dogs are working in extreme environmental conditions, or for a lengthy (14 days) deployment.

Fat: More Than Just Energy

The roles of fat in the canine diet are multiple, and although energy is a primary function for dietary fat, it has a critical role important in cell structure, membrane function, the and cyclooxygenase and lipoxygenase enzyme pathways that mediate inflammation, and adipose tissue is a major endocrine organ important in all aspects of energy and metabolism.[40–43]

In the first 20 to 30 minutes of intense (sprint) exercise, the primary substrate used by cells for energy is from stored carbohydrate (glycogen). When lower-intensity exercise is maintained beyond that time, fat provides energy through beta-oxidation, and protein is used for gluconeogenesis, and ultimately, for glucose oxidation as energy.[9,10,37] To rephrase, at lower-intensity work levels (30%–50% of Vo_2 max), fat is the primary substrate, and as the intensity of work increases to 80% to 90% of Vo_2 max (which is typical of anaerobic work such as sprinting), energy utilization is almost entirely muscle glycogen.[9,10] In a highly conditioned dog, fat usage at moderate-intensity work (30%–70% Vo_2 max) can provide sustained energy for several hours, which is something that is not possible with glucose as the energy substrate, even with increased carbohydrate consumption.[10] Thus, fat must be used as the source of sustained energy for canine diets in dogs working at moderate intensity for an intermediate time, and in all endurance athletes. This physiologic situation is distinctly different from that observed in human endurance athletes, where the focus for sustaining energy for work is on repletion of glycogen through carbohydrates. Multiple studies have demonstrated the incredible adaptation to fat oxidation in sled dogs, allowing them to consume fat in their diets as high as 60% to 70% ME (or higher), which allows them to use fat for energy over days of continuous work, and to preserve muscle glycogen.[23,25,41,44] In all canines, increasing fat in their diet must be introduced slowly over 1 to 3 months to allow gastrointestinal, mitochondrial, and metabolic adaptation at the same time as increases in utilization are occurring.[23] To date, there are few studies that evaluate fat sources (saturated fats, polyunsaturated fatty acids [PUFA], and medium-chain triglyceride [MCT] oils) for their effects on performance or for use as functional fats. Nevertheless, there appears to be no metabolic benefit to replacing saturated fats with either MCT or PUFA in canine diets from a performance perspective.[37,44] However, the use of long-chain PUFA, as either plant-based oils (corn, safflower, canola) or omega-3 (marine) oils, may impact olfactory function, reduce inflammation, and improve rehabilitation of working canines, and as such, should receive further research attention.[39–41,45,46]

Carbohydrates and Dietary Fibers: Canine Athletes Have Different Needs

Carbohydrates are present in diets as a source of immediate energy as glycogen in muscle and liver, and to provide glucose to the select organs with a preference for it as fuel (eg, brain, kidneys). With the exception of the diet for a lactating bitch, there is no requirement for carbohydrates in the canine diet; however, carbohydrates come in many forms aside from the starches used for energy. In particular, complex carbohydrates that make up dietary fibers are important components in the canine diet for maintenance of the normal gastrointestinal microbiome and function.[27]

Dietary carbohydrates and muscle glycogen are the clear choice for energy for muscle work in the short-term, high-intensity work of sprinting (<20 minutes, high-speed work as may be seen in working protection canines). However, for dogs whose energy demands are for more moderate-intensity, longer-duration activities (as with many S&R or detection canines working a large area), studies show that fat and energy obtained from protein metabolism are the preferred substrates (searching, hunting, and so forth).[9,10,22,28] Thus, protection canines may be fed a diet that is more similar to an active pet dog: targeting a profile containing a modest to increased amount of protein (22%–24% protein ME), to maintain muscle strength and function, a lower level of fat provided as energy to help maintain an ideal body condition (15%–18% fat ME), and the remainder being complex carbohydrates (eg, 30%–50% ME). Conversely, disaster canines (detection canines) that will have moderate-intensity, longer-duration work cycles over multiple days (or longer), will require diets with higher protein (eg, protein at 24%–28% ME), higher fat (eg, 20%–25% ME, or even higher in certain working conditions), and more modest amounts of carbohydrate (eg, 20%–30% ME). In circumstances where dogs are performing repetitive, intense, but short-term (<20 minutes) sprint activities that need a source of immediate energy, a carbohydrate supplement may be fed immediately after the intense exercise activity. The highly digestible carbohydrate maltodextrin or similar supplements provide maximal glucose availability to the muscle cells for replenishing glycogen.[47] Dogs working moderate-intensity, but intermediate to long work cycles, will require additional energy to sustain work throughout the day that is not carbohydrate based. One way to meet this need is to feed a small amount of high-protein/high-fat meal (eg, 3 oz canned recovery food or cat food) every 4 to 6 hours during rest and rehydration periods. All diets fed to working canines should have highly digestible ingredients to reduce the risk of stress diarrhea that is common during high-intensity work. Recent studies show carbohydrates from certain grain groups are a component of dysbiosis or "stress" diarrhea that can occur in many working dogs during deployment.[48–51] Thus, diet selection for a working dog requires individualization, not only for the work tasking of that canine but also to determine the balance of ingredients that will lead to a healthy, stable gastrointestinal tract.[48,50] As work on the role of the intestinal microbiome and its critical role in health and disease expands, this will also play a greater role in decision making about what defines optimal nutrition in working canines.[49,50,52]

Dietary Fiber, Vitamins and Minerals, and Electrolytes in Support of Working Canines

Complex carbohydrates present in diets as dietary fiber are important in gastrointestinal health and function in 2 important ways. First, soluble fiber sources (eg, fermentable fibers) are essential to a healthy intestinal and colonic microbiome and maintenance of colonic epithelial cell health.[27,53,54] Soluble fibers serve as substrate for digestion by healthy commensal bacteria (eg, prebiotics) and thus can help prevent stress diarrhea.[48,50,51] The second type of dietary fiber important in intestinal health is the family of insoluble dietary fibers (eg, nonfermentable fibers), of which dietary cellulose is an example. This group of fibers is important in enhancing normal gastrointestinal motility; they provide a bulking effect that increases the transit of foods through both the small and the large intestine (reducing food digestibility and important in weight loss), and, as bulking agents in the colon, are essential to normal defecation and preventing constipation.[27,53,54] Both soluble fiber and insoluble fiber are essential to some degree in the standard canine diet, but there have been few studies to date assessing the optimal concentrations of each type of fiber in a working canine diet. However, diets containing soluble fiber to support intestinal microbiome health would be expected to be beneficial in helping reduce the incidence of "stress" diarrhea.[48,50,51] A minimal amount (<3% dry matter) of insoluble fiber should be the target of a working canine diet, to reduce fecal volume and maximize nutrient digestibility.

Vitamins, minerals, and electrolytes are critical dietary components for the working canine because they are vital in almost all chemical reactions and transmembrane transport systems in energy utilization.[10,27] In addition, during exercise, there is an increased need to support the metabolic pathways required in tissue synthesis and repair, and the increased utilization of these nutrients during states of metabolic acidosis and protection from oxidative damage that occurs as a result of the metabolism of fats for energy.[10,27] However, there are no studies to date documenting the need to increase the levels of any of these nutrients above what is present in a complete and balanced diet, or via supplementation of the diets of dogs fed balanced foods. Furthermore, supplementation of a balanced diet not only may cause imbalance but also can result in interactions or intolerances between these minerals or nutrients that are detrimental.[10] Finally, it is a common situation in many kennels or within the working dog community for these canines to be fed some aspect of their diet from noncommercial (homemade or raw) rations consisting of primarily animal meat and fat sources. In these situations, not only is it important to make sure the handlers are fully aware of the food safety issues that are presented by this feeding method[55] but also recommendations should be made to assure the diet is complete and balanced with addition of appropriate levels of vitamins, minerals, and electrolytes under the supervision of a board-certified nutritionist (www.acvn.org/directory).

Nutrition and Function: Olfaction, Heat Tolerance, and Supplements in Working Dogs

The increasing importance and numbers of working canines in our daily lives have resulted in greater interest in optimizing their health and performance. Some areas of scientific investigation, such as the role of supplements in prevention and management of injury and management of rehabilitation from injury, which is a fact of their lifestyle, have been ongoing for many years. The role of nutrition and nutritional supplements in management and prevention of injury and orthopedic disease has been a focus of many recent reviews and is the subject of specialists who now focus on sports medicine and rehabilitation in canine athletes.[10,37,41,45,46] The interested reader is referred to these sources for additional information and a detailed review of the use of omega 3 fatty acids, glucosamine and chondroitin, antioxidants (vitamin E and vitamin C), and other nutraceuticals. As a point of note, it is generally recommended by veterinarians and lay persons alike, that working dogs (across all types of work) should be supplemented, if not contraindicated, with veterinary-approved glucosamine and chondroitin supplements, and additional amounts of marine fish oils (omega 3 fatty acids) to mitigate the wear and tear on joints and reduce associated inflammation and those deleterious effects on joint function. To date, there is a large body of scientific evidence demonstrating that supplementation with marine source omega 3 fish oils is beneficial in reducing inflammation and improving oxidant status.[45,56,57] However, although evidence supporting use of glucosamine and chondroitin remains controversial and studies are conflicting, their use may also be beneficial in many dogs and is not expected to be harmful, and thus, recommendations for use continue.[58–62]

There are many important physical characteristics that make a detection canine a highly valuable team member, but the dog's prodigious ability to use their nose to detect minute amounts of odor is perhaps their most valuable contribution (see Chapter 7: Special Senses). There are a variety of factors that may impact the working canine's olfactory capabilities, including the following: the canine anatomy, health of the nose and nasal cavity, presence of systemic diseases, pharmaceuticals, conditioning and training, hydration, nutrition, and the nasal and intestinal microbiota.[7] Jenkins and coauthors[7] recently reviewed this fascinating subject in detail, and particularly the complex and interrelated role of the microbial ecosystem of the body in this process, and the interested reader is referred to this paper for additional detail. Interestingly, there is clear evidence that dogs that are highly conditioned for exercise have a significant improvement in their odor-detection capabilities.[9] The relationship of diet and the microbiome is a complex and undeniable relationship; however, the role of diet and microbiome effects on canine olfaction remains to be clearly elucidated. The only study to date that has reported a specific diet effect on olfaction capability was from Angle and coworkers,[8] who noted a modest improvement in odor detection when canine diets were supplemented with long-chain PUFA. The understanding of the role of nutrients in optimizing olfaction and odor detection clearly requires additional attention.

As discussed in the earlier sections on energy requirements of working canines, the targets for the appropriate amount of energy for work are based on energy needs for muscle work and the duration, frequency, and intensity of the work. However, what has not been evaluated or tested is the added energy requirement needed for canines to maintain the mental focus and attention required to do detection work.[7] There is mounting evidence that diets containing increased amounts of fats as energy for brain cells (MCT oils) and increased but carefully considered concentrations of antioxidant nutrients (omega 3 fatty acids [eg, fish oil], increased B vitamins, vitamin E, and selenium) can result in increased mental focus and acuity in aging canines.[63] The use of differing fat sources and nutrients with increased antioxidant properties on mental alertness and function has been a source of intense interest in companion dog owners, but the effects have not been studied in working canines.

Finally, although water balance has not been discussed in this article, hydration is critical to maintenance of canine muscle function and endurance. In addition, there is clear evidence that maintaining adequate hydration of the working canine is also critical to optimal nasal membrane function and odor detection.[64] Decreased membrane fluidity owing to dehydration results in altered odorant receptor function and decreased transduction of the neural signal to the brain.[7] In multiple field studies, dogs often do not increase their voluntary consumption of water while working, a fact observed in disaster canine studies.[17] There have been several strategies used over the years to increase hydration in working canines, including administration of subcutaneous fluids and adding different substances to water, ranging from electrolytes to sugar combinations.[65] Rehydration of canines in the field by subcutaneous fluid administration is not ideal, as the volume of fluid required to rehydrate most working dogs is large (>1 L in some cases) and is not always readily or repeatedly accepted. Furthermore, in the study by Otto and coworkers,[65] hydration using the subcutaneous methods resulted in increased creatinine levels, an indicator of either lack of complete hydration or of muscle damage. In addition, repeated administration of fluids subcutaneously in canines in field conditions may increase the risk of inadvertent exposure to contaminants present on the skin or coat. The studies by Otto clearly revealed that oral rehydration strategies containing additional electrolytes were highly effective, as dogs would voluntarily consume more water with the additive than simply water alone.[65] In the author's experience with disaster S&R canines working in hot, humid environments, water baiting with a small amount (2–3 tbsp) of a canned high-protein/high-fat food (recovery diet or cat food) added to water has resulted in complete consumption of offered water during their standard recovery period. This approach, similar to adding electrolytes to water, has led to increased voluntary consumption of water and maintenance of hydration in dogs as assessed by mucous membrane moisture and skin turgor. Furthermore, over a long work cycle, the "water baiting" approach provides protein and fat energy in a highly digestible, non-kibble form whereby energy replenishment for maintenance of muscle work and odor detection is needed.

SUMMARY

Nutritional decisions and selecting diets with the appropriate types and amounts of nutrients for any animal are complicated but are made more difficult by the fact that all living beings are unique, and their nutritional needs are as well. The process of nutritional decision making is perhaps even more challenging in a working canine, not only because of their highly variable work conditions but also by the increasing evidence that all aspects of nutrition may impact the quality of this work, not just the impact on muscle work and function but also olfactory sensitivity and gut microbiome stability. Nevertheless, this review has offered guidelines for the nutrition of working canines that, it is hoped, will be a useful starting point to finding the optimal balance of nutrients and energy for support of their working needs and long-term health.

CLINICS CARE POINTS

- Selecting appropriate nutrition for working canines is critical to ensuring optimal performance in protection or detection work.
- Canine athletes use protein and fat for energy and maintenance of intermediate- to long-duration work, in contrast to other species (humans), who use carbohydrate loading and glycogen storage for maintenance of energy for muscle function.

- Working protection (police/protection) canines typically work in short, intense bursts of activity, requiring increased protein for maintenance of muscle mass, but more carbohydrate and less fat for energy to perform their mission.
- Detection canines must often perform their work in environmentally intense areas, at moderate-intensity levels over multiple days, intermediate-intensity and -duration work that requires significant increases in protein and fat to maintain muscle function, mental acuity, and olfaction detection capabilities.

DISCLOSURE

Dr. Zoran is a member of the Purina Advisory Board as a subject matter expert who meets annually with other subject matter experts to provide scientific and clinician feedback to Nestle Purina Petcare. This relationship had no impact on the development, writing, or information provided in this article.

REFERENCES

1. Americans with Disabilities Act 1990 (Section 35.136).
2. American Veterinary Medical Association. Service, emotional support and therapy animals. Available at: https://www.avma.org/resources-tools/animal-health-welfare/service-emotional-support-and-therapy-animals. Accessed December 1, 2020.
3. Gengler B. 'Service dogs, therapy dogs, and working dogs, oh my!', *Advance-Titan (Oshkosh, WI)*, p. 4. 2019. Available at: http://search.ebscohost.com/login.aspx?direct=true&db=plh&AN=138737665&site=eds-live. Accessed December 1, 2020.
4. ASB Technical Report 025, First Edition. Crime scene/death investigation – dogs and sensors terms and definitions. AAFS Standards Board, LLC. 2017. Available at: http://www.asbstandardsboard.org/wp-content/uploads/2019/05/025_TR_e1_2017.pdf. Accessed December 1, 2020.
5. Mullin RA, Witzel AL, Price J. Maintenance energy requirement of odor detection, explosive detection and human detection working dogs. Peer J 2015;3:e767.
6. Jones KD, Downend AB, Otto CM. Search-and-rescue dogs: an overview for veterinarians. J Am Vet Med Assoc 2004;225(6):854–60.
7. Jenkins EK, DeChant MT, Perry EB. When the nose doesn't know: canine olfactory function associated with health, management, and potential links to microbiotia. Front Vet Sci 2018;5:56.
8. Angle TC, Wakshlag JJ, Gillette RL, et al. The effects of exercise and diet on olfactory capability in detection dogs. J Nutr Sci 2014;3:e44.
9. Wakshlag J, Schmalberg J. Nutrition for working and service dogs. Vet Clin North Am Small Anim Pract 2014;44:719–40.
10. Toll PW, Gillette RL, Hand MS. The canine athlete. In: Hand MS, Thetcher CD, Rremillard RL, et al, editors. Small animal clinical nutrition. 5th Edition. Marceline, MO: Walsworth Publishing; 2010. p. 323–57.
11. Hill RC, Bloomberg MS, Legrand-Defretin V, et al. Maintenance energy requirements and the effects of diet on performance in racing greyhounds. Am J Vet Res 2000;61:1566–73.
12. Reynolds AJ, Fuhrer L, Dunlap HL, et al. Effect of diet and training on muscle glycogen storage and utilization in sled dogs. J Appl Physiol 1995;79:1601–7.
13. Kienzle E. Energy. In: National Research Council (NRC), editor. Nutrient requirements of dogs and cats. Washington, DC: National Academies Press; 2006. p. 29–48.

14. Reinhardt GA. Nutrition for sporting dogs. In: Dee JF, Bloomberg MS, Taylor RA, editors. Canine sports medicine and surgery. Philadelphia: WB Saunders Co; 1998. p. 348–56.
15. Ordway GA, Floyd DL, Longhurst JC, et al. Oxygen consumption and hemodynamic responses during graded treadmill exercise in the dog. J Appl Physiol 1984;57:601–7.
16. Ahlestrom O, Redman P, Speakman J. Energy expenditure and water turnover in hunting dogs in winter conditions. Br J Nutr 2011;106:S158–61.
17. Gordon LE. Injuries and illnesses among Federal Emergency Management Agency–certified search-and-recovery and search-and-rescue dogs deployed to Oso, Washington, following the March 22, 2014, State Route 530 landslide. J Am Vet Med Assoc 2015;247:901–8.
18. Maxwell LC, Barclay JK, Mohrman DE, et al. Physiologic characteristics of skeletal muscles in dogs and cats. Am J Physiol 1977;233:C14–8.
19. Wakshlag J, Cooper BJ, Wakshlag RR, et al. Biochemical evaluation of mitochondrial respiratory chain enzymes in canine skeletal muscle. Am J Vet Res 2004;65: 480–4.
20. Gunn HM. Differences in the histochemical properties of skeletal muscles of different breeds of horses and dogs. J Anat 1978;127:615–34.
21. Schmidt-Nielsen J. Scaling: why animal size is so important. Cambridge (United Kingdom): Cambridge University Press; 1984.
22. Hill RC, Lewis DD, Scott KC, et al. The effects of increased protein and decreased carbohydrate in the diet on performance and body condition in racing greyhounds. Am J Vet Res 2001;62:440–7.
23. Reynolds AJ, Fuhrer L, Dunlap HO, et al. Lipid metabolite responses to diet and training in sled dogs. J Nutr 1994;124:2754S–9S.
24. McClelland G, Zwingelstein G, Taylor CR, et al. Increased capacity for circulatory fatty acid transport in a highly aerobic mammal. Am J Physiol 1994;266:R1280–6.
25. McKenzie EC, Hinchcliff KW, Valberg SJ, et al. Assessment of alterations in triglyceride and glycogen concentrations in muscle tissue of Alaskan sled dogs during repetitive. Am J Vet Res 2008;69(8):1097–103.
26. Downey RL, Kronfeld DS, Banta CA. Diet of beagles affects stamina. J Am Anim Hosp Assoc 1980;16:262–7.
27. Gross KL, Jewell DE, Yamka RM, et al. Macronutrients. In: Hand MS, Thatcher CD, Remillard RL, et al, editors. Small animal clinical nutrition. Topeka, KS: Mark Morris Institute; 2010. p. 49–106.
28. Kronfeld DS, Hammel EP, Ramberg CF, et al. Hematological and metabolic responses to training in racing sled dogs fed medium, low and zero carbohydrate. Am J Clin Nutr 1977;30:419–30.
29. Davenport GM, Altom EK. Effect of diet on hunting performance of English pointers. Vet Ther 2001;2:10–23.
30. Laflamme DP. Development and validation of a body condition score system for dogs. A clinical tool. Canine Pract 1997;22:10–5.
31. Baker JA, Davis MS. Effect of conditioning on exercise induced hyperthermia and post exercise cooling in dogs. Comp Exerc Phys 2018;14:91–7.
32. Robbins PJ, Ramos MT, Zanghi BM, et al. Environmental and physiological factors associated with stamina in dogs exercising at high ambient temperatures. Front Vet Sci 2017;4:144.
33. Sakurai T, Izawa T, Kizaki T, et al. Exercise training decreases expression of inflammation-related adipokines through reduction of oxidative stress in rat white adipose tissue. Biochem Biophys Res Commun 2009;379:605–9.

34. Gonzalez-Gil AM, Elizondo-Montemayor L. The role of exercise in the interplay between myokines, hepatokines, osteokines, adipokines and modulation of inflammation for energy substrate redistribution and fat mass loss: a review. Nutrients 2020;12:1899.

35. Freeman LM, Sutherland-Smith J, Prantil LR, et al. Quantitative assessment of muscle in dogs using a vertebral epaxial muscle score. Can J Vet Res 2017; 81:255–60.

36. Rogers O. Protein and amino acids. In: National Research Council (NRC), editor. Nutrient requirements of dogs and cats. Washington, DC: National Academy Press; 2006. p. 111–45.

37. Wakshlag JJ. The role of nutrition in canine performance and rehabilitation. In: Zink MC, Van Dyke JB, editors. Canine sports medicine and rehabilitation. 1st ed. Ames, IA: John Wiley and sons; 2013. p. 60–81.

38. Querengasesser A, Iben C, Leibetseder J. Blood changes during training and racing in sled dogs. J Nutr 1994;124:2760S–4S.

39. Ober J, Gillette RL, Angle TC, et al. The effects of varying concentrations of dietary protein and fat on blood gas, hematologic, serum chemistry, and body temperature before and after exercise in Labrador retrievers. Front Vet Sci 2016;3:59.

40. Bauer JE. Facilitative and functional fats in diets of cats and dogs. J Am Vet Med Assoc 2006;229:680–4.

41. Bauer JE. Fats and fatty acids. In: National Research Council (NRC), editor. Nutrient requirements of dogs and cats. Washington, DC: National Academy Press; 2006. p. 81–110.

42. Kil DY, Swanson DS. Endocrinology of obesity. Vet Clin North Am Small Anim Pract 2010;40:205–19.

43. Zoran DL. Obesity in dogs and cats: a metabolic and endocrine disorder. Vet Clin North Am Small Anim Pract 2010;40:221–39.

44. Reynolds AJ, Hayek MG, Lepine AJ, et al. The role of fat in the formulation of performance rations: focus on fat sources. In: Carey DP, Reinhart GA, editors. Recent advances in canine and feline nutrition: 1998 iams nutrition symposium proceedings vol II. Wilmington, OH: Orange Frazer Press; 1998. p. 277–81.

45. Burri L, Wyse C, Gray SR, et al. Effects of dietary supplementation with krill meal on serum pro-inflammatory markers after the Iditarod sled dog race. Res Vet Sci 2018;121:18–22.

46. Vassalotti G, Musco N, Lombardi P, et al. Nutritional management of search and rescue dogs. J Nutr Sci 2017;6:e44.

47. Wakshlag JJ, Kalifelz FA, Barr SC, et al. Effects of exercise on canine skeletal muscle proteolysis: an investigation of the ubiquitin proteasome pathway and other metabolic markers. Vet Ther 2002;3:215–25.

48. Chiofalo B, DeVita G, Presti VL, et al. Grain free diets for utility dogs during training work: evaluation of the nutrient digestibility and faecal characteristics. Anim Nutr 2019;5:297–306.

49. Wernimont SM, Radosevich J, Jackson MI, et al. The effects of nutrition the gastrointestinal microbiome in cats and dogs: impact on health and disease. Front Microbiol 2020;11:1266.

50. MacLeay JM, Jewell DE, Suchodolski JS. The effects of nutrition on the gastrointestinal microbiome of cats and dogs: impact on health and disease. Front Microbiol 2020;11:1266.

51. Yaguiyan-Colliard L, Grandjean D. Digestive issues of working and athletic dogs. Vet Focus 2013;23:9–13.

52. Singh R, Sharma L. Nutrigenomics: a combination of nutrition and genomics: a new concept. J Physiol Nutr Phys Ed 2019;4:417–21.
53. Lattimer JM, Haub MD. Effects of dietary fiber and its components on metabolic health. Nutrients 2010;2:1269–89.
54. DeGodoy MRC, Kerr KR, Fahey GC. Alternative dietary fiber sources in companion animal nutrition. Nutrients 2013;5:3099–117.
55. Davies RH, Laws JR, Wales AD. Raw diets for dogs and cats: a review with particular reference to microbiological hazards. J Small Anim Pract 2019;60:329–39.
56. Bauer JE. The essential nature of dietary omega 3 fatty acids in dogs. J Am Vet Med Assoc 2016;249:1267–72.
57. Roush JK, Dodd CE, Fritsch DA, et al. Multicenter veterinary practice assessment of therapeutic effects of omega 3 fatty acids on osteoarthritis in dogs. J Am Vet Med Assoc 2010;236:59–66.
58. McCarthy G, O'Donovan J, Jones B, et al. Randomized, double-blind, positive-controlled trials to assess the efficacy of glucosamine/chondroitin sulfate for the treatment of dogs with osteoarthritis. Vet J 2007;174:54–61.
59. Bhathai A, Spryszak M, Louizos C, et al. Glucosamine and chondroitin use in canines for osteoarthritis: a review. Afr Vet J 2017;7:36–49.
60. Vandeweerd JM, Coisnon C, Clegg P, et al. Systematic review of the efficacy of nutraceuticals to alleviate clinical signs of osteoarthritis. J Vet Intern Med 2012;26:448–56.
61. Comblain F, Serisier S, Barthelemy N, et al. Review of dietary supplements for the management of osteoarthritis in dogs in studies from 2004-2014. J Vet Pharm Ther 2015;39:1–15.
62. Johnson KA, Lee AH, Swanson KS. Nutrition and nutraceuticals in the changing management of osteoarthritis for dogs and cats. J Am Vet Med Assoc 2020;256:1335–41.
63. Pan Y, Landsberg G, Mougeot I, et al. Efficacy of a therapeutic diet on dogs with signs of cognitive dysfunction syndrome (CDS): a prospective double blinded placebo controlled clinical study. Front Nutr 2018;5:127.
64. Marchal S, Bregeras O, Puanx D, et al. Rigorous training of dogs leads to high accuracy in human scent matching to sample performance. PLoS One 2016;11:963.
65. Otto CM, Hare E, Nord JL, et al. Evaluation of three hydration strategies in detection dogs working in a hot environment. Front Vet Sci 2017;4:174.

Current Rules and Regulations for Dogs Working in Assistance, Service, and Support Roles

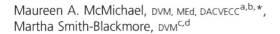

Maureen A. McMichael, DVM, MEd, DACVECC[a,b,]*,
Martha Smith-Blackmore, DVM[c,d]

KEYWORDS

- Canine • K-9 • Law enforcement K-9 • Service dog • Assistance dog
- Emotional support animal • Therapy animal • Search and rescue dog

KEY POINTS

- Numerous federal and state agencies have implemented legislation via administrative regulations to control public access for working dogs, to enforce specific protections, to allow certain permissions, and to define specific working dog activities.
- The Department of Justice enforces the Americans with Disabilities Act that allows subsets of service animals into public places and has the most stringent definitions. It does not provide allowances for emotional support animals (ESAs) or therapy animals and only covers dogs and miniature horses.
- The Department of Housing and Urban Development enforces housing allowances under the Fair Housing Act (FHA). The FHA, having a more lenient definition of service animals, allows ESAs and multiple species beyond dogs and miniature horses.
- The Department of Transportation provides guidelines for airline carriers through the Air Carrier Access Act (ACAA) in regard to air travel for working dogs. The ACAA was updated in January of 2021, and the major change is the removal of ESAs from the previous allowances.
- Veterinarians should be aware of the most recent regulations to assist pet owners with access and necessary documentation.
- There may be increased criminal responsibility for maltreatment of working dogs in some locations.

[a] Department of Clinical Sciences, College of Veterinary Medicine, Auburn University, Auburn, AL 36849, USA; [b] Carle Illinois College of Medicine, University of Illinois, Champaign, IL, USA; [c] Animal Law and Policy Program, Harvard Law School, Harvard University, Cambridge, MA, USA; [d] Cummings School of Veterinary Medicine, Tufts University, 419 Boston Avenue, Medford, MA 02155, USA
* Corresponding author.
E-mail address: mam0280@auburn.edu

Vet Clin Small Anim 51 (2021) 821–837
https://doi.org/10.1016/j.cvsm.2021.04.003
0195-5616/21/© 2021 Elsevier Inc. All rights reserved.

INTRODUCTION

Veterinarians encounter dogs represented as working dogs in practice with increasing frequency; it is essential that veterinarians be familiar with up-to-date legal and logistical guidelines for dogs working in service, assistance, and support roles (**Table 1**). Veterinarians may find themselves in tenuous positions when asked to provide certain documentation for clients. When a client asks for a letter stating that an animal is used for service, assistance, therapy, or emotional support, understanding such designations is essential but can be confusing. Definitions, in some cases, overlap and may apply to dogs only, to dogs and miniature horses, or to a variety of species. Some categories of working dogs are permitted to accompany their handler in places where pets are not allowed and they may have specific protections under the Americans with Disabilities Act (ADA), the Department of Housing and Urban Development (HUD) Fair Housing Act (FHA), or the Air Carrier Access Act (ACAA). In regard to service animals, the ADA guarantees equal access to public spaces for individuals with disabilities that limit or impair activities (mental or physical) assisted by a service dog (or miniature horse). A review of these laws and regulations may give veterinarians some guidance on how agencies verify whether claims are legitimate or not, what questions can be asked of a client, and what questions should be avoided.

In addition to the guidelines that offer some categories of working dogs protected access, there is recent legislation in several states that allows nonveterinary professionals to legally provide prehospital emergency care and/or transportation to some service animals, apparently superseding the veterinary practice act of that state. For a thorough review of that subject, Palmer L, Operational Canines, in this issue.

This article updates the definitions, legal restrictions, and protections as well as highlighting the veterinarian's role in attending to these animals and their handlers' needs.

DEFINITIONS

There are 4 definitions that generally are used to describe dogs working in service, assistance, and support roles: assistance animal, service animal, emotional support animal (ESA), and therapy animal. These definitions were created by the agencies regulating them and, in some cases, they overlap (eg, are accepted by 2 or more agencies), whereas in other cases they may not. Although search and rescue (S&R) dogs are considered service animals by most definitions, they are not covered by the ADA, FHA, or ACAA, because they are not used to assist a person with a disability. The legalities covering S&R canines are discussed at the end of this article.

Assistance Animal

Assistance animals are the broadest category, as defined by various legislative bodies.[1] It refers to any animal (no species limitations identified) that provides assistance or emotional support or performs tasks or work for a person with a disability. It encompasses, for the purposes of federal housing requirements, the categories of service animal and ESA and is not limited to specific species. For instance, HUD states that "there are 2 types of assistance animals: (1) service animals, and (2) other trained or untrained animals that do work, perform tasks, provide assistance, and/or provide emotional therapeutic support for individuals with disabilities."[2]

Service Animal

The service animal category, as defined by title II and title III of the ADA, originally was restricted to dogs but has been updated to include miniature horses.[3] These are the only 2 species currently covered under the ADA guidelines. This definition of a service

Working Dog Categories and Access

Category of Working Animal	Allowed Species—Works for	Regulatory Authority and Examples	Specialized Training Needed	Documentation Needed	Questions that May be Asked	Airline Rules
Assistance animal (umbrella term includes both service animals and ESAs)	Service animals are dogs or miniature horses. ESAs are a broad range of species that are commonly kept in households (exceptions for "unique animals" if the person can prove the need). Assists person with a disability	HUD/FHA	No specific training needed	For housing: proof of disability benefits, housing voucher, health care provider letter of support confirming a disability-related need for that particular species of animal	If disability is obvious, none. If disability is not apparent: (1) Is the animal required due to a disability? (2) What work or task is the animal trained to perform?	Assistance animal is an umbrella term for service animal and ESA. Service animals are treated, as discussed later. If an ESA, it is treated as a pet.
Service animal	Dog or miniature horse only Assists person with a disability	DOJ/ADA ACAA Guide dog, guide horse, seeing eye dog, hearing or signal dog, psychiatric service dog, SSigDOG, seizure response dog	Must be trained to perform a specific task for the handler specifically related to their disability. Permitted to accompany the handler anywhere in public	Identification cards, written documentation, harnesses/tags, credible verbal assurance from the handler with a disability	(1) Is the animal a service animal? (2) Does the handler have a disability? An airline is expected to determine if the animal presents a threat to the health or safety of passenger or will cause a disruption to airline service	Animal Air Transportation Health Form (the veterinarian fills out only the animal health section of this form); DOT Service Animal Behavior and Training Assessment Form; Animal Relief Attestation Form for flights longer than 8 h. Also requires documentation from human health practitioner

(continued on next page)

Table 1
(continued)

Category of Working Animal	Allowed Species— Works for	Regulatory Authority and Examples	Specialized Training Needed	Documentation Needed	Questions that May be Asked	Airline Rules
SDIT	Dogs. Exposed to the same or similar experiences they will be expected to perform in when they are fully trained	ADA does not cover SDITs but the FHA does include them for housing purposes. All states but 5 allow same or similar public access as fully trained service animals.	In training	None in states where permitted, but for access in public places, appropriate vests, a health certificate from a veterinarian and identification cards are helpful.	None specified	Pet flight rules apply ACAA does not allow SDITs as assistance animals
ESA	No species limits. Assists person with an emotional need through companionship	FHA	No specific training needed/ allowed in housing but not in public places	For housing, documentation from a qualified physician, psychiatrist or other mental health practitioner for a specific disability	Landlords may ask for current documentation (within 12 mo) that the ESA is required for the mental health of the individual.	Pet flight rules apply. ACAA no longer allows ESAs in cabins as service animals.

Therapy animal	No species limits Works for the benefit of individuals other than the handler	None—works by individual permissions and arrangements. May be a companion for a child in court, in airports to calm travelers, enrichment for hospital	Varies for assisted living patients	Depends on the private arrangement	None specified. A health certificate from a veterinarian may be helpful.	Pet flight rules apply.
S&R	Generally canine	FEMA or states. Works by individual permissions and arrangements	S&R training	Depends on the arrangement. Health and training certificates are helpful.	Handler and K-9 should travel in uniform. Vests, identification cards advised	Various airlines have their own policies.

animal requires that a dog or miniature horse be trained to perform specific tasks or do specific work for the benefit of an individual with a recognized disability, and the tasks or work must be directly related to the disability. This definition includes disabilities of the physical (eg, seizures and wheelchair), sensory (eg, blindness and deafness), psychiatric (eg, posttraumatic stress disorder [PTSD]), and intellectual or other mental health categories. Types of work or tasks that may be provided for by the service animal include, but are not limited to, interrupting a pattern of behavior (eg, early patterns of PTSD that if interrupted may prevent full-blown panic attacks), alerting individuals to approaching persons (eg, for deaf individuals), assistance with navigation (eg, for the sight impaired), retrieving items (eg, medications and communication devices), assistance with movement or balance, and providing rescue work.

Examples of service animals given by the ADA include the following;

A guide dog or seeing eye dog[4] is a carefully trained dog that serves as a travel tool for persons who have severe visual impairments or are blind.

A hearing or signal dog is a dog that has been trained to alert a person who has a significant hearing loss or is deaf when a sound occurs, such as a knock on the door.

A psychiatric service dog is a dog that has been trained to perform tasks that assist individuals with disabilities to detect the onset of psychiatric episodes and lessen their effects. Tasks performed by psychiatric service animals may include reminding the handler to take medicine, providing safety checks or room searches, or turning on lights for persons with PTSD, interrupting self-mutilation by persons with dissociative identity disorders, and keeping disoriented individuals from danger.

A sensory signal dog or social signal dog (SSigDOG) is a dog trained to assist a person with autism. The dog alerts the handler to distracting repetitive movements common among those with autism, allowing the person to stop the movement (eg, hand flapping).

A seizure response dog is a dog trained to assist a person with a seizure disorder. How the dog serves the person depends on the person's needs. The dog may stand guard over the person during a seizure or the dog may go for help. A few dogs have learned to predict a seizure and warn the person in advance to sit down or move to a safe place.

Under title II and title III of the ADA, service animals are limited to dogs. Entities must make reasonable modifications in policies, however, to allow individuals with disabilities to use miniature horses if they have been individually trained to do work or perform tasks for individuals with disabilities.[5]

To qualify as a service animal for protections under the ADA, the animal must be a dog or miniature horse and must perform specific tasks or jobs for the benefit of the individual directly related to their disability. This is the key distinction between a service animal and other categories of working animals. Some examples of disparate definitions of the term, *service animal*, include Alabama's, which defines it as "any dog that is individually trained to work or perform tasks for the benefit of an individual with disability" and Alaska, which defines service animal as "a dog guide or another animal..." This difference means that a person with a service animal other than a dog would be allowed to visit public places in Alaska but not Alabama. It is essential that veterinarians know the definitions for their state as well as the federal acts.

The ADA does not specify any training standards for any category of service animal or ESA.

Emotional Support Animal

ESAs are any species that provides physical, psychological, and/or emotional support through companionship. These animals are not trained specifically to perform any task or work related to a disability. This category, as defined previously by the ACAA (ESAs previously were classified as service animals) and the FHA (classified as assistance animals), requires that the use of the animal is supported by documentation from a qualified physician, psychiatrist, or other mental health practitioner for the specific disability. Unlike for the ADA, landlords are permitted to ask for current documentation (issued within the past 12 months) that the ESA is required for the mental health of the individual. This is the biggest distinction between service animals covered under the ADA (eg, a person cannot ask about the extent or nature of a disability) and ESAs covered under the FHA, where documentation of the need for a specific animal for that specific disability is required. The ACAA no longer allows ESAs in cabins as service animals.

Therapy Animal

A therapy animal (any species) is controlled by the handler but working for the benefit of others, as opposed to a service animal or ESA, which is for the benefit of the handler. Therapy animals participate in a form of therapy considered animal-assisted therapy which may occur in a variety of settings, including public schools, assisted living facilities, airports, courts of law, and many others. The animal-assisted therapy can be for an individual (eg, as a companion for a child in court) or for groups (eg, to calm travelers at an airport). Therapy animals can enter the buildings where they "work" due to private arrangements, but they are not covered explicitly under the ADA for access to public buildings. A search for this category did not yield any other federal or state legislation that specifically allows therapy dogs access to the public places where they work.

CURRENT RESTRICTIONS (LAWS, REGULATIONS, ORDINANCES, AND SO FORTH)

In general, restrictions or immunity from restrictions, falls into 3 categories: where the working dog is allowed to go, housing allowances, and air travel.

Where a Canine Is Allowed

This category, where a canine is allowed to go, includes public transportation (excluding air travel), public restaurants and buildings (eg, schools), and private buildings, such as offices. In general, this category includes any place that a human handler is able to go. The ADA provides protection for service dogs (and miniature horses) that allow them to accompany their handler to these public spaces. A service animal, according to the ADA, is a dog or miniature horse that is trained to perform specific tasks or do specific work for the benefit of an individual with a recognized disability and the tasks or work must be related directly to the disability. The definition includes disabilities of the physical (eg, seizures and wheelchair), sensory (eg, blindness and deafness), psychiatric (eg, PTSD), and intellectual or other mental health categories. Because the ADA does not cover ESAs, canines providing emotional support are not specifically protected to accompany their handler to public places. S&R canines are discussed separately.

Housing Allowances

HUD is the agency that governs housing restrictions and/or allowances under the FHA. HUD defines an assistance animal as one that "works, provides assistance, or performs tasks for the benefit of a person with a disability or provides emotional support for a person with a physical or mental impairment that substantially limits at least one major life activity or bodily function."[2] For the purposes of housing, the FHA is more lenient in the definition than the ADA, allowing potential renters to request housing for a broader range of disabilities. The ADA does not provide access for support or other assistance animals, whereas the FHA does make this allowance.

How the FHA differs from the ADA is that housing providers are allowed to ask for documentation. If the need for a service animal is obvious (eg, a blind person with a seeing eye dog or a dog helping to pull a wheelchair), a landlord should grant accommodation without question. If the disability is not apparent (eg, anxiety disorders), however, or the need for that particular animal is not apparent, the housing provider is advised to ask 2 specific questions: (1) whether the animal is required due to a disability and (2) what work or task the animal has been trained to perform. Housing providers cannot ask about the nature or extent of the disability and should ask for documentation only if the disability is not apparent. If these questions are not answered satisfactorily, the person requesting accommodations is expected to provide documentation. The FHA requires that housing requests include reliable documentation of a disability as well as the need for that particular species of service animal for accommodation. Reliable documentation includes statements of disability benefits, housing vouchers, or health care providers' letters of support.[2] The documentation must include confirmation of a disability related need for a particular species of animal.

Unlike the ADA, the FHA allows for a broad range of species that commonly are kept in households, including dogs, cats, small birds, rabbits, hamsters, gerbils, fish, turtles, or other small domesticated animals. Exceptions that fall outside of this list are known as "unique animals" (eg, capuchin monkeys). Exceptions for unique animals are made if the person can prove the need.[6] Capuchin monkeys are uniquely helpful in performing tasks due to their opposable thumbs and are used to assist people with paralysis by providing assistance, such as opening medication bottles.

Air Travel

The Department of Transportation (DOT) publishes guidelines under the ACAA, which previously had been more lenient than the ADA in regard to assistance animals traveling on airplanes. Guidelines had used the same terms as the FHA to include ESAs as service animals but recently have been updated. In February of 2020, the DOT published a notice of proposed rulemaking with proposed changes to the ACAA service animal rule.[7] Significant changes proposed included a new definition of service animal that eliminates ESAs as well as a requirement that completed documentation must be submitted in advance of travel. The new definition states that a service animal for purposes of the ACAA is "a dog that is individually trained to do work or perform tasks or do specific work for the benefit of an individual with a recognized disability and the tasks or work must be directly related to the disability." It includes disabilities of the physical (eg, seizures and wheelchair), sensory (eg, blindness and deafness), psychiatric (eg, PTSD), and intellectual or other mental health categories. The changes specifically state that "airlines are not required to recognize ESAs as service animal," recommending they be treated as pets. It also recognizes dogs as the only species to qualify as service animals. There now is a maximum of 2 service animals per passenger. Additional changes included 3 forms that were to be filled out in advance and submitted to the airline;

1. Animal Air Transportation Health Form—to be filled out by a veterinarian stating the animal is in good health
2. DOT Service Animal Behavior and Training Assessment Form—to be filled out by the handler/owner
3. Animal Relief Attestation Form—to be filled out by the handler/owner for flights in excess of 8 hours. The form attests to the animal's ability to relieve itself in a sanitary manner or that it would not need to during the duration of the flight.

Only the Animal Air Transportation Health Form must be completed by a veterinarian. During the comment period for the proposed rule change, there were requests for extensions, with more than 19,000 comments received. The main concerns expressed were the requirement to fill out the forms in advance (ie, putting people with disabilities at a disadvantage) and the elimination of the ESA category. The DOT stated in the comments that the elimination of ESAs was due to the fact that they may not undergo the same rigorous training with regard to public behavior as service dogs do. The revised ACAA was passed in January 2021 and does not require the passenger to submit the forms in advance (eg, they can use the kiosk and do not have to book flights in advance).[8] As of January 11, 2021, 4 airlines (ie, Alaska, American, Delta, and United) have stated they no longer allow ESAs or therapy animals to travel in cabins for free. These animals are treated as pets. Qualified service dogs still will be allowed to travel in cabins for free.

For passengers with a qualified service animal, airlines are expected to allow dogs in cabins for travel based on evidence, such as identification cards, written documentation, harnesses, and/or tags or the credible verbal assurance from the handler with a disability. Similar to the FHA, the ACAA allows airlines to ask (1) whether the animal is a service animal and (2) if the individual handler has a disability. They also are expected to determine if the animal presents a threat to the health/safety of passengers or will cause a disruption to the airline service. Airline personnel are to ask only for documentation if a passenger's verbal assurance is not credible and the airline cannot in good faith determine whether the animal is a service animal or an ESA.

Service Dogs in Training

It is important that service dogs in training (SDITs) are exposed to the same or similar experiences they are expected to perform in when they are fully trained. The ADA does not cover SDITs but the FHA does include them for housing purposes. States may make individual laws allowing SDITs access to public facilities. Currently, all states but 5 allow this category the same or similar access that fully trained service animals have in regard to public access. The new proposed ACAA does not allow SDITs except as pets.[8]

SEARCH AND RESCUE CANINES

Legislation affecting access to public spaces for S&R canines has been divided into Federal Emergency Management Agency (FEMA) deployed canines and regional/state/local (nonfederal) working canines for clarity. Many working canines perform in both categories but for purposes of legislation the categories are separate. Multiple attempts to contact FEMA for clarification on written legislation for access to public places for working dogs that are deployed was unsuccessful. Individual airlines have varied acceptance policies for S&R canines.

Working dog handlers that have deployed for FEMA have stated that there are allowances as long as the handler and canine are in uniform and the handler has credentials that allow for access to public transportation (Deb Zoran, DVM, PhD, personal communication, unpublished data, 2021). In many instances, the teams use pet-friendly hotels or stay in public buildings (eg, high schools and convention centers). In some cases, the dogs are kept in vehicles (eg, law enforcement K-9s) during meal times or when they are not permitted to be left alone in a room.

For non-FEMA work, which often is at the state level or county level, several states have published specific legislation allowing access to public places. States that have public access laws for S&R canines include California, Connecticut, Maine, New

Hampshire, Pennsylvania, Texas, and Vermont (Appendix A). In general, these laws include some non-S&R categories, such as law enforcement and firefighter canines. These laws make it illegal to deny service or access or to charge extra for access or service for the canine specifically.

Some states have S&R legislation embedded within the disability legislation or buried in other areas, making keeping track of these laws challenging. Arizona and Kentucky make it illegal to charge a fee to license law enforcement or S&R canines (Appendix B).

OTHER RULES AND REGULATIONS
State Laws

States have the ability to modify or expand some federal laws and several states have modified laws pertaining to assistance animals. A legally accepted assistance animal in 1 state may not be eligible for the same access or benefits afforded to that category in another state.

The Animal Legal and Historical Center is a project of the Michigan State University College of Law. The goal, according to the Web site, is to bring together the legal aspects pertaining to animals in the United States. According to the Web site, the goals of this center are

- To provide a Web library of legal and policy materials as related to animals
- To provide expert explanation of the materials for both lawyer and nonlawyers
- To provide a historical perspective about social and legal attitudes toward animals and how the present perspective was reached

Theirs is the most comprehensive overview of individual state laws that exists and covers numerous aspects of legalities regarding animals for the understanding of lawyers and lay people.[9]

Theft and Criminal Acts

Laws that specifically protect assistance animals from theft and criminal acts are present in all but 6 states as of 2019. Most of this legislation protects law enforcement canines and S&R canines. Specific legislation can be found in Appendix C. In addition, many states make it a criminal act to fraudulently claim the right to have a service animal. These laws may be helpful for veterinarians to remind clients as well as explain their own liability related to fraudulently endorsed certificates.

Identification of the Working Dog

Identification and verification of the working animal are not standardized and, in many cases, certificates that appear to be legal are available for a small fee online. Other paraphernalia, used to legitimize the working nature of a dog, such as vests, collars and tags, also are available from illegitimate credentialing organizations for a fee. The lack of standardization makes it difficult for the public and for veterinarians to know which animals are protected under various governmental regulations.

WHAT VETERINARIANS NEED TO KNOW

Currently, the only documentation veterinarians can be expected to fill out are a health certificate and, in some cases, a form attesting to the demeanor of the dog. Comments on the proposed rulemaking for the revisions to the ACAA expressed concern about veterinarians having to attest to the demeanor of the dog on airplanes.

Veterinarians, specifically, mentioned the difficulty of predicting behavior of any animal, particularly in unfamiliar, crowded, loud public places.

Concerns about liability, should a dog bite someone, are valid. The current rules include having a handler/owner fill out the form attesting to the dog's demeanor, with the veterinarian filling out only the health certificate. If in the future veterinarians are expected to fill out forms on the demeanor of the dog, the expectation is that the dog is calm, obedient, and would not become aroused in the presence of crowds or other animals. One attorney has advised that veterinarians not sign attestations for a dog's future behavior (Raphael Moore, JD, LLM General Counsel, Veterinary Information Network, Personal Communication, 2020).

SUMMARY

Three federal agencies, Department of Justice (DOJ) (ADA), HUD (FHA), and DOT (ACAA), have created guidelines to establish access to public places for service animals. Individual states have the ability to modify the FHA guidelines and individual airlines have the ability to modify the ACAA to some degree. These guidelines are specific for people with disabilities and do not specify access for S&R canines.

Because the nuances of the legislation are changing rapidly and are complex, there likely are entities that believe they need a veterinarian's assurances that an assistance animal is legitimate. With the exception of health certificates, veterinarians should not feel obligated to either attest to the demeanor of the animal or verify the legitimacy of a specific working dog. From a veterinarian's point of view, it is difficult to predict an animal's behavior in challenging circumstances.

CLINICS CARE POINTS

- Local, state, and national legislation changes frequently and veterinarians are advised to remain up to date on the changes by accessing real time data via individual Web sites (eg, ADA.gov) or the American Veterinary Medical Association legal updates (eg, in particular, the state updates [https://www.avma.org/advocacy/state-local-issues/state-legislative-updates]).

- Excellent resources exist for veterinarians to access up-to-date information on specific government Web sites (eg, ADA.gov, HUD.gov, and federalregister.gov) or under specific rules (eg, https://www.federalregister.gov/documents/2020/12/10/2020-26679/traveling-by-air-with-service-animals).

- Additionally, the Animal Legal and Historical Center, Michigan State University College of Law (https://www.animallaw.info/topic/table-state-assistance-animal-laws) maintains an up-to-date Web site on all aspects of animal law and is a vital resource for veterinarians.

DISCLOSURES

The authors report no conflicts of interest. This document represents current rules and regulations as of the time of this writing. Local, state, and national legislation changes frequently and veterinarians are advised to remain up to date on the changes by accessing real time data via individual or collective Web sites discussed in this article.

REFERENCES

1. Available at: https://www.hud.gov/sites/dfiles/FHEO/documents/19ServiceAnimal NoticeFHEO_508.pdf. Accessed January 10, 2021.
2. Available at: https://www.hud.gov/sites/dfiles/PA/documents/HUDAsstAnimalNC1-28-2020.pdf.

3. Available at: https://www.ada.gov/pubs/ada.htm.
4. Available at: https://www.seeingeye.org/.
5. Available at: https://adata.org/guide/service-animals-and-emotional-support-animals.
6. Part IV: Type of Animal. Available at: https://www.hud.gov/sites/dfiles/PA/documents/HUDAsstAnimalNC1-28-2020.pdf. p 12.
7. Available at: https://www.transportation.gov/briefing-room/us-department-transportation-announces-final-rule-traveling-air-service-animals.
8. Available at: https://www.regulations.gov/document?D=DOT-OST-2018-0068-12959.
9. Available at: https://www.animallaw.info/topic/table-state-assistance-animal-laws.

APPENDIX A

State search and rescue canine access

1. Texas

V.T.C.A., Health & Safety Code § 785.001 - .005
  https://www.animallaw.info/statute/tx-dogs-rescue-chapter-785-search-and-rescue-dogs.
  § 108.002. Certain Charges or Security Deposits Prohibited
  A commercial lodging establishment or restaurant may not require the payment of an extra fee or charge or a security deposit for a service canine that accompanies an individual to the establishment or restaurant if:

(1) The individual is:
  (A) A peace officer or firefighter assigned to a canine unit; or
  (B) A handler of a search and rescue canine participating in a search and rescue operation under the authority or direction of a law enforcement agency or search and rescue agency; and
(2) The individual is away from the individual's home jurisdiction while in the course and scope of duty because of:
  (A) A declared disaster; or
  (B) A mutual aid request or mutual aid training.

Credits
Added by Acts 2011, 82nd Leg., ch. 579 (H.B. 3487), § 1, eff. Sept. 1, 2011. Redesignated from V.T.C.A., Bus. & C. § 106.002 by Acts 2013, 83rd Leg., ch. 161 (S.B. 1093), § 22.001(4), eff. Sept. 1, 2013.
  V. T. C. A., Bus. & C. § 108.002, TX BUS & COM § 108.002

2. Pennsylvania

https://www.animallaw.info/statute/pa-dog-law-chapter-8-dogs-consolidated-dog-laws#s602.
  Pennsylvania: § 459-602. Dogs used for law enforcement* * *

(c) Illegal to deny facilities or service due to dog use.—It shall be unlawful for the proprietor, manager or employee of a theater, hotel, motel, restaurant or other place of entertainment, amusement or accommodation to refuse, withhold from or deny to any person, due to the use of a working police dog, detection dog or search and rescue dog used by any State or county or municipal police or sheriff's department or agency, fire department, search and rescue unit or agency or handler under the supervision of those departments, either directly or indirectly, any of the accommodations, advantages, facilities or privileges of the theater, hotel, motel, restaurant or other place of public entertainment, amusement or accommodation. Any person who violates any of the provisions of this subsection commits a misdemeanor of the third degree.

3 P.S. § 459-602

3. Maine

Maine's law is a bit strange because it is hidden in laws that relate to the powers of the Fish and Game department. This is being added to the Michigan Animal Law Web site soon.

Title 12. Conservation. Part 13. Inland Fisheries and Wildlife. Subpart 2. Department Organization. Chapter 903. Department of Inland Fisheries and Wildlife. Subchapter 2. Commissioner: Powers and Duties.

12 M.R.S.A. § 10105

§ 10105. Other powers

4-A. Search and rescue dogs. A person assisting the commissioner under subsection 4 with a search and rescue dog certified by or in training with an organization recognized by the Bureau of Warden Service may be accompanied by the search and rescue dog in a place of public accommodation without being required to pay an extra charge or security deposit for the search and rescue dog. The owner of the search and rescue dog is liable for any damages done to the premises by that animal. For purposes of this subsection, "place of public accommodation" has the same meaning as in Title 5, section 4553, subsection 8, paragraph A.

Also see § 164-B. Immunity from civil liability for assistance given to law enforcement dogs, search and rescue dogs and service dogs

https://www.animallaw.info/statute/me-assistance-animal-assistance-animalguide-dog-laws#s164B

4. Vermont

https://www.animallaw.info/statute/vt-assistance-animal-assistance-animalguide-dog-laws#s4502

§ 4502. Public accommodations

(k) A police officer, a firefighter, or a member of a rescue squad, search and rescue squad, first response team, or ambulance corps who is accompanied by a service dog shall be permitted in any place of public accommodation, and the service dog shall be permitted to stay with its master. For the purposes of this subsection, "service dog" means a dog owned, used, or in training by any police or fire department, rescue, or first response squad, ambulance corps, or search and rescue organization for the purposes of locating criminals and lost persons, or detecting illegal substances, explosives, cadavers, accelerants, or school or correctional facility contraband.

5. Connecticut

§ 53-330a. Access to public transportation and places of public accommodation for volunteer canine search and rescue teams.

https://www.animallaw.info/statute/ct-assistance-animals-connecticut-assistance-animalguide-dog-laws#s53_330a

6. California

California: § 54.25. Peace officer or firefighter assigned to canine unit; handler of search and rescue dog; duty away from home jurisdiction; discrimination; civil fine https://www.animallaw.info/statute/ca-assistance-animal-california-assistance-animalguide-dog-laws#s5425

7. New Hampshire

167-D:4 Service Animals May Accompany.

167-D:5 Application of RSA 167-D:4 to Search and Rescue Dogs.

The provisions of RSA 167-D:4 shall also apply to dogs involved in search and rescue missions at the request of a government agency when such dogs are in the course of, or traveling to or from the scene of, their official duties.

https://www.animallaw.info/statute/nh-assistance-animals-assistance-animalguide-dog-laws#sD5

APPENDIX B

Additional search and rescue canine legislation

Arizona

A. A city or town may not charge an individual who has a disability and who uses a service animal as defined in § 11-1024, a person that trains a service animal as defined in § 11-1024 or an individual who uses a search and rescue dog a license fee for that dog.

B. An applicant for a license for a search and rescue dog shall provide adequate proof satisfactory to the enforcement agent that the dog is a search and rescue dog.

https://www.animallaw.info/statute/az-assistance-animal-arizonas-assistance-animalguide-dog-laws#s32.

Kentucky

39F.040 Specialized squad using search dogs; requirements; organization of general rescue squad.

Gives some requirements for handlers of SAR dogs

https://www.animallaw.info/statute/ky-dog-laws-also-includes-cats-ferrets-kentucky-consolidated-dog-laws-license-impound-bite#s39F.

APPENDIX C

State search and rescue anticruelty laws

Alabama

§ 13A–11 to 261. Harassment of, interference with, etc., duties of police animals, search and rescue animals, or handlers; causing physical harm or death; entering containment area; restraining, taunting, endangering, etc.

https://www.animallaw.info/statute/al-cruelty-alabama-consolidated-cruelty-statutes#s261.

Arkansas

A.C.A. § 5 to 54 to 126.

§ 5-54-126. Killing or injuring search and rescue dogs or animals used by law enforcement

https://www.animallaw.info/statute/ar-dog-consolidated-dog-laws#s554126.

California

§ 600. Horses or dogs used by peace officers or volunteers; willful and malicious harm or interference; punishment; restitution
https://www%2eanimallaw%2einfo%2fstatute%2fca%2dservice%2danimal%2d%26sect%3b%2d600%2dhorses%2dor%2ddogs%2dused%2dpeace%2dofficers%2dwillful%2dand%2dmalicious%2dharm%2dor.

Connecticut

§ 53 to 247. Cruelty to animals. Animals engaged in exhibition of fighting. Intentional injury or killing of police animals or dogs in volunteer canine search and rescue teams
https://www.animallaw.info/statute/ct-cruelty-consolidated-cruelty-laws#s247.

Florida

843.19. Offenses against police canines, fire canines, SAR canines, or police horses
https://www.animallaw.info/statute/fl-police-dog-84319-offenses-against-police-canines-fire-canines-sar-canines-or-police.

Georgia

Ga. Code Ann., § 16 to 11 to 107.
    § 16-11-107. Harming a law enforcement animal.

Idaho

§ 18-7039. Killing and otherwise mistreating police dogs, police horses, search and rescue dogs and accelerant detection dogs
https://www.animallaw.info/statute/id-dog-consolidated-dog-laws#s7039.

Illinois

70/2.01d. Search and rescue dog.
    70/4.03. Teasing, striking or tampering with police animals, service animals, accelerant detection dogs, or search and rescue dogs prohibited
https://www.animallaw.info/statute/il-assistance-animals-assistance-animalguide-dog-laws.

Indiana

35-46-3-11.3 Search and rescue dog; mistreatment or interference
https://www.animallaw.info/statute/cruelty-consolidated-cruelty-statutes#s11_3.

Kansas

21-6416. Harming or killing certain dogs
https://www.animallaw.info/statute/ks-assistance-animal-consolidated-assistance-animal-laws#s21_6416.

Massachusetts

M.G.L.A. 272 § 77A Willfully injuring police dogs and horses https://www.animallaw.info/statute/ma-cruelty-consolidated-cruelty-statutes#s77A.

Michigan

M.C.L.A. 750.50c.
    750.50c. Intentionally killing, causing physical harm to, harassing, or interfering with police dog, police horse, or search and rescue dog

https://www.animallaw.info/statute/mi-service-animal-chapter-750-michigan-penal-code-michigan-penal-code-0.

Minnesota

609.596. Killing or harming public safety dog
https://www.animallaw.info/statute/mn-cruelty-consolidated-cruelty-statutes#s596.

Montana

45-8-209. Harming a police dog—penalty—definition
https://www.animallaw.info/statute/mt-cruelty-consolidated-cruelty-statutes#s209.

New Jersey

2C:29-3.1. Purposeful infliction of harm on animal owned or used by law enforcement agency or interference with law enforcement officer using such animal; "search and rescue dog" defined
https://www.animallaw.info/statute/nj-dogs-consolidated-dog-laws#s2C_29_3_1.

North Carolina

§ 14-163.1. Assaulting a law enforcement agency animal or an assistance animal
https://www.animallaw.info/statute/nc-assistance-animals-assistance-animalguide-dog-laws#s14_163_1.

North Dakota

§ 12.1-17-09. Killing or injury of law enforcement support animal—Definition—Penalty
https://www.animallaw.info/statute/nd-dogs-consolidated-dog-laws#s12_1_17_09.

Oregon

O. R. S. § 30.822.
30.822. Theft of or injury to search and rescue animal or therapy animal; attorney fees
https://www.animallaw.info/statute/or-damages-30822-theft-or-injury-search-and-rescue-animal-or-therapy-animal-attorney-fees

Pennsylvania

§ 5531. Definitions
"Police animal." An animal, including, but not limited to, dogs and horses, used by the Pennsylvania State Police, a police department created by a metropolitan transportation authority operating under 74 Pa.C.S. Ch. 17 (relating to metropolitan transportation authorities), a police department created under the act of April 6, 1956 (1955 P.L. 1414, No. 465),2 known as the Second Class County Port Authority Act, the Capitol Police, the Department of Corrections, a county facility or office or by a municipal police department, fire department, search and rescue unit or agency or handler under the supervision of the department, search and rescue unit or agency in the performance of the functions or duties of the department, search and rescue unit or agency, whether the animal is on duty or not on duty. The term shall include, but not be limited to, an accelerant detection dog, bomb detection dog, narcotic detection dog, search and rescue dog and tracking animal.
§ 5548. Police animals
https://www.animallaw.info/statute/pa-cruelty-consolidated-cruelty-statutes#s5548.

Rhode Island

Gen.Laws 1956, § 4-1-30.1
§ 4-1-30.1. Cruelty to public safety—Dogs and horses
https://www.animallaw.info/statute/ri-cruelty-chapter-1-cruelty-animals#s30_1.

Tennessee

§ 39-14-205. Intentional killing; police dogs; justifiable killing
https://www.animallaw.info/statute/tn-cruelty-consolidated-cruelty-statutes#s205.

Utah

§ 76-9-307. Injury to service animals—Penalties
https://www.animallaw.info/statute/ut-assistance-animal-assistance-animalguide-dog-laws#s76_9_307.

Washington

9.91.175. Interfering with search and rescue dog
https://www.animallaw.info/statute/wa-dog-consolidated-dog-laws#s991175.

Wyoming

§ 6-5-211. Injuring or killing a police dog, fire dog, search and rescue dog or police horse prohibited; penalties
https://www.animallaw.info/statute/wy-dog-consolidated-dog-laws#s6_5_211.

Canine Special Senses

Considerations in Olfaction, Vision, and Audition

Melissa Singletary, DVM, PhD, DACVPM*, Lucia Lazarowski, PhD

KEYWORDS

- Olfaction • Audition • Vision • Sensory systems • Working dog • Detection canine

KEY POINTS

- The sensory arm of the central nervous system is composed of various multimodal sensory systems and the collective integration of sensory information is important for a full and robust appreciation of the surrounding environment. This environmental awareness is vital for canine partners trained to perform tasks that can be critical in nature, such as explosives detection or guiding the visually impaired.
- Ensuring key sensory systems of olfaction, vision, and audition are intact, functioning, and undisrupted by medical conditions or treatments is an important consideration in the working dog. Dysfunction in these key sensory systems may have significant impacts on working performance and may compromise efficacy.
- Extensive impact studies on performance in working dogs under a wide variety of conditions that may be diagnosed or induced are needed. Insights from clinical reports, other vertebrate studies, and human literature are used to highlight areas for consideration.

INTRODUCTION

For any living creature, environmental awareness is key for survival. Various sensory systems have evolved to provide this critical capacity to sense their environment. Some examples involve chemosensory systems, such as taste and smell, whereas others involve detection of waves of electromagnetic radiation in sensing of light, detection of waves of acoustic resonance in sensing sounds, and mechanoreception in sensing touch and pressure. Humans have harnessed the sensory systems of the dog to train for task-oriented work, such as their superior sense of smell in detection work and augmenting human sensory systems in individuals needing support from a guide or assistance dog. The social disposition of canines makes use of working dogs a successful and powerful relationship.

Department of Anatomy, Physiology and Pharmacology, Canine Performance Sciences Program, College of Veterinary Medicine, Auburn University, 104 Greene Hall, AL 36849, USA
* Corresponding author.
E-mail address: mas0028@auburn.edu

Vet Clin Small Anim 51 (2021) 839–858
https://doi.org/10.1016/j.cvsm.2021.04.004
vetsmall.theclinics.com
0195-5616/21/© 2021 Elsevier Inc. All rights reserved.

Rapid detection, input, and processing of environmental surroundings are critical in working dogs, based on task, and require the key sensory systems of olfaction, vision, and audition to be intact, functioning, and undisrupted by medical conditions or treatments. A reduction in the abilities to sense and respond to the environment may have serious implications on overall performance and task demands, compromising their objective, whether detection of an explosive or detection of oncoming traffic.

This review highlights 3 major sensory systems: olfaction, vision, and audition. The quick recognition and treatment of conditions having an impact on these systems can maintain a working dog in service or reduce the overall time they are out of service, thereby conserving resources and preserving their objective. Although not discussed in this section, consideration for physical performance, conformation, musculoskeletal and associated proprioception, and somatosensation also plays an important role in working dog function. Although these 3 key sensory systems are discussed separately throughout this article, it is an important note that they are multimodal systems and work in tandem for an optimized sensory capability.

OVERVIEW OF CANINE OLFACTION

Dogs are highly dependent on their sense of smell to navigate the world around them. Unlike humans, who are predominantly visual navigators, dogs' superior sense of smell has made then an invaluable resource throughout history. As such, detection canines are specialized for multiple odor-based tasks, and this is an area of active capabilities research across the industry. These fields include specialties, such as search and rescue, narcotics, explosives, medical (eg, cancer detection), pests, biological threats, conservation, ecology, agriculture, electronics, human remains, and tracking. These detection canines are employed across the spectrum of federal, state, and local governments; the Department of Defense; private entities; and civilian nonprofit organizations, to highlight a few.

The successful use of canines in olfactory-based tasks is attributable to multiple characteristics and advantages both anatomically and physiologically. In particular, the specialized olfactory neuroepithelium covers a large surface area[1] and is densely packed with olfactory receptor cells, which collectively express approximately 825 different odorant receptors.[2,3] The olfactory system is subdivided into the main olfactory system, which predominately processes volatile odorants, and the accessory olfactory system, the vomeronasal, which predominately processes pheromones. The air is filled with odors that represent the environmental landscape through scents that canines recognize and interpret. The odors enter through the nares to traverse the nasal passages toward the olfactory recess destined for the olfactory neuroepithelia, where they are processed for odor recognition (**Fig. 1**).[1] This dedicated olfactory recess is not found in humans and is an advantage likely contributing to the increased olfactory acuity in dogs. This recess receives upwards of 20% of the inspired air, whereas active sniffing is estimated to direct approximately 2.5 times more air to the olfactory recess per unit of time.[4] The neuroepithelia lines the scroll-like projections, termed the *ethmoid labyrinth*, and the most caudal section of the nasal septum.[1] This delicate maze serves to substantially increase the total surface area of the receptive field, measured at more than 200 cm^2 and providing a notable advantage in the dog's sense of smell and odorant detection capabilities.[1,5]

Unlike sound and light waves, odorants are chemical signals that can remain in a location for longer periods of time. A dog is able to smell not only what is actively happening in a snapshot of time but also what happened in an area for a period of

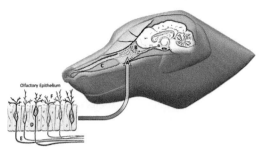

Fig. 1. Olfactory neuroepithelium and nasal anatomy. A, olfactory epithelium; B, olfactory bulb; C, nasal cavity; D, supporting cells (tan); E, projection axons from olfactory sensory neurons (blue, green, and orange); and F, olfactory mucosa, receptive field and dendritic processes of olfactory sensory neurons.

time afterward. The deposition of odor molecules throughout the neuroepithelial receptive field creates a pattern, which has been indicated as a means of enhancing odor discrimination that may provide localization information related to an odor source.[1]

Once odorants arrive at the neuroepithelium, they encounter the odorant receptors (G-protein coupled receptors-GPCRs), and, if recognized at the odorant-receptor interface, the olfactory sensory neuron depolarizes, resulting in an action potential. With millions of olfactory receptor neurons in the olfactory epithelium, a significant amount of input is transmitted, modified, and presented to form an odor profile. The signal initiated in the neuroepithelium is transmitted to the olfactory bulb and subsequent areas of the brain within the olfactory pathway to ultimately be perceived as an odor. The olfactory system is evolutionarily older than that of vision and is considered to be a more primal system, especially because it does not require the same thalamic relay to access the prefrontal cortex and limbic system as other sensory systems.[6,7] This feature makes olfaction a powerful sensory system, with direct connections to select areas of the brain involved in emotion and memory.[8–10]

Anosmia, a complete loss of smell, and hyposmia, a partial loss, can have profound effects on animals that specialize in odor detection.[11] Recognition and appreciation of these conditions are limited in dogs, and hyposmia may be underrepresented due to the difficulty of clinical identification and the high degree of compensation due to receptive redundancy. Hyposmia and anosmia are appreciated more readily in humans with the accessibility and use of psychophysical testing.[12] A multitude of factors are known to influence olfaction in humans but have not been studied in dogs. Hyposmia can be categorized broadly into 3 areas[13]:

1. Conductive—result of a disruption in the access of an odorant to the olfactory epithelium[14]
2. Sensory loss—result of olfactory epithelial damage[14–16]
3. Neural hyposmia—result of central or peripheral nervous system damage and/or disruption to the olfactory neural pathway[13]

The human literature identifies more than 200 different causes for olfactory dysfunction or loss of smell overrepresented by sinonasal disease, infectious disease, and traumatic injury[12,17] (**Table 1**).

Multiple factors can influence olfactory performance, including environmental (eg, humidity, temperature, and barometric pressures), physiologic (fitness level, age, and nutrition), and likely others, such as microbiota, that are underexplored.

Table 1
Categories of conditions that have been identified as associated with olfactory dysfunction; collective highlights from human and animal literature Select olfactory dysfunction-associated conditions from human and animal literature.

Categories	Select Examples	References
Metabolic and endocrine diseases	Hypothyroidism, Cushing's syndrome, diabetes mellitus	Bromley,[96] 2000
Neurologic diseases and disorders	Granulomatous meningoencephalitis	Myers,[16] 1990
Neurodegenerative diseases	Alzheimer's disease and Parkinson's disease	Deems et al,[17] 1991
Trauma	Traumatic brain injury and head trauma	Bromley,[96] 2000
Inflammation and olfactory epithelium damage	Nasal irritants and allergens	Deems et al,[17] 1991
Obstructive localized lesions	Nasal tumors and polyps	Seiden and Duncan[14], 2001; Malaty and Malaty[15], 2013; Myers,[16] 1990
Infectious disease	Viral, bacterial, and fungal infections	Myers,[20,21] 1988
Medication Induced	High-dose metronidazole and high-dose steroids	Ezeh et al,[30] 1992; Jenkins et al,[97] 2018

[a]This table highlights a select number of conditions and does not represent an exhaustive list of conditions reported across veterinary and human medicine.

Dietary and nutritional supplements have shown varying degrees of influence on olfaction. In a study by Angle and colleagues,[18] supplementation with corn oil showed an improvement on olfaction, whereas a study by Altom and colleagues[19] showed supplementation with coconut oil representing 8% of a 16% fat diet was associated with olfactory impairment. Further studies are needed to make recommendations on dietary supplements and olfactory function.

Olfactory deficits were reported in dogs with canine distemper and canine parainfluenza virus infection.[20,21] Conditions described in the human literature are not well documented in the veterinary literature and limit understanding of the specific impact on canine odor-detection performance. Many conditions may compromise olfaction, and a careful evaluation should be considered with suspected diseases and disorders (eg, upper respiratory disease and head trauma) in a working dog.[22]

The impact a condition or intervention has on olfaction may be transient and sensation returns to normal within a period of time or acute with long-lasting effects or can become chronic. The olfactory system is unique in its regenerative capability, whereby individual olfactory sensory neurons can regenerate in generally 45 days to 60 days by means of its resident stem cell population in the olfactory epithelium.[23] This regenerative capacity allows the olfactory system to recover from insults providing some resiliency.

The olfactory neuroepithelium is protected by a mucous layer, which is affected by air quality. A higher relative humidity corresponds with increased performance by dogs in detection-based work in some reports.[24] This may be due to the humidity maintaining the moisture within the air, which is supportive of the mucosal barrier and odorant transport. Higher humidity, however, also is a risk factor in working dogs when considered in conjunction with higher temperatures, which increase the risk for overexertion and heat stress, thus having a detrimental effect on perfor-mance.[25,26] Thermoregulation is a critical consideration in overall health and olfactory function. The compensatory mechanisms used by dogs under high heat, such as increased rate of panting, also is likely to decrease olfactory function and perfor-mance.[27] Establishment of health-based work cycles accounting for environmental conditions is an important tool to maintaining overall health and performance as well as olfactory function. Additionally, detection dogs may work in austere or extreme environments with poor air quality/air flow, increased exposure to particulates, poten-tial toxins, or respiratory irritants that may have an impact on olfactory function. Little research is available on occupational exposures in working dogs, specifically the im-pacts relative to olfactory performance and function. Until further data are available, considerations for what may be harmful to olfactory function in humans also should be considered for the canine counterpart.[28] Due to the nature of their work, exposure to toxins unintentionally or intentionally, explosives powders and precursors, or pharmaceutical-based agents (eg, synthetic opioids and synthetic marijuana) may occur. Prompt recognition and reversal administration can be life-saving with expo-sures to potent synthetic opioids, such as fentanyl and carfentanil. In a study by Essler et. al, reversal of fentanyl (intravenous administration) with naloxone (intranasal or intramuscular [IM] administration) in a clinical trial did not demonstrate impairment of olfactory acuity at 2 hours, 24 hours, or 48 hours postreversal to detection of a uni-versal detection calibrant.[29] Avoiding intranasal medications or vaccinations should be considered in routine preventative care. Published studies evaluating the effects of intranasal vaccine administration on olfaction and performance, particularly in working dogs, are lacking in the literature, although this is an area of current study. Un-til further studies are available, it is reasonable that the transient local inflammation in nasal passageways could have an impact on olfaction, albeit short term; therefore, un-less otherwise indicated, selection of an effective alternative vaccine administration should be considered, if available (eg, intraoral or subcutaneous).

When treating a working dog, the potential impact of pharmaceuticals and nutra-ceuticals on performance in several areas, including olfaction, should not be over-looked. Some medications may have a direct localized effect on olfactory tissues or may have an effect through systemic delivery.

Two studies evaluated pharmaceuticals reported to cause hyposmia in humans directly in dog populations. The first was conducted by Ezeh and colleagues,[30] which evaluated the effects of high-dose steroids on overall olfactory function reporting high-dose dexamethasone (Cushing syndrome–inducing levels), and hydrocortisone in combination with deoxycorticosterone acetate (DOCA), both resulted in diminished ol-factory capability. Low-dose steroids (anti-inflammatory), however, are a treatment of humans with hyposmia under certain conditions and have been reported to restore some olfactory function.[31–33] It is likely that this effect could be seen in dogs due to the anti-inflammatory properties of low-dose steroids if the insulting cause of olfactory dysfunction was inflammatory or exacerbated by inflammation. Steroids have sys-temic impact on the performance of a working dog, however, and careful consider-ation for use should be given.

The second study, conducted by Jenkins and colleagues,[34] evaluated the effects of 2 antimicrobials, doxycycline and high-dose metronidazole, which are reported to cause hyposmia in humans. Only the high-dose metronidazole, demonstrated a decrease in ol-factory performance with standard doses of doxycycline, showing no measurable effect.

The biomedical literature contains references to olfactory dysfunction and deficits, but there are few reports that identify olfactory enhancement, such as those reported with zinc nanoparticles,[35–37] although zinc in other forms, such as zinc oxide, zinc gluconate, and zinc sulfate, has shown negative impacts on olfaction when administered intranasal or in experimental studies with olfactory sensory neurons.[38–40] Therefore the delivery mechanism and composition of medications and nutraceuticals can result in variation of their subsequent effects.

Most reports predominantly found in human literature reference a detrimental effect of pharmaceuticals (for extensive review, see Doty and colleagues[41] and Lötsch and colleagues[42]). Alternatively, some medications have been evaluated for their use in treatment of olfactory disorders. For a more extensive review of medications used to treat olfactory disorders, see Whitcroft and colleagues,[12] which provides a summary of human studies reporting the use of medications for treatment of anosmia. It is unknown if similar effects occur in dogs due to limited available studies in the species. Care should be taken when administering medications that may have an impact on olfactory and cognitive function in working dogs.

OVERVIEW OF CANINE VISION

Vision is a key sense in working dogs, especially for tasks augmenting human sensory systems, such as those performed by guide dogs and assistance dogs for safe navigation and alerting/danger avoidance behavior. For more specific tasks and roles that guide dogs and assistance dogs play, see the article on assistance and service dogs. Generally, there is significant anatomic similarity between humans and dogs, but the differences are notable, especially when considering how to interpret working dog behavior and situational expectations. Dogs are quadrupeds and, therefore, are much lower to the ground than bipedal humans, which provides a vastly different scenery in a given landscape. The handler may see the upper portion of a crowd with heads and faces, whereas the working dog sees the lower portion, of shoes and legs. This difference in perspective should be considered when assessing the impact of disturbances on normal vision.

Canine vision is considered poor in comparison to human vision, although there are instances where specialized features allow for task-specific enhancements. Vision in the canine is thought to be less specialized for acuity and more for motion detection, with an increased function under low light conditions.[38,43]

Light waves penetrate the clear cornea at the front of the eye. Through the cornea, light waves move through the aqueous humor or the anterior chamber passing through the opening of the iris (pupil) and are focused before passing through the lens. The biconvex crystalline structure of the lens in dogs is suspended behind the iris by the ciliary body, which contains muscular attachments capable of altering the lens confirmation. The flexible and dynamic nature of the lens allows for accommodation (ie, adjustment from flatter to a more rounded confirmation), thereby changing the field of focus for differing distances. Posterior to the lens, light waves move through the vitreous chamber to the retina (**Fig. 2.**).[44] In the retina, photoreceptor cells (rods and cones) are found. The light interacts with the photoreceptive layer of cells in the retina activating a signal cascade of neuronal activation in the ganglion cells, whose axons converge at the back of the eye to form the optic disk, which is the beginning of the optic nerve. This region of the retina is what is visible during a fundic examination. The optic nerve exits the eye and travels through the optic chiasm, where fibers may decussate between the left and right sides to a varying extent and emerge as the optic tracts. These optic tracts continue relaying information along the optic pathway to the higher cognitive areas of the brain for visual processing.[44] Prey animals commonly have laterally placed eyes, with a significant level of decussation at the optic chiasm, whereas eyes with forward and front placement (more common to predators including canids) show a lower level

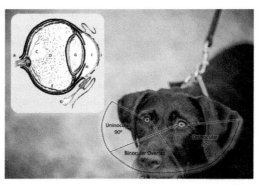

Fig. 2. Canine eye anatomy and field of vision (binocular vs monocular). A, optic nerve; B, convergence of axons representing the blind spot situated below the fovea; C, tapetum lucidum; D, nontapetal retina; E, retina cross-section; F, ciliary body; G, lens; H, iris; I, anterior chamber; J, cornea; and K, gland of the third eyelid.

of decussation at the optic chiasm.[44–46] Eye placement also has an impact on the range of visual field in the horizontal plane, where dogs are reported to show a range of 60° to 70° greater field of view than humans.[44] This may mean dogs have a larger horizontal scanning vantage but with reduced depth perception due to the decreased degree of binocular vision (see **Fig. 2**).[44]

The specialized light-reflective, choroid-covered, tapetum lucidum represents approximately 30% of the fundus in dogs and other species.[47–50] This common adaptation allows dogs to see in low light more easily by increasing retinal sensitivity compared with humans, who are absent this structure.[51,52]

Dogs exhibit dichromatic vision expressing 2 forms of light-sensitive photo pigments in the retinal cells pertaining to color vision in comparison to humans, who have trichromatic vision and express 3 forms.[44] Although this is likened to human red/green color blindness (deuteranopia), dogs are capable of discriminating colors by brightness intensities and distinguish red and green from gray.[53–55] The visual spectrum in dogs allows for differentiation of hues in the blue spectrum (430–485 nm) and yellow spectrum (500–620 nm) (**Fig. 3**).[44,56–58] Due to multiple factors,

Comparative Schematic of Visible Color Hues: Human and Canine

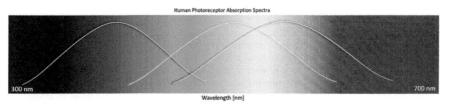

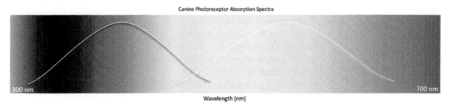

Fig. 3. Comparative canine retinal anatomy (Lower) and visual spectrum to human (Upper).

including a UV-transparent lens and a specific cone sensitivity to sections of the UV-spectrum, dogs likely are able to appreciate UV light as a blue-violet color.[59]

Numerous conditions have an impact on vision, including visual obscuring lesions, such as cataracts, glaucoma, uveitis, intraocular hemorrhage, and anterior lens luxation.[60] Conditions related to the cornea or orbital structures can result in diminished visual field, decreased range of globe movement, or decreased palpebral fissure due to pain, swelling, and inflammation.[61] A wide variety of ophthalmic conditions may diminish visual acuity or function, some of which are amenable to medical intervention. Any condition associated with temporary or permanent blindness or intraocular or orbital pain (bilateral or unilateral) benefits from quick recognition and prompt treatment. **Table 2** highlights select medical considerations for vision in working dogs. Consultation or referral to a board-certified veterinary ophthalmologist (American College of Veterinary Ophthalmologists [ACVO]) also may be considered in a working dog with eye disease of significant consequence. Breeding colonies should consult routinely with ophthalmologists for genetic screening and routine examinations (for further information on breeding colonies, see the articles, Breeding Program Management and Production and Reproductive Management).

Exposure of potentially harmful substances may be an occupational concern. Decontamination procedures should include adequate attention to the eyes, including generous flush with ophthalmic solution. Care should be taken to manage resulting waste solution and prevent cross-contamination with other areas or surfaces and use of appropriate personal protective equipment (see the article on Operational Canines for more information on decontamination).

For a more comprehensive review of comparative canine vision, see Barber and colleagues.[62]

Table 2
Select medical considerations in vision for working dogs

Categories	Select Examples	References
Ophthalmic medications	Ophthalmic medications may have side effects on ocular conditions, such as those containing corticosteroids, which can delay corneal healing and exacerbate infectious disease or ulceration. Topical nonsteroidal anti-inflammatory drugs share similar cautions and are contraindicated with glaucoma.	Grahn et al,[98] 2009
Systemic medications	Some systemic medications have been reported to have ocular side effects, such as ivermectin-induced blindness. Limited information is available in animals, but ocular adverse effects have been identified in humans to select systemic drugs.	Plummer,[60] 2016; Epstein and Hollingsworth,[99] 2013; Santaella et al,[100] 2017
Breeding animals	Eye examination certification: Companion Animal Eye Registry (through Orthopedic Foundation for Animals) establishes criteria based on the Blue Book for examinations performed by board-certified (ACVO) ophthalmologist.	King et al,[101] 2019

[a]This table highlights a select number of considerations with relevance to working dogs.

OVERVIEW OF CANINE AUDITION

Sound is not constrained by barriers to the same extent as vision, because sound is less impeded by objects than light. This makes sound an important sensory system for navigation, threat detection, and environmental awareness under a wide range of circumstances. Auditory dysfunction can be caused by multiple insults or conditions, but acoustic damage varies by factors, such as the type of stimulus involved, exposure duration, interval duration, frequency, comorbidities, and the characteristics of the noise involved.[63] An example of the impact these factors have on the potential for damage comes from the recommendations for noise exposure in humans, where a 3-dB amplitude increase results in an approximate doubling of the sound energy, which requires a reduction in exposure time to mitigate damage.[64] High-amplitude sound waves are associated more commonly with noise-induced damage or noise-induced hearing loss (NIHL), and affected regions in the cochlea typically are at or above those frequencies associated with the noise exposure.[63]

Dogs are considered to have greater sensitivity to sound, especially at higher frequencies.[65] Infrasound is below human detectable levels (<20 Hz) and ultrasound above it (>20,000 Hz).[66] Small rodents and insects are detectable in the ultrasonic range by carnivores, although are undetected by human ears.[67–69] High frequency is important for sound localization.[70] Dogs are reported to be capable of detecting sounds much farther than the distance of human detection. Wolves are reported to hear another wolf's howl from a distance of 6 miles to 10 miles, depending on the terrain.[71–73] Dogs also are capable of using sound to equate additional qualities, such as size, with regard to conspecifics and other animals.[74] A low growl can indicate how large the individual is, because production of vocal communications are generated at frequencies that can have a physical relationship to size.[75,76]

The external ear is important for passive amplification through collecting, funneling, and amplifying selective wavelengths.[77] The pinna, highly cartilaginous and flexible, and anatomic orientation can contribute to this amplification.[78] This mobility of the pinna aids in sound localization.[79] The general pinna vertical features, such as erectness or floppiness, also have an impact on audition. Erect ears are assumed to be especially good at localizing sound at longer distances due to their orientation and accessible funnel-like anatomic properties, but generally this difference from floppy-eared dogs is negligible.[80] Any alteration through injury (eg, lacerations and aural hematoma) or surgery (eg, ear cropping) may impair the normal function of sound localization.[81] The muscle attachments also allow for fine pinna movement and control for orientation and improved hearing sensitivity, especially at higher frequencies.[80,82,83] The external ear forms an L-shaped canal acting as a resonance tube until reaching the tympanic membrane, which covers the opening to the tympanic bulla and middle ear. The middle ear contains 3 ear ossicles—malleus, incus, and stapes—acting as sound amplifiers, converting the wave energy that disturbs the tympanic membrane into mechanical energy through the vibration of these ossicles.[84] The stapes is embedded in the oval window, which represents the opening to the inner ear. The inner ear consists of 2 main sensory apparatuses, the cochlea and the vestibular system. Although critically important to normal ambulation and function as it pertains to proprioception and balance, especially in working dogs, the vestibular system is outside the scope of this review.

The functional unit of the cochlea is the organ of Corti, which contains the sensory hair cells responsible for signal transduction to the cochlear nerve (**Fig. 4**). The hair cells sit atop the basilar membrane, which rests between the scala media and the scala tympani (see **Fig. 4**). This basilar membrane is narrow and stiff at the base

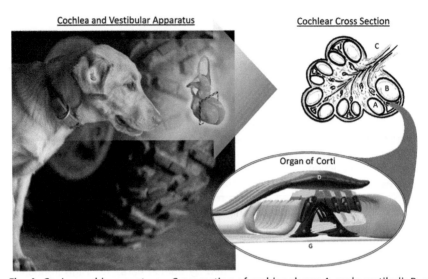

Fig. 4. Canine cochlear anatomy. Cross-section of cochlea shows A, scala vestibuli; B, scala. tympani; C, cochlear nerve; zoomed in section within the scala media illustrates the organ of Corti with D, tectorial membrane; E, inner hair cell; F, row of outer hair cells; and G, basilar membrane.

and extends wider with increasing flexibility as it reaches the apex. The hair cells contain cilia, stereocilia, and kinocilia, which are organized in a stairstep fashion, with the stereocilia ascending toward the single kinocilia, and are connected by tip links that allow for mechanical opening and closing of associated potassium ion channels. The tectorial membrane binds the cilia of the hair cells, and, when the basilar membrane is deflected due to the traveling fluid wave, the hair cells become bent, opening their ion channels and depolarizing the cells. The hair cells are specialized and release vesicles of neurotransmitter to adjacent cochlear nerve dendrites when depolarized. The basilar membrane qualities in width and stiffness create a gradient from base to apex that relate to peak frequency responsiveness of high frequency at the base and low frequency at the apex, referred to as a tonotopic organization (**Fig. 5**).

Regarding hearing protection in working dogs, which is a consideration for occupational exposures to loud noises, such as gunfire, traffic, large event venues, noisy kennels, or busy airports, a more extensive review is needed. The requirement for alertness to perform task-specific objectives many times negates the ability to consistently provide hearing protection. There are innate adaptive responses present that are a natural first-line defenses in dogs to provide protection to the auditory system. These include functions of muscular attachments to the tympanic membrane, the inner ear ossicles, and the outer hair cells. These mechanisms stiffen respective membranes thereby reducing movement. These protective mechanisms are limited, however, and sudden loud noises may transduce before these mechanisms can be responsive. A 50-ms to 100-ms delay is reported to occur before some of these reflexive mechanisms can be initiated and, therefore, is not an effective means of protection for short-pulse, sudden-impact type noises.[80,81] Damage to the hair cells is considered permanent, and frequency-specific hearing loss can occur due to shearing of the hair cell cilia. Therefore, a dog may suffer from hearing loss that is not readily recognizable with normal day-to-day noise volumes and is limited to a more specific decibel range.

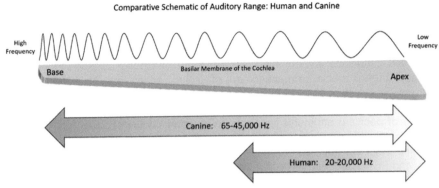

Fig. 5. Canine auditory spectrum. A comparative schematic of the auditory range between humans and canines. Basilar membrane is illustrated from base to apex in its width from narrow to wide in association with the corresponding sensitivity to frequencies of high to low.

An example of multimodal sensory optimization is the relationship between auditory localization and orientation of visual field through directed head movement and the highly integrated areas of signal processing.[85,86] When a sound source is identified, head orientation and, therefore, visual field are adjusted in the direction of the sound.[87] The auditory system is important to directing attention and providing key awareness for spatial orientation responses, although, especially in working dogs, there likely is a task-based prioritization that occurs with use of olfactory and visual cues for these responses as well. The attentiveness to sounds is more alerting at higher frequencies compared with lower frequencies, which may be attributable to the salient nature of higher frequency sounds.[88]

The auditory system is important in dogs, especially to performance of working dogs and suitability for work. This could reference ability to respond to verbal cues or detect the sound of an approaching vehicle. Although not representative for all dogs, some reports suggest hearing loss may be associated with behaviors in dogs that are of concern in relation to performance, such as aggression, increased startle and stress-related responses, and training difficulties.[80,89,90] A loss of hearing or impairment of hearing may result in a working dog being unsuitable for continued service and considered for retirement. Severity of hearing loss and task-specific requirements of the working dog may allow for continued service or limited service with clearly outlined protocols for limitations of use. An example of modified use through hand gestures and defined work environment limitations is referenced in Schneider and colleagues,[91] for a detection dog (a 6-year-old springer spaniel) in the United Kingdom. More detailed reviews of managing deafness in dogs has been published by Scheifele and colleagues,[92] Becker 2017,[93] and Strain and colleagues.[80]

In a recent extensive review on canine audition, Barber and colleagues[81] note the lack of specific and targeted data on noise sensitivities and standards of practice in dogs and conclude that, until such information becomes available, dogs should be considered as sensitive to sound and susceptible to noise-related damage or NIHL as humans under similar circumstances. Therefore, if it is recommended for a handler to use hearing protection in a specific context, then it is likely that the same considerations for limiting exposure should be considered in the accompanying working dog, especially during transport and times where full alertness is not required to be on task.

Numerous etiologies can result in hearing impairment or loss and some conditions may benefit from quick recognition and medical intervention. A highlight of medical considerations for hearing in working dogs can be found in **Table 3**. Some conductive disorders, such as otitis externa, otitis media, and cerumen accumulation, are treated more readily with quick recognition and intervention. The sequela for long-standing untreated conditions, however, can result in permanent or intensive interventions. Other conductive conditions are not highlighted but are described by Schiefle and colleagues,[92] in their article on management of canine hearing loss. Unlike conduction deafness, which refers to an inability to transmit sound waves or attenuation of sound intensities, sensory hearing loss may be accompanied by cochlear distortions due to damage of cochlear structures (eg, hair cells). Most congenital disorders likely are selected against in purpose-bred working dog lines; however, in breeding colonies it is an important consideration for selection (see articles, Breeding Program Management, and Production and Reproductive Management). Reduced hearing associated with age (presbycusis) may occur, but the average working dog still is relatively young and many are retired before 10 years of age. Lesions along the cochlear nerve pathway between the cochlea and the brainstem may result in a neural-based hearing loss.[92]

Table 3
Medical considerations relating to audition

Categories	Select Examples	References
Ototoxic medications	Aminoglycosides, diuretics, and cisplatin	Oishi et al,[94] 2012
Conductive disorders	Inflammation, cerumen accumulation, otitis, tympanic membrane rupture, hyperplasia, neoplasia	Scheifele et al,[92] 2012
Sensory disorders	Presbycusis, ototoxicity, NIHL, congenital deafness	
Neural disorders	Acoustic neuroma, acoustic neuritis, multiple sclerosis	

[a]This table highlights a select number of considerations with relevance to working dogs. Represents collective highlights.

Careful consideration should be made when using medications that are reported to have ototoxicity in working dogs. These include aminoglycosides (eg, gentamycin, streptomycin, neomycin, and amikacin), a concern for adults and also pregnant dogs, because they may lead to subsequent hearing impairment in the litter.[94] Diuretics, such as furosemide, are reported to result in mostly a transient ototoxicity, an important limitation to discuss with the handler or owner when considering this medication. Careful monitoring of patients on potentially ototoxic medications may allow for quick recognition and response preventing permanent hearing damage. The additional consideration of supplementation with select antioxidants, discussed in more detail by Oishi and colleagues,[94] in their article reviewing ototoxicity in dogs and cats, may be of benefit.

EVALUATION CONSIDERATIONS AND METHODS

A basic neurologic examination is key for early recognition of conditions that may affect key sensory systems in working dogs. It is important to include the handler in routine examinations to reinforce normal conditions and responses in their dog making early indicators of abnormal more apparent and provide a quicker referral for veterinary care. A limited neurologic examination included in routine screenings can be helpful to the practitioner. More common than not, olfactory function is not a classic sensory system evaluated in general practice and often is not included on cranial nerve examination templates. This is a critical capability in many working dogs, however, especially detection canines. Testing for olfactory function can be difficult, but the most common test is a blinded treat test, a crude test of the innate food-driven response to an appreciable quantity of odor. In performing this test, it is important to isolate the sensory system being tested to olfaction and, therefore, minimize visual input by blindfolding the animal or hiding the food object out of visual sight, such as held in 1 fist of 2 fists presented palm side down, and reducing any tactile stimulation of inadvertently touching the vibrissae or creating air current when adjusting and presenting the test. Reducing any noise that could orient the animal toward the presenting odor also should be avoided. Because this test relies on a food-driven behavioral response, it may not always indicate olfactory dysfunction in animals that are satiated, ill, or generally lack food motivation. More detailed threshold testing or imaging (eg, computed tomography [CT] or magnetic resonance imaging [MRI]) may be conducted at research facilities or specialty practices and teaching hospitals. Working dogs with specific detection training, however, commonly have detailed training records and a general history of performance or recent variations in performance in odor-based training should be taken during examination. Although not required for veterinarians to have a full understanding of the terminology and training techniques, general trends or deviations from an individual's normal performance metrics, such as in the rate of odor-target finds, misses, false alerts, and duration time of search, can be useful. For a glossary of terminology, see the American Academy of Forensic Sciences Standards Board Technical Report, *Dogs and Sensors: Terms and Definitions*.[95]

All testing, including the blinded auditory stimulus (acoustic startle), should be conducted to best isolate the sensory system being tested and eliminate the ability of the animal to compensate using other sensory clues (eg, visual and tactile). Common evaluation methods of sensory function for other modalities are listed in **Table 4**.

Table 4
Evaluation methods for key sensory function in olfaction, vision, and audition

Sensory System	In-clinic Evaluations (Specialized Equipment Not Required)	Specialty Practice or Research Program (Specialized Equipment or Expertise Needed)
Olfaction	Controlled odor presentation	Electroencephalogram Odor threshold testing
Vision	Menace response Obstacle course Visual tracking Pupillary light reflex Dazzle reflex Ophthalmic and retinal examination Schirmer tear test Intraocular pressure Fluorescein stain	Electroretinogram Ocular ultrasound MRI or CT
Audition	Controlled auditory stimulus Otoscopic examination	Brainstem auditory evoked response

It is key to acquire a full history, because many indications of issues with any of these key areas may be observed more subtly as changes in performance or recent adaptations/variations in performance.

DISCUSSION

Although these key sensory systems are discussed separately, they are multimodal, and the collective integration of sensory information from the key sensory systems is important for a full and robust appreciation of the surrounding environment. Each sensory signal not only has to be detectable but also has to be processed through subsequent neural pathways to be functionally recognized to attain a compositional meaning. Any deficiencies along this pathway may result in a variation of outcomes, such as change in odor detection threshold, odor perception, or lack of input altogether from the source. In the pet population, slight reduction in the normal function of these sensory systems may go un-noticed and have little impact on an animal's daily functioning due to redundancy in the system and compensation. In working dogs, however, these sensory systems are relied on heavily and even partial disruption could reduce the effectiveness of the dog for its task. Thus, it is important to consider an extensive history, including inquiring on performance and training history, perform a detailed examination, including key neurologic and ophthalmic tests and evaluations, and provide guidance in a return-to-work strategy when conditions are diagnosed and treatment plans are issued. The personal and financial investment in a working dog is significant and replacement is not classically an expedient process, which makes keeping a working dog in service a high priority.

SUMMARY

Developing a treatment plan in a working dog should account for any potential impacts medications or therapies will have on their subsequent performance. A plan that limits deleterious effects on performance while meeting the medical needs of the patient is optimal and a clear plan that outlines limitations and side effects is important in supporting a dog's safe return to work. Additional evaluations addressing key sensory systems, such as olfactory threshold and discrimination testing, should be considered before return to work if the treatment or medications used are associated with sensory loss or dysfunction.

CLINICS CARE POINTS

- Veterinarians play a critical role in the health of working dogs and careful evaluation of key sensory systems can improve early diagnosis and treatment of conditions that otherwise may compromise the performance of a working dog.

- It is helpful to provide a clearly outlined treatment plan and consider any potential limitations on performance due to diagnosis and prognosis, medications, or procedures.

- Considerations for limiting exposure and minimizing risk to occupational hazards, such as loud noises, respiratory irritants, and ocular hazards, should be applied to humans and their canine counterparts when feasible under operational objectives.

- A loss of vision, hearing, or sense of smell may result in a working dog being unsuitable for work due to compromised performance. Continuation of service is based on the severity and duration of sensory loss and consideration for return to work should be based on careful sensory-specific evaluations.

- Many conditions are amenable to treatment with quick recognition and response by the handler and veterinarian, which maintains the mission and reduces time out of work for the canine.

DISCLOSURE

No disclosures to report.

ACKNOWLEDGMENTS

The authors would like to acknowledge as thank Dr Eleanor (Missy) Josephson, Dr Brandon Brunson, and Dr Paul Waggoner for their kind review of this article.

REFERENCES

1. Craven BA, Paterson EG, Settles GS. The fluid dynamics of canine olfaction: Unique nasal airflow patterns as an explanation of macrosmia. J R Soc Interface 2010;7(47):933–43. https://doi.org/10.1098/rsif.2009.0490.
2. Nei M, Niimura Y, Nozawa M. The evolution of animal chemosensory receptor gene repertoires: roles of chance and necessity. Nat Rev Genet 2008;9(12): 951–63. https://doi.org/10.1038/nrg2480.
3. Niimura Y, Matsui A, Touhara K. Extreme expansion of the olfactory receptor gene repertoire in African elephants and evolutionary dynamics of orthologous gene groups in 13 placental mammals. Genome Res 2014;24(9):1485–96. https://doi.org/10.1101/gr.169532.113.
4. Rygg AD, Van Valkenburgh B, Craven BA. The influence of sniffing on airflow and odorant deposition in the canine nasal cavity. Chem Senses 2017;42(8): 683–98. https://doi.org/10.1093/chemse/bjx053.
5. Lawson MJ, Craven BA, Paterson EG, et al. A Computational Study of Odorant Transport and Deposition in the Canine Nasal Cavity: Implications for Olfaction. Chemical Senses 2012;37(6):553–66.
6. Kay LM, Sherman SM. An argument for an olfactory thalamus. Trends Neurosci 2007;30(2):47–53. https://doi.org/10.1016/j.tins.2006.11.007.
7. Shepherd GM. Perception without a thalamus: How does olfaction do it? Neuron 2005;46(2):166–8. https://doi.org/10.1016/j.neuron.2005.03.012.
8. Kanter ED, Haberly LB. NMDA-dependent induction of long-term potentiation in afferent and association fiber systems of piriform cortex in vitro. Brain Res 1990; 525(1):175–9. https://doi.org/10.1016/0006-8993(90)91337-G.
9. Rajmohan V, Mohandas E. The Limbic System. Acta Psychiatr Scand 1982; 66(2):11–4. https://doi.org/10.1111/j.1600-0447.1982.tb00316.x.
10. Sokolowski K, Corbin JG. Wired for behaviors: From development to function of innate limbic system circuitry. Front Mol Neurosci 2012;5(APRIL):55. https://doi.org/10.3389/fnmol.2012.00055.
11. Smith DV, Duncan HJ. Primary Olfactory Disorders: Anosmia, Hyposmia, and Dysosmia, . Science of Olfaction. New York, NY: Springer; 1992. p. 439–66. https://doi.org/10.1007/978-1-4612-2836-3_16.
12. Whitcroft KL, Hummel T. Clinical Diagnosis and Current Management Strategies for Olfactory Dysfunction. JAMA Otolaryngol Neck Surg 2019;145(9):846. https://doi.org/10.1001/jamaoto.2019.1728.
13. Henkin RI. Drug-Induced Taste and Smell Disorders: Incidence, Mechanisms and Management Related Primarily to Treatment of Sensory Receptor Dysfunction. Drug Saf 1994;11(5):318–77. https://doi.org/10.2165/00002018-199411050-00004.
14. Seiden AM, Duncan HJ. The diagnosis of a conductive olfactory loss. Laryngoscope 2001;111(1):9–14. https://doi.org/10.1097/00005537-200101000-00002.

15. Malaty J, Malaty IAC. Smell and taste disorders in primary care. Am Fam Physician 2013;88(12):852–9.

16. Myers LJ. Dysosmia of the dog in clinical veterinary medicine. ID - 19902214966. Prog Vet Neurol 1990;1(2):171–9.

17. Deems DA, Doty RL, Settle RG, et al. Smell and Taste Disorders, A Study of 750 Patients From the University of Pennsylvania Smell and Taste Center. Arch Otolaryngol - Head Neck Surg 1991;117(5):519–28. https://doi.org/10.1001/archotol.1991.01870170065015.

18. Angle CT, Wakshlag JJ, Gillette RL, et al. The effects of exercise and diet on olfactory capability in detection dogs. J Nutr Sci 2014;3:e44. https://doi.org/10.1017/jns.2014.35.

19. Altom EK, Davenport GM, Myers LJ, Cummins KA. Effect of dietary fat source and exercise on odorant-detecting ability of canine athletes. Res Vet Sci 2003;75(2):149–55. https://doi.org/10.1016/S0034-5288(03)00071-7.

20. Myers LJ, Hanrahan LA, Swango LJ, Nusbaum KE. Anosmia associated with canine distemper. Am J Vet Res 1988;49(8):1295–7.

21. Myers LJ, Nusbaum KE, Swango LJ, Hanrahan LN, Sartin E. Dysfunction of sense of smell caused by canine parainfluenza virus infection in dogs. Am J Vet Res 1988;49(2):188–90. http://www.ncbi.nlm.nih.gov/pubmed/2831762.

22. Otto C. The Anatomy of the Canine Nose, effects of disease on olfaction. In: Canine Olfaction Science and Law. Boca Raton (FL): CRC Press; 2016. p. 33–44.

23. Costanzo RM. Regeneration of Olfactory Receptor Cells. Ciba Foundation Symposium, 160, 2007. p. 233–48. https://doi.org/10.1002/9780470514122.ch12.

24. Conover MR. Predator-Prey Dynamics: The Role of Olfaction. Boca Raton, Florida: CRC Press; 2007.

25. Andress M, Goodnight ME. Heatstroke in a military working dog. US Army Med Dep Journal; 2013. p. 34–7. http://www.ncbi.nlm.nih.gov/pubmed/23277443.

26. Patrick JR, Meghan TR, Brian MZ, et al. Environmental and Physiological Factors Associated With Stamina in Dogs Exercising in High Ambient Temperatures. Frontiers in Veterinary Science 2017;4:144.

27. Gazit I, Terkel J. Explosives detection by sniffer dogs following strenuous physical activity. Appl Anim Behav Sci 2003;81(2):149–61. https://doi.org/10.1016/S0168-1591(02)00274-5.

28. Hayes JE, McGreevy PD, Forbes SL, Laing G, Stuetz RM. Critical review of dog detection and the influences of physiology, training, and analytical methodologies. Talanta 2018;185:499–512. https://doi.org/10.1016/j.talanta.2018.04.010.

29. Essler JL, Smith PG, Berger D, et al. A Randomized Cross-Over Trial Comparing the Effect of Intramuscular Versus Intranasal Naloxone Reversal of Intravenous Fentanyl on Odor Detection in Working Dogs. Animals 2019;9(6):385. https://doi.org/10.3390/ani9060385.

30. Ezeh PI, Myers LJ, Hanrahan LA, Kemppainen RJ, Cummins KA. Effects of steroids on the olfactory function of the dog. Physiol Behav 1992;51(6):1183–7. https://doi.org/10.1016/0031-9384(92)90306-M.

31. Blomqvist EH, Lundblad L, Bergstedt H, Stjärne P. Placebo-controlled, randomized, double-blind study evaluating the efficacy of fluticasone propionate nasal spray for the treatment of patients with hyposmia/anosmia. Acta Otolaryngol 2003;123(7):862–8.

32. Golding-Wood DG, Holmstrom M, Darby Y, Scadding GK, Lund VJ. The treatment of hyposmia with intranasal steroids. J Laryngol Otol 1996;110(2):132–5. https://doi.org/10.1017/s0022215100132967.

33. Heilmann S, Huettenbrink KB, Hummel T. Local and systemic administration of corticosteroids in the treatment of olfactory loss. Am J Rhinol 2004;18(1):29–33. https://doi.org/10.1177/194589240401800107.

34. Jenkins EK, Lee-Fowler TM, Angle TC, Behrend EN, Moore GE. Effects of oral administration of metronidazole and doxycycline on olfactory capabilities of explosives detection dogs. Am J Vet Res 2016;77(8):906–12. https://doi.org/10.2460/ajvr.77.8.906.

35. Jia H, Pustovyy OM, Wang Y, et al. Enhancement of Odor-Induced Activity in the Canine Brain by Zinc Nanoparticles: A Functional MRI Study in Fully Unrestrained Conscious Dogs. Chem Senses 2016;41(1):53–67. https://doi.org/10.1093/chemse/bjv054.

36. Singletary M, Hagerty S, Muramoto S, et al. PEGylation of zinc nanoparticles amplifies their ability to enhance olfactory responses to odorant. PLoS One 2017;12(12):1–20. https://doi.org/10.1371/journal.pone.0189273.

37. Moore CH, Pustovyy O, Dennis JC, Moore T, Morrison EE, Vodyanoy VJ. Olfactory responses to explosives associated odorants are enhanced by zinc nanoparticles. Talanta 2012;88:730–3. https://doi.org/10.1016/j.talanta.2011.11.024.

38. Alexander TH, Davidson TM. Intranasal Zinc and Anosmia: The Zinc-Induced Anosmia Syndrome. Laryngoscope 2006;116(2):217–20. https://doi.org/10.1097/01.mlg.0000191549.17796.13.

39. Hagerty S, Daniels Y, Singletary M, et al. After oxidation, zinc nanoparticles lose their ability to enhance responses to odorants. BioMetals 2016;29(6):1005–18. https://doi.org/10.1007/s10534-016-9972-y.

40. McBride K. Does Intranasal Application of Zinc Sulfate Produce Anosmia in the Mouse? An Olfactometric and Anatomical Study. Chem Senses 2003;28(8):659–70. https://doi.org/10.1093/chemse/bjg053.

41. Doty RL, Bromley SM. Effects of drugs on olfaction and taste. Otolaryngol Clin North Am 2004;37:1229–54. https://doi.org/10.1016/j.otc.2004.05.002, 6 SPEC.ISS.

42. Lötsch J, Knothe C, Lippmann C, Ultsch A, Hummel T, Walter C. Olfactory drug effects approached from human-derived data. Drug Discov Today 2015;20(11):1398–406. https://doi.org/10.1016/j.drudis.2015.06.012.

43. McGreevy P, Grassi TD, Harman AM. A Strong Correlation Exists between the Distribution of Retinal Ganglion Cells and Nose Length in the Dog. Brain Behav Evol 2004;63(1):13–22. https://doi.org/10.1159/000073756.

44. Miller PE, Murphy CJ. Vision in dogs. J Am Vet Med Assoc 1995;207(12):1623–34. http://www.ncbi.nlm.nih.gov/pubmed/7493905.

45. Herron MA, Martin JE, Joyce JR. Quantitative study of the decussating optic axons in the pony, cow, sheep, and pig. Am J Vet Res 1978;39(7):1137–9.

46. Byosiere SE, Chouinard PA, Howell TJ, Bennett PC. What do dogs (Canis familiaris) see? A review of vision in dogs and implications for cognition research. Psychon Bull Rev 2018;25(5):1798–813. https://doi.org/10.3758/s13423-017-1404-7.

47. Lesiuk TP, Braekevelt CR. Fine structure of the canine tapetum lucidum. J Anat 1983;136(Pt 1):157–64. http://www.ncbi.nlm.nih.gov/pubmed/6833116.

48. Ollivier FJ, Samuelson DA, Brooks DE, Lewis PA, Kallberg ME, Komáromy AM. Comparative morphology of the tapetum lucidum (among selected species). Vet Ophthalmol 2004;7(1):11–22. https://doi.org/10.1111/j.1463-5224.2004.00318.x.

49. Yamaue Y, Hosaka YZ, Uehara M. Spatial relationships among the cellular tapetum, visual streak and rod density in dogs. J Vet Med Sci 2015;77(2): 175–9. https://doi.org/10.1292/jvms.14-0447.

50. YAMAUE Y, HOSAKA YZ, UEHARA M. Macroscopic and Histological Variations in the Cellular Tapetum in Dogs. J Vet Med Sci 2014;76(8):1099–103. https://doi.org/10.1292/jvms.14-0132.

51. Hebel R. Distribution of retinal ganglion cells in five mammalian species (pig, sheep, ox, horse, dog). Anat Embryol (Berl) 1976;150(1):45–51. https://doi.org/10.1007/BF00346285.

52. Peichlcu L. Topography of ganglion cells in the dog and wolf retina. J Comp Neurol 1992;324(4):603–20. https://doi.org/10.1002/cne.903240412.

53. Rosengren A. Experiments in colour discrimination in dogs. Acta Zool Fenn 1969;121:1–19.

54. Byosiere SE, Chouinard PA, Howell TJ, Bennett PC. The effects of physical luminance on colour discrimination in dogs: A cautionary tale. Appl Anim Behav Sci 2019;212:58–65. https://doi.org/10.1016/j.applanim.2019.01.004.

55. TANAKA T, WATANABE T, EGUCHI Y, YOSHIMOTO T. Color Discrimination in Dogs. Nihon Chikusan Gakkaiho 2000;71(3):300–4. https://doi.org/10.2508/chikusan.71.300.

56. Jacobs GH, Deegan JF, Crognale MA, Fenwick JA. Photopigments of dogs and foxes and their implications for canid vision. Vis Neurosci 1993;10(1):173–80. https://doi.org/10.1017/S0952523800003291.

57. Neitz J, Geist T, Jacobs GH. Color vision in the dog. Vis Neurosci 1989;3(2): 119–25. https://doi.org/10.1017/S0952523800004430.

58. Siniscalchi M, D'Ingeo S, Fornelli S, Quaranta A. Are dogs red–green colour blind? R Soc Open Sci 2017;4(11). https://doi.org/10.1098/rsos.170869.

59. Douglas RH, Jeffery G. The spectral transmission of ocular media suggests ultraviolet sensitivity is widespread among mammals. Proc R Soc B Biol Sci 2014; 281(1780). https://doi.org/10.1098/rspb.2013.2995.

60. Plummer CE. Diagnosing Acute Blindness in Dogs. Today's Vet Pract 2016;18–23. December.

61. Renwick PW, Petersen-Jones SM. Orbital and Ocular Pain. In: Peiffer RL, Petersen-Jones SMBT-SAO, Fourth E, editors. Small Animal Ophthalmology. Edinburgh: W.B. Saunders; 2009. p. 203–52. https://doi.org/10.1016/B978-070202861-8.50011-7.

62. Barber ALA, Mills DS, Montealegre- ZF, Ratcliffe VF, Guo K, Wilkinson A. Functional Performance of the Visual System in Dogs and Humans: A Comparative Perspective. Comp Cogn Behav Rev 2020;15:1–44. https://doi.org/10.3819/CCBR.2020.150002E.

63. Ryan AF, Kujawa SG, Hammill T, Le Prell C, Kil J. Temporary and Permanent Noise-induced Threshold Shifts. Otol Neurotol 2016;37(8):e271–5. https://doi.org/10.1097/MAO.0000000000001071.

64. Lynch ED, Kil J. Compounds for the prevention and treatment of noise-induced hearing loss. Drug Discov Today 2005;10(19):1291–8. https://doi.org/10.1016/S1359-6446(05)03561-0.

65. Lipman EA, Grassi JR. Comparative Auditory Sensitivity of Man and Dog. Am J Psychol 1942;55(1):84. https://doi.org/10.2307/1417027.

66. Pye JD, Langbauer WR. Ultrasound and Infrasound, . Animal Acoustic Communication. Berlin, Heidelberg: Springer; 1998. p. 221–50. https://doi.org/10.1007/978-3-642-76220-8_7.

67. Brudzynski SM, Fletcher NH. Rat ultrasonic vocalization: short-range communication. Handbook of Behavioral Neuroscience, Vol 19. Elsevier; 2010. p. 69–76.
68. Powell RA, Zielinski WJ. Mink response to ultrasound in the range emitted by prey. J Mammal 1989;70(3):637–8.
69. Peterson EA, Heaton WC, Wruble SD. Levels of auditory response in fissiped carnivores. J Mammal 1969;50(3):566–78. https://doi.org/10.2307/1378784.
70. Fay RR, Popper ANTA-TT-. In: NV-1 o, Fay RR, Popper AN, editors. Comparative Hearing: Mammals, Vol 4. New York, NY: Springer New York; 1994. https://doi.org/10.1007/978-1-4612-2700-7.
71. Harrington FH, Mech LD. Wolf vocalization, . Wolf and Man. Elsevier; 1978. p. 109–32. https://doi.org/10.1016/B978-0-12-319250-9.50014-1, 1978:109-132.
72. Henshaw RE, Stephenson RO. Homing in the Gray Wolf (Canis lupus). J Mammal 1974;55(1):234–7. https://doi.org/10.2307/1379281.
73. Mech LD, Boitani L. Wolves: Behavior, Ecology, and Conservation. Chicago Illinois: University of Chicago Press; 2003.
74. Faragó T, Pongrácz P, Á Miklósi, Huber L, Virányi Z, Range F. Dogs' Expectation about Signalers' Body Size by Virtue of Their Growls. In: Giurfa M, editor. PLoS One 2010;5(12):e15175. https://doi.org/10.1371/journal.pone.0015175.
75. Bowling DL, Garcia M, Dunn JC, et al. Body size and vocalization in primates and carnivores. Sci Rep 2017;7(1):41070. https://doi.org/10.1038/srep41070.
76. Riede T, Fitch T. Vocal tract length and acoustics of vocalization in the domestic dog (Canis familiaris). J Exp Biol 1999;202(20):2859–67.
77. Fletcher NH, Fahey P. Acoustic Systems in Biology. Phys Today 1993;46(7):79. https://doi.org/10.1063/1.2808977, 79.
78. Heffner HE, Heffner RS. High-Frequency Hearing. The Senses: A Comprehensive Reference, 3, 2008. p. 55–60. https://doi.org/10.1016/B978-012370880-9.00004-9.
79. Njaa BL, Cole LK, Tabacca N. Practical Otic Anatomy and Physiology of the Dog and Cat. Vet Clin North Am - Small Anim Pract. 2012;42(6):1109–26. https://doi.org/10.1016/j.cvsm.2012.08.011.
80. Strain GM. In: Strain GM, editor. Deafness in Dogs and Cats. Wallingford: CABI; 2011. https://doi.org/10.1079/9781845937645.0000.
81. Barber ALA, Wilkinson A, Montealegre -ZF, Ratcliffe VF, Guo KMDS. A Comparison of Hearing and Auditory Functioning Between Dogs and Humans: Pre-Publication Proof. Comp Cogn Behav Rev 2020;15:1–50. https://doi.org/10.3819/CCBR.2020.150005E.
82. Phillips DP, Calford MB, Pettigrew JD, Aitkin LM, Semple MN. Directionality of sound pressure transformation at the cat's pinna. Hear Res 1982;8(1):13–28. https://doi.org/10.1016/0378-5955(82)90031-4.
83. Gorlinskiĭ IA, Babushina ES. Directionality of sound perception in the external ear of the dog. Biofizika 1985;30(1):133–6.
84. Hemilä S, Nummela S, Reuter T. What middle ear parameters tell about impedance matching and high frequency hearing. Hear Res 1995;85(1-2):31–44. https://doi.org/10.1016/0378-5955(95)00031-X.
85. Sterbing-D'Angelo SJ. Evolution of sound localization in mammals. Evolution of Nervous Systems, 3, 2007. p. 253–60. https://doi.org/10.1016/B0-12-370878-8/00074-4.
86. Heffner HE, Heffner RS. The evolution of mammalian sound localization. Acoustics Today 2016;35(12):20–7.
87. Heffner HE. Auditory awareness. Appl Anim Behav Sci 1998;57(3-4):259–68. https://doi.org/10.1016/S0168-1591(98)00101-4.

88. Huber A, Barber ALA, Faragó T, Müller CA, Huber L. Investigating emotional contagion in dogs (Canis familiaris) to emotional sounds of humans and conspecifics. Anim Cogn 2017;20(4):703–15. https://doi.org/10.1007/s10071-017-1092-8.

89. Venn RE, McBrearty AR, McKeegan D, Penderis J. The effect of magnetic resonance imaging noise on cochlear function in dogs. Vet J 2014;202(1):141–5. https://doi.org/10.1016/j.tvjl.2014.07.006.

90. Baker MA. Evaluation of MR safety of a set of canine ear defenders (MuttMuffs®)at 1T. Radiography 2013;19(4):339–42. https://doi.org/10.1016/j.radi.2013.07.004.

91. Schneider DC, Foss KD, De Risio L, Hague DW, Mitek AE, McMichael M. Noise-Induced Hearing Loss in 3 Working Dogs. Top Companion Anim Med 2019;37:100362. https://doi.org/10.1016/j.tcam.2019.100362.

92. Scheifele L, Clark JG, Scheifele PM. Canine Hearing Loss Management. Vet Clin North Am Small Anim Pract 2012;42(6):1225–39. https://doi.org/10.1016/j.cvsm.2012.08.009.

93. Becker SC. *Living with a Deaf Dog 2nd Edition*. Wenatchee, WA: Dogwise Publishing; 2017. 9781617812118.

94. Oishi N, Talaska AE, Schacht J. Ototoxicity in dogs and cats. Vet Clin North Am Small Anim Pract 2012;42(6):1259–71. https://doi.org/10.1016/j.cvsm.2012.08.005.

95. AAFS Standards board LLC. BAS. Crime Scene/Death Investigation – Dogs and Sensors Terms and Definitions. ASB Tech Rep 2017;025. First Edit. 025_TR_e1_2017.pdf (aafs.org) accessed 2.11.2021.

96. Bromley SM. Smell and taste disorders: A primary care approach. Am Fam Physician 2000;61(2):427–36.

97. Jenkins EK, DeChant MT, Perry EB. When the Nose Doesn't Know: Canine Olfactory Function Associated With Health, Management, and Potential Links to Microbiota. Front Vet Sci 2018;5(MAR). https://doi.org/10.3389/fvets.2018.00056.

98. Grahn BH, Wolfer J. Therapeutics. In: Peiffer RL, Petersen-Jones SMBT-SAO, Fourth E, editors. Small Animal Ophthalmology. Edinburgh: W.B. Saunders; 2009. p. 50–66. https://doi.org/10.1016/B978-070202861-8.50008-7.

99. Epstein SE, Hollingsworth SR. Ivermectin-induced blindness treated with intravenous lipid therapy in a dog. J Vet Emerg Crit Care 2013;23(1):58–62. https://doi.org/10.1111/vec.12016.

100. Santaella RM, Fraunfelder FW. Ocular adverse effects associated with systemic medications: Recognition and management. Drugs 2007;67(1):75–93. https://doi.org/10.2165/00003495-200767010-00006.

101. King A, Huey JH, Barrie K, et al. The Blue Book: Ocular Disorders Presumed to Be Inherited in Purebred Dogs. 12th Edition. American College of Veterinary Ophthalmologists; 2019. Blue Book | Orthopedic Foundation for Animals | Columbia, MO (ofa.org). Accessed February 11, 2021.

Sports Medicine and Rehabilitation in Working Dogs

Meghan T. Ramos, VMD[a],*, Brian D. Farr, DVM[a,b],
Cynthia M. Otto, DVM, PhD, DACVEC, DACVSMR[a]

KEYWORDS

- K-9 • Canine • Physical fitness • Injury prevention • Return to work

KEY POINTS

- Working dog sports medicine integrates the handler, trainer, and veterinarian to provide performance enhancement, injury prevention, and return to work after injury or illness.
- Wellness and preventive medicine for working dogs emphasize work-related nutrition, nutritional supplements, body composition optimization, behavioral enrichment, and injury recovery.
- Rehabilitating a working dog requires handler involvement, accommodating the dog's temperament, creatively modifying exercises and restrictions, and returning the dog to job performance or providing advice for alternative working options or retirement.

INTRODUCTION

Canine sports medicine is a recent addition to veterinary specialty services and has evolved predominantly from surgery and physical rehabilitation, where the focus has been on restoring mobility to companion dogs. Working dog sports medicine is the seamless pursuit of optimizing performance, preventing injury, and mitigating performance-degradation factors. Sports medicine truly is a core component of the comprehensive care of working dogs. Working dog rehabilitation involves a tailored approach to modify training and work while returning the dog to a safe and functional operational level. When integrated together, working dog sports medicine and rehabilitation take a whole dog approach to developing, maintaining, and regaining physical, mental, and behavioral performance.

---

[a] Penn Vet Working Dog Center, Clinical Sciences and Advanced Medicine, School of Veterinary Medicine, University of Pennsylvania, 3401 Grays Ferry Avenue, Philadelphia, PA 19146, USA;
[b] Army Medical Department Student Detachment, 187th Medical Battalion, Medical Professional Training Brigade, Joint Base San Antonio - Fort Sam Houston, San Antonio, TX, USA
* Corresponding author.
E-mail address: megramos@upenn.edu

Vet Clin Small Anim 51 (2021) 859–876
https://doi.org/10.1016/j.cvsm.2021.04.005
vetsmall.theclinics.com
0195-5616/21/© 2021 Elsevier Inc. All rights reserved.

Working dogs are different from sporting dogs and companion dogs, and working dog sports medicine and rehabilitation must be different as a result. Working dogs are tactical athletes that use their body and rely on optimal fitness to complete their job. Their health and fitness are essential to keeping themselves (eg, urban search and rescue dogs on unstable surfaces and military or law enforcement dogs performing patrol or apprehension) and the people around them (eg, their handlers and/or the community that they serve) safe. A bomb detection dog returning to work too quickly after an upper respiratory infection may have compromised detection of its trained explosive odor. Similarly, a dual-purpose law enforcement dog with substandard hip stability that slips and falls while chasing a criminal may allow that person to escape or to turn and injure or kill the handler or other law enforcement officers.

Veterinary sports medicine and rehabilitation traditionally have focused primarily on treating disease and secondarily preventing injury. Veterinarians providing sports medicine and rehabilitation for working dogs, however, could adopt the model established for human tactical and competitive athletes.[1,2] These elite human athletes benefit from an integrated team of sports psychologists to guide mental preparation and performance, sports nutritionists to fuel performance, sport-specific or job-specific strength and conditioning coaches to enhance physical performance, and sports medicine physicians and physical therapists to promote wellness, optimize training, and treat and recover from injury. Although most organizations utilizing working dogs do not have the full spectrum of these resources, veterinarians can integrate with the working dog handler, trainer, and other specialists to provide many of the same services.

This article discusses wellness, physical fitness, and rehabilitation for the working dog. Although brief by necessity, the authors hope to highlight key points and direct the readers to further resources.

WELLNESS FOR WORKING DOGS

Keeping the working dog healthy involves much more than what is needed for the typical companion animal. This article addresses the sports medicine perspective on working dog nutrition, supplements, body composition (both fat and musculature), and the impact of various environmental and job factors. The effects of behavior on performance and how various routine preventative, diagnostic, and therapeutic modalities could have an impact on performance are covered. Finally, a range of other working dog–specific preventive medicine and sports medicine topics are covered, and this article finishes with highlighting the role of regular evaluation in maintaining performance.

SPORTS MEDICINE NUTRITION

The essentials of working dog nutrition are covered in Debra L. Zoran's article, "Nutrition of Working Dogs: Feeding for Optimal Performance and Health," in this issue. In this section, the interplay between nutrition and sports medicine and rehabilitation is highlighted.

Nutrition and Performance

The timing of nutrition is a consideration for working dogs. Some dogs may benefit from preactivity, during-activity, or postactivity modifications to their feeding. Dogs performing repeated days of short-duration and intermediate-duration events may benefit from postactivity supplementation with a carbohydrate-based supplement.[3,4] Dogs at risk for gastric dilatation-volvulus should not be fed immediately before (within

60–90 minutes) moderate-intensity to high-intensity activity, and they should not be fed immediately after (within 30 minutes of completing) those activities.[5] In addition, feeding multiple smaller meals per day and using options to slow the rate of eating should be considered.[5] Finally, although feeding convenience and consistency are priorities for many handlers, some dogs may benefit from emerging research on intermittent fasting.[6]

Like human athletes, the energy and macronutrient needs of working dogs may change.[7] Dogs not actively working or training due to operational requirements or handler obligations (eg, nondog training or vacation) should have their food adjusted to avoid gaining body fat. Similarly, dogs entering a period of increased training or work (eg, extended deployment) should have their food adjusted to avoid catabolizing muscle mass for energy. Dogs recovering from illness, injury, or procedures should be evaluated carefully to ensure they are receiving the proper nutrients for recovery while avoiding excess calories that would make the return-to-work process more difficult.

Nutritional Supplements

Many canine nutritional supplements exist, and working dog handlers typically are interested in options to increase or sustain their dog's performance or health. When approached by a handler with questions regarding a particular supplement, the authors recommend asking questions outlined in **Box 1**. When evaluating a particular supplement, the factors outlined in **Box 2** should be considered.

Joint health often is the primary reason working dog handlers want to supplement. Although the evidence still is growing, products with glucosamine hydrochloride,[8] chondroitin sulfate, or avocado soybean unsaponifiables should be considered.[9] Supplementation with omega-3 fatty acids for their anti-inflammatory properties also may be of benefit for working dogs.[10] Fish oil is inexpensive but may be difficult or unpleasant to feed. In addition, the altered platelet function and detrimental effects on wound healing should be considered.[10] Supplementing L-carnitine has been shown to increase the performance and recovery of working dogs.[11,12] Supplementation with corn oil has been shown to increase olfactory performance,[13] whereas supplementation with coconut oil has been shown to decrease olfactory performance.[14]

Body Composition

Working dogs are tactical athletes who use their body to complete their job.[15] Thus, the body they bring to the job and its composition are crucial. The 2 main factors are the amount of body fat and the amount of muscle.

Body fat

Appropriate levels of body fat are highly correlated with health and longevity in dogs and also with athletic performance in humans.[16–19] Maintaining a lean body

---

Box 1
Questions for handler regarding nutritional supplements

What food are you currently feeding, and does it fit your dog's nutritional requirements?

Have you optimized the amount and timing of their nutrition?

Are you trying to fix (eg, treat) or prevent an issue?

What specific goal are you trying to achieve (eg, joint health, addition of "missing" dietary element)?

Box 2
Nutritional supplement considerations

What are the primary active ingredients?

Do any of them have evidence to support the label claims?

Does this product and/or the ingredients function to enhance performance or prevent or treat disease?

Has this specific formulation been evaluated?

Is giving this product financially sustainable for the handler and/or organization?

Are there any potential consequences from stopping this product?

---

composition likely is the single most important factor in overall health and a major contributor to athletic performance for dogs and humans. Body fat primarily is a function of the calories provided to the dog and the balance of that energy expended on the activities performed. Both of these factors are managed by the handler, so great care should be taken to educate them on their role in maintaining their dog's lean body composition.[20]

Body fat can be measured in several ways, including laboratory methods (eg, dual-energy x-ray absorptiometry and deuterium oxide dilution), morphometric measurement, and semi-subjective evaluation (eg, body condition score [BCS]).[21,22] Most working dog veterinarians do not have access to laboratory methods or require that level of precision. Training a handler to accurately perform BCS via the 9-point system is essential, and this method can be supplemented by pictures evaluated via telehealth.[23,24] The authors recommend handlers evaluate and record a BCS on a monthly basis with in-person or telehealth evaluation by a veterinarian every 3 months to 6 months. Feeding amounts then should be adjusted to maintain the desired body composition.

Most working dogs should maintain a lean body composition with a BCS of 3.5 to 4.5/9, although some dogs may be involved in careers where a different BCS is necessary.[23,25] Dogs performing in extremely hot conditions or performing highly body weight–dependent activities (eg, extended locomotion) may benefit from a lower BCS (3–3.5/9). Conversely, dogs performing in cold climates with constant (eg, swimming) or intermittent (eg, game bird retrieving) exposure to cold water may benefit from the insulating effects of a slightly higher BCS (4.5–5.5/9).[26]

Musculature

Appropriate muscle mass also is crucial for working dog performance. Musculature is positively associated with health and performance and inversely with injury rate.[27–29] As with BCS, there are several methods to assess musculature, including quantitative magnetic resonance measurements, ultrasonography of the epaxial muscles, and a muscle condition scoring (MCS) system.[30,31] Working dog handlers, trainers, and veterinarians need a version of the MCS expanded to include musculature beyond adequate. The authors propose expanding the standard MCS to include musculature that is not associated with disease. In this system, an MSC of 3/5 would be typical of a companion dog performing at the recreational level. Similar to human tactical athletes, the authors believe all working dogs need more developed musculature (eg, 3.5–5/5) to perform and limit injury.[32] Working dogs performing primarily moderate to long-duration endurance activities (eg, search and rescue, tracking/trailing, or single purpose detection) likely need an MCS of 3.5/5 (similar to a triathlete); those performing a balance of endurance and strength or power activities (eg, dual-purpose patrol and detection dogs) likely need an MCS of 4/5 (similar to a decathlete); and those performing primarily strength or power activities (eg, single purpose patrol) likely need an MCS of 4.5 to 5/5 (similar to a football running back or linebacker).

BEHAVIOR, STRESS, ENRICHMENT, AND RECOVERY

Minimizing stress and optimizing recovery are crucial to sustaining performance. Many working dogs are highly energetic and motivated to work (often called high-drive) and can have a difficult time settling. Some dogs are housed in kennels, are transported long distances or durations in vehicles, and can spend much of their lives relatively inactive but required to work at a moment's notice. This section briefly addresses some of the more common interactions between behavior and performance.

Housing

Working dog housing can affect behavior and performance.[33,34] Dogs may live with the handler and each night be housed indoors or in an outdoor kennel. This form of housing likely is the least stressful, provides the greatest potential for recovery, and allows for the greatest nonwork interaction with and oversight by the handler. One downside of at-home housing is the lack of oversight by veterinarians or leadership. Although not as important for seasoned handlers, less-experienced handlers may benefit from home visits or telehealth evaluations. Other dogs are housed in kennels when not training or working with their handlers. Although kennel design and management differ widely, kenneled dogs may have increased environmental stress, decreased ability to implement recovery recommendations, interaction with rotating caretakers, and periods without close observation. Kennel housing, however, typically allows for greater oversight of working dog management and the implementation of systematic interventions.

Regardless of the housing situation, veterinarians in the United States should refer to the Animal Welfare Act (or country-specific guidance) and carefully consider the following housing factors listed in **Box 3**.

Behavioral Enrichment

The implementation of enrichment strategies for kenneled working dogs, outlined in **Table 1**, should be considered.[35–41]

With all enrichment options, the duration of effectiveness, the simplicity of the intervention for handlers or caretakers, and the durability and risk of inadvertent injury should be considered carefully.

Box 3
Working dog housing factors

Kennel size (including allowances for proper sitting and sleeping posture)

Kennel surface (ease of sanitation balanced with pressure distribution)

Prevalence of kennel-related issues including spinning, jumping, chewing, callus formation, and dermatologic issues.

Effect of kenneling on passive environmental acclimation

Table 1	
Enrichment for working dogs	
Type	**Strategy**
Social	Group housing, arranged play groups with compatible dogs, and non-work human interaction
Physical	Bedding options, options to be indoors or outdoors, and a variety of toys
Sensory	A variety of music. Consider pheromone treatment. Be cautious of the potential interaction between olfactory enrichment and odor detection ability
Nutritional	Puzzle feeders

Transportation

Many working dogs spend significant time in vehicles while traveling to or from training or deployment. Human tactical athlete research indicates a relationship between vehicle exposure and spinal musculature fatigue,[42] and working dogs may experience a similar effect. Working dog veterinarians should consider the following vehicle-related factors (**Box 4**) to determine if a working dog will be able to perform.

Timing

Shift work is common for many military and law enforcement working dogs, and this format also can be used during search and rescue operations. Shift work is taxing on the body and results in fatigue, alterations to the circadian rhythm and sleep cycles, reduced mental performance, and sleepiness.[43–45] Working dog veterinarians should consider strategies to enhance sleep and consider isolating group kenneled dogs on different shifts from visual and auditory interruptions from people and dogs.[46,47] Physical fitness and career-specific training also should be adjusted relative to shift work.

PREVENTATIVES, THERAPEUTICS, AND DIAGNOSTICS

This section highlights some of the more frequent effects common preventatives, therapeutics, and diagnostics may have on working dog performance.

Preventatives

Vaccination, although crucial for prevention of infectious disease, causes a systemic immunologic effect. Working dog veterinarians should consider the timing of vaccines

Box 4
Working dog vehicle-related factors
Effect of confinement in smaller-than-usual kennel on posture and recovery
Effect of kennel or vehicle surface on recovery and callus formation
Effect of confinement on heat injury (if doors are accidently closed or the climate control system fails)
Effect of confinement on acclimation (if maintained in a climate controlled environment)
Effect on behavior of having people approach the vehicle or of being around activity without being engaged

relative to intense training or deployment and the potential local effects (eg, muscle soreness with intramuscular vaccination, fascial irritation with subcutaneous vaccination, and the potential for altered olfaction with intranasal vaccination).

Therapeutics

Common therapeutics also may affect performance. Intramuscular injections may cause temporary lameness. Metronidazole administration can degrade the detection threshold for up to 10 days after administration in some dogs.[48] Although this effect was not seen with doxycycline administration, the effect of other therapeutics on olfaction is not known, and working dog veterinarians should avoid unnecessary intervention for uncomplicated or minor issues.

Diagnostics

Many working dogs require sedation for diagnostic imaging, and some working dogs require sedation for examination. Although these procedures are relatively benign medically, working dog veterinarians should be aware of and educate handlers on the immediate effects (eg, nausea and inappetence) and longer-lasting effects (eg, joint discomfort from manipulation) that may impair performance. Handlers should be made aware that dogs recovering from sedation should not return to work immediately because of residual effects of sedation on balance, cognition, and proprioception. Most dogs are recovered and ready for training or operational use by 12 hours to 24 hours, but this may vary with sedation protocols.

HANDLER-LEVEL PREVENTATIVE INTERVENTIONS

Veterinarians should be sure that working dog handlers are familiar and proficient with several important preventative interventions.

Paw Care

Paw, pad, and nail injuries are common in working dogs, and a significant injury can sideline a working dog for days to weeks. Paws and pads can be lacerated, abraded, punctured, or burned, and long nails can be torn or fractured. Working dog veterinarians should educate handlers to regularly inspect their dog's pads for proper conditioning and to maintain nail length through physical activity or trimming/grinding. Pads that are too soft can be conditioned through walking or pulling a load on rough surfaces, and just-in-time toughening can be accomplished by topical sprays, such as Pad-Tough (Creative Science, Missouri). Pads that either are too tough or cracked or about to be exposed to hot surfaces, snow/ice, or water can be softened and protected by applying a wax-based product, such as Musher's Secret (Preservo Products, Quebec, Canada). Paws, pads, and nails also should be inspected regularly after training or deployment, so injuries can be quickly identified and remedied.

Post-training/Work Examinations

In addition to inspecting their dog's feet after training or deployment, working dog handlers should be taught to perform a brief examination of their dog's integumentary and musculoskeletal systems (**Table 2**). Simply observing their dog walk, sit, and jump into a vehicle can help a handler identify musculoskeletal issues. Similarly, a thorough nose-to-tail sweep with bare hands or light-colored gloves can aid in detecting wounds sustained or foreign bodies in the skin or coat. The end goal is rapid identification and resolution of issues that could affect performance.

Table 2		
Post-training/work examination		
Body System	**Brief Examination Components**	
Musculoskeletal	Observe the dog in the following activities	Walking Trotting Sitting Jumping into and out of the car
Integument	Bare hand sweep of the entire body to look for injuries	Abrasions Lacerations Foreign bodies Paw pad injuries

IMPORTANCE OF CANINE STRUCTURE AND POSTURE

Canine structure is the anatomic arrangement of the musculoskeletal system.[49] Following closure of the growth plates of the appendicular skeleton the ability to change or improve the structure of a dog is limited to development of the skeletal muscles or surgical intervention.[50–52] Canine posture is the alignment or carriage of the body as a whole or parts and is determined by the interaction between the musculoskeletal and nervous systems.[53,54] Posture is evaluated in both static positions (sit, stand, and down) and athletic movements (running, jumping, and climbing).[54,55] Unlike structure, a dog's static and athletic posture may be improved by simple interventions, such as therapeutic exercise.[51,56]

Structure and posture are indispensable aspects of physical fitness and performance of working dogs.[56] In order to critically evaluate structure and posture, a thorough understanding of the normal anatomic structure of common working dog breeds (eg, Labrador Retrievers, Belgian Malinois, and German Shepherds) is necessary. Evaluation of a working dog requires a multimodal approach to assess the muscles, tendons, ligaments, bones, joints, nerves, vasculature, fascia, and other connective tissues. Systematic palpation of all musculoskeletal components coupled with a dynamic movement assessment of transitional (sit-to-stand and down-to-stand) movements provides a compressive overview of structure and posture of a working dog.

Identifying and promoting proper posture in both the sit and down positions (**Fig. 1**) may make the difference between a long working career and early retirement for a working dog patient.[55,57] Posture determines the carriage of the body at rest and during athletic movement.[53,54] Studies in human sports medicine demonstrate that correct posture during athletic movement and static positioning has positive effects on both athletic ability and overall health.[53–55] Human athletes and working dogs are similar in that postural changes typically are not recognized by the patient but rely on the perspective of an observer, such as an athletic trainer for humans or a handler or veterinarian for working dogs. Observation of postural changes frequently are early indicators of muscular or neurologic weakness, pain, or injury.[56,57] Common working dog postural changes are kyphosis or lordosis (**Fig. 2**), abduction of a limb, and lateral rotation of a paw (**Fig. 3**). Postural changes frequently are the first signs observed in hip and elbow dysplasias, lumbosacral abnormalities, iliopsoas strains, and cranial cruciate ligament tears.

While performing the structural and postural evaluation, it is important to consider the interbreed and intrabreed structural variations and common working dog injuries. The most apparent and well-studied anatomic structural and postural variation among

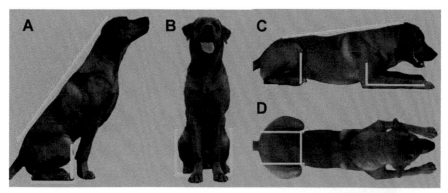

Fig. 1. Represents the proper posture in the sit and down positions. (*A*) Shows the proper sit position. Note the straight line from the head to the base of the tail. The stifle is dorsal to or just cranial to the digits. (*B*) Shows a square sit in which the hips, stifle, and digits are within the same sagittal plane. (*C*) Shows the proper posture down position. Note the straight line from the head to the base of the tail. The forelimb is flexed at the elbow and shoulder. The stifle is dorsal to or just cranial to the digits. (*D*) Shows the dorsal view of a proper posture down. Ipsilateral limbs are aligned in the sagittal plane, and the hindlimb digits are obscured by the stifles. All photos are original images taken by Kasey Seizova at the Penn Vet Working Dog Center.

working dogs is the angulation of pelvic limbs, which is determined by structure of the axial and long bones and influenced by the interplay of the skeletal muscles, tendons, ligaments, and nerves.[56,58,59] Structural and postural evaluation of the pelvic limb are important because the pelvic limbs play the primary role in locomotor dynamics of athletic type movements (sprinting and jumping).[60–62] Working dogs perform repetitive, high-energy, propulsive, and quick change in direction athletic movements throughout their career. Both the physical demands on and the structure and postural relationship of the pelvic limbs of working dogs likely contribute to chronic injuries and degenerative conditions that lead to early retirement in military working dogs.[63–66] A recent

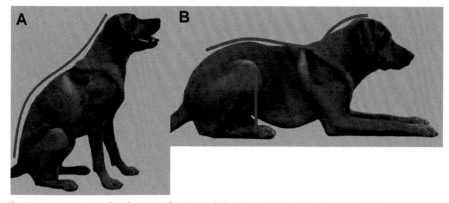

Fig. 2. Demonstrates kyphosis in the sit and down positions. (*A*) demonstrates kyphosis in a sit as highlighted by the red line. (*B*) Highlights a kyphotic spine in a down position. Note the stifles are not over the hind limb digits in both images. All photos are original images taken by Kasey Seizova at the Penn Vet Working Dog Center.

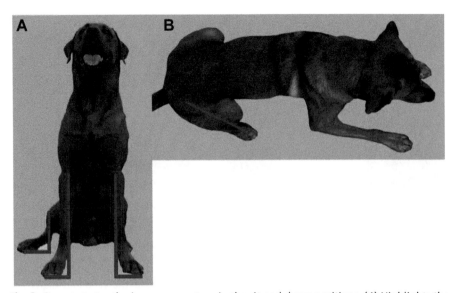

Fig. 3. Demonstrates the improper posture in the sit and down positions. (*A*) Highlights the abduction of the right hind limb paw and stifle. The image demonstrates the lateral deviation of the forelimbs as seen by the forepaws. (*B*) Highlights the abduction of the forelimb and hindlimb in a down position. All photos are original images taken by Kasey Seizova at the Penn Vet Working Dog Center.

study of different working dog breeds classified pelvic limb structure into 3 distinct groups.[67] The German Shepherd dogs clustered together with the most angulated pelvic limb and the Doberman Pinschers clustered together with the least angulated or most straight pelvic limb.[67] A majority of the Belgian Malinois clustered together in the moderately angled group, whereas the Labradors were distributed between the least angulated and moderately angulated.[67] These findings may provide further insight as to why some breeds excel at specific athletic tasks and careers. Pelvic limb structure also has been associated with some orthopedic disorders.[50,68] For example, a pelvic limb with little angulation (straight) posture is suggested as a predisposing factor in the development of stifle disorders.[67,68]

The ability to critically evaluate the structure and posture of a working dog is beneficial. Recognition of postural changes of kyphosis, abduction, and pelvic rounding can serve as early signs of pain, injury, arthritic changes, or dysplasia. Monitoring for progression or regression of posture can serve as a gauge for recovery from injury or postoperative orthopedic procedures, such as cranial cruciate ligament repairs. Once veterinarians are confident in this skill set, they can begin teaching working dog handlers to understand appropriate posture and recognize subtle changes. Incorporating these simple and inexpensive practices and establishing relationships with working dog handlers through education may lead to longer working careers and life span of working dogs.

WORKING DOG PHYSICAL FITNESS
Foundational Fitness for Working Dogs

Working dogs inherently develop muscle during their career specific training and active lifestyles. Without a targeted fitness plan, however, the dog experiences disproportionate muscle development as a result of naturally bearing approximately two-thirds of their weight on their forelimbs during normal physical activity.[56] A canine physical fitness plan should consist of activities that complement, enhance, and fill in the missing components that are not addressed during career specific skill training sessions.[69] Canine physical fitness encompasses both health-related and skill (athletic ability)-related components **(Table 3)**.[57,69] Definitions for each modality are provided in **Table 4**. Implementation of a foundational fitness program should be executed prior to advanced programs to ensure that the working dog has proper form before attempting advanced exercises. A foundational fitness program focuses on components required to perform basic physical tasks, such as running, jumping (up and down), navigating unstable surfaces, and quickly or abruptly changing direction.[57] Focusing on these areas of fitness establishes the muscles of the core (spine and abdominals), hind limbs, and supporting soft tissue structures that are not primarily engaged during routine physical activities.[64,66,70] Once a foundation fitness program is completed, such as the Penn Vet Working Dog Center Fit to Work Foundation Fitness Program,[57] career-oriented fitness program should be pursued.

Advanced Physical Fitness Programs

Formalized canine fitness programs specific to working dogs are few and far between. Many established programs within working dog kennels are not readily available to the public. Stringent time and logistical constraints of many working dog organizations make implementation of a fitness program difficult. Therefore, the development or recommendation of a program should be time-efficient and financially reasonable. The program should include a warm-up, repetition or duration circuit exercises, and a cool-down regimen. The plan should include safety guidelines for all exercises. There are several resources available for canine physical fitness programs, ranging from high-intensity interval training, to resistance sled dragging, to underwater treadmills, and to equipment-based fitness. Prior to implementation, all considered programs should be reviewed for balance of fitness components and practicality.

Recovery from Injury for a Working Dog

Following serious injury, illness, or surgery, the working dog likely requires a minimum of 2 weeks out of work and, depending on the procedure, often much longer. Similar to a professional human athlete, disruption of their athletic routine requires a comprehensive recovery plan prior to returning to work. Recovery from an injury or illness for a working dog is considered a success if the dog can perform all career-related activity safely and proficiently. Depending on the career of the dog, this could include navigating dangerous terrain, pursuing a criminal, or demonstrating that an event venue is free of explosives. As illustrated throughout this article, a plethora of information must be considered prior to clearing a dog for active duty. The rehabilitative and sports medicine approach to a working dog recovery plan consists of 4 distinct sequential phases: activity restriction, rehabilitation, return to work, and maintenance. The length of each phase depends on the extent of the injury or illness and compliance of the handler.

Table 3 Canine physical fitness	
Health-related	Cardiorespiratory endurance, muscular endurance, muscular strength, stability, and mobility
Skill-related	Agility, balance, speed, and power

Table 4
Physical fitness components

Term	Definition
Stability	The ability to maintain the forelimb, hindlimb, and spine (cervical, thoracic, lumbosacral) in optimal positions for power generation and injury prevention. Activities requiring stability include but are not limited to jumping up or down, sprinting, braking, turning, or moving over uneven or unstable surfaces.
Cardiorespiratory short- duration endurance	The ability to sustain high-intensity anaerobic activity for a short period (less than 2 minutes). Activities requiring anaerobic endurance include but are not limited to sprinting and short pulling or dragging.
Cardiorespiratory long-duration endurance	The ability to sustain low-intensity aerobic activity for a prolonged period (greater than 2 minutes). Activities requiring aerobic endurance include but are not limited to walking, trotting, and prolonged pulling.
Muscular Strength	The ability of a muscle group to exert maximal force. Activities requiring muscular strength include but are not limited to dragging, pulling, and navigating obstacles.
Muscular endurance	The ability of a muscle group to maintain contraction (isometric, concentric, eccentric) required for the specific activity. Activities requiring muscular endurance include but are not limited to holding body weight in space and squatting.
Power	The ability of a muscle group to exert maximal force in a short period of time. Activities requiring muscular power include but are not limited to sprinting (initial acceleration) and jumping.
Speed	The ability to move the body quickly over distance. The predominant activity- requiring speed is sprinting (after initial acceleration).
Balance	The ability to maintain equilibrium while stationary or moving. Activities requiring balance include but are not limited to turning, navigating obstacles, or moving over uneven or unstable surfaces.
Mobility	The ability to move the body without limitation from joints, muscles, tendons, or other connective tissues.
Agility	The ability to change the position of the body in space with speed and accuracy. Activities requiring agility include but are not limited to turning, navigating obstacles, crawling, and jumping.

Activity restriction

The first phase of recovery is the activity restriction. For surgical procedures, the sutures and integrity of the procedure are most vulnerable during this time. For medical conditions, rest often is required for appropriate healing. During this time, the handler should be provided strict and very specific guidelines on what they may and may not do and for how long. Advising the handler to implement mentally stimulating activities, described previously, are alternatives to exercise during this recovery period. Antianxiety or sedation medications may be concerning for working dog handlers due to perceived impact on future performance. The impact of failed activity restriction and benefits of pharmacologic sedation, however, should be discussed. In addition, other nonpharmacologic techniques to decrease anxiety should be included in the plan. An example of an activity restriction guidelines for neuter and gastropexy is outlined in **Table 5.**

Table 5
Activity restriction guidelines for neuter and gastropexy

Timeline after Surgery	Activity	
	Permitted	Restricted
Day 1–7	• Maximum 5 minutes on-leash fecal and urinary relief walks only—once the dog relieves itself, bring the dog back inside • May perform sit and down, paying attention to form • The Elizabethan collar must be worn at all times • Administer medications as prescribed	• Avoid stairs • No free time off-leash outside • No jumping into vehicles, onto furniture or people • No playing retrieve, tug, or with other dogs • No odor detection, agility, advanced obedience, searching, or criminal apprehension.

Day 8–14	• Stretching—cookie stretches bows, and counter stretches
	• May perform sit and down, paying attention to form
	• Massage and skin rolling around incisions
	• 5–10 minutes on-leash walks
	  ○ 3–5 times per day
	• On-leash stairs
	• May do 3 minutes on-leash odor work.
	  ○ Odor placed no higher than chest height, for food reward only.
	• The Elizabethan collar must be worn at all times
	• Administer medications as prescribed
		• No free time off leash outside
		• No jumping into vehicles, onto furniture or people
		• No playing retrieve, tug, or with other dogs
		• No agility, advanced obedience, searching, or criminal apprehension

Rehabilitation
The second phase of a recovery plan is the rehabilitation. The goal of this phase is to return the dog to performance of basic physical tasks, such as controlled running, jumping, and changing direction. The duration and exercises pursued in this phase are dependent on the severity of the inciting injury, illness, or surgery. All dogs enter this phase with some degree of muscle atrophy from disuse during the activity restriction phase. During this time, it is critical for handlers to understand the dog's limitations and identify subtle signs of discomfort, such as reluctance to attempt the rehabilitation exercises, early termination of the exercises, lip licking, and stress yawning. The handler should be provided strict and specific guidelines on approved activities, such as stretching, posture re-enforcement, body weight stability exercises, low-impact range of motion, and transition (sit-to-stand and down-to-stand) movements. For optimal compliance, an open line of communication between the handler and veterinarian should be established for consultation on clearances of specific activities.

Return to work
The return-to-work phase is specific to a dog's career. The goal of this phase is to re-establish the strength, endurance, and skill-related components of physical fitness. The dog should begin a customized physical fitness plan, as described previously.

During this phase, the dog should be introduced to controlled and low-impact training of career activities, such as obedience, odor work, agility, and criminal apprehension. A collaborative effort between the veterinarian, handler, and trainer is required to determine the progression of all career-related activities or whether the dog is able to safely and effectively return to its original career or a modified career or needs to be retired.

Maintenance

Maintenance is the most important phase and a lifelong commitment to fitness and injury prevention. This phase includes regular (quarterly, biannual, or annual) appointments to adjust and assess the dog's fitness and adapt the plan to the current needs. For dogs with chronic conditions, like arthritis, dysplasia, or lumbosacral instability, the plan needs to be dynamic. For healthy or fully recovered dogs, the focus is on maintaining musculature, mobility, and injury prevention.

SUMMARY

Canine sports medicine and rehabilitation recently has evolved to embody the optimization of performance, injury prevention, and mitigation of musculoskeletal degeneration. This article discusses the diverse factors and considerations of working dog wellness and injury prevention. The importance of recognizing normal and abnormal posture and anatomic structure for performance evaluation and early indication of musculoskeletal injury. The need for canine physical fitness programs is highlighted and the paradigm of crate rest and medications challenged, with a 4-phase recovery plan that enables informed decisions on whether a working dog can return to work safely. The topics presented in this article are a brief overview into sports medicine and rehabilitation of working dogs. Further research of these elite canine athletes is necessary to address the remaining gaps in knowledge.

CLINICS CARE POINTS

- Working dogs require thorough wellness care to support and improve their overall performance and longevity.
- Involvement and education of the handler are necessary for routine wellness, implementation of fitness, and return-to-work protocols.
- The sports medicine approach through posture and structure may lead to earlier diagnosis and treatment monitoring for musculoskeletal injuries.
- Sports medicine and rehabilitation for working dogs is a relatively new area of research with research gaps that currently are addressed by extrapolating from human sports medicine studies.

DISCLOSURE

The authors do not have any commercial or financial conflicts of interest regarding the material presented in this article. Dr M.R. Ramos and Dr C.M. Otto are employed by the Penn Vet Working Dog Center (PVWDC). Dr B.D. Farr is employed by the U.S. Army. The PVWDC currently receives funding from Pennsylvania Emergency Management Agency, Pennsylvania Game Commission, National Institutes of Health, Department of Homeland Security, US Department of Agriculture, Kleberg Foundation, and Zoetis. The sports medicine and rehabilitation residency at the PVWDC at the time of publication is sponsored by Dechra. Donors to the PVWDC are Dechra, Nestle-

Purina, Royal Canin, Nutramax, Boehringer-Ingelheim, Merial, Merck, and Respond Systems. The PVWDC previously was funded by Nestle-Purina, Virox, and Red Arch Cultural Heritage Law & Policy Research Foundation. Dr B.D. Farr previously received funding through the Army Medical Department Student Detachment. The views and information presented are those of the author (Farr) and do not represent the official position of the U.S. Army Medical Center of Excellence, the U.S. Army Training and Doctrine Command, or the Department of Army, Department of Defense, or U.S. Government.

REFERENCES

1. Grier T, Anderson MK, Depenbrock P, et al. Evaluation of the US Army Special Forces tactical human optimization, rapid rehabilitation, and reconditioning program. J Spec Oper Med Peer Rev J SOF Med Prof 2018;18(2):42–8.
2. Dijkstra HP, Pollock N, Chakraverty R, et al. Managing the health of the elite athlete: a new integrated performance health management and coaching model. Br J Sports Med 2014;48(7):523–31.
3. McKenzie EC, Hinchcliff KW, Valberg SJ, et al. Assessment of alterations in triglyceride and glycogen concentrations in muscle tissue of Alaskan sled dogs during repetitive prolonged exercise. Am J Vet Res 2008;69(8):1097–103.
4. Reynolds AJ, Carey DP, Reinhart GA, et al. Effect of postexercise carbohydrate supplementation on muscle glycogen repletion in trained sled dogs. Am J Vet Res 1997;58(11):1252–6.
5. Hill RC. The nutritional requirements of exercising dogs. J Nutr 1998;128(12 Suppl):2686S–90S.
6. Leung YB, Cave NJ, Heiser A, et al. Metabolic and immunological effects of intermittent fasting on a ketogenic diet containing medium-chain triglycerides in healthy dogs. Front Vet Sci 2020;6:480.
7. Loftus JP, Yazwinski M, Milizio JG, et al. Energy requirements for racing endurance sled dogs. J Nutr Sci 2014;3:e34.
8. McCarthy G, O'Donovan J, Jones B, et al. Randomised double-blind, positive-controlled trial to assess the efficacy of glucosamine/chondroitin sulfate for the treatment of dogs with osteoarthritis. Vet J 2007;174(1):54–61.
9. Boileau C, Martel-Pelletier J, Caron J, et al. Protective effects of total fraction of avocado/soybean unsaponifiables on the structural changes in experimental dog osteoarthritis: inhibition of nitric oxide synthase and matrix metalloproteinase-13. Arthritis Res Ther 2009;11(2):R41.
10. Bauer JE. Therapeutic use of fish oils in companion animals. J Am Vet Med Assoc 2011;239(11):1441–51.
11. Varney JL, Fowler JW, McClaughry TC, et al. L-Carnitine metabolism, protein turnover and energy expenditure in supplemented and exercised Labrador Retrievers. J Anim Physiol Anim Nutr 2020;104(5):1540–50.
12. Varney JL, Fowler JW, Gilbert WC, et al. Utilisation of supplemented l-carnitine for fuel efficiency, as an antioxidant, and for muscle recovery in Labrador retrievers. J Nutr Sci 2017;6:e8.
13. Angle CT, Wakshlag JJ, Gillette RL, et al. The effects of exercise and diet on olfactory capability in detection dogs. J Nutr Sci 2014;3:e44.
14. Altom EK, Davenport GM, Myers LJ, et al. Effect of dietary fat source and exercise on odorant-detecting ability of canine athletes. Res Vet Sci 2003;75(2):149–55.

15. Pryor RR, Colburn D, Crill MT, et al. Fitness characteristics of a suburban special weapons and tactics team. J Strength Cond Res 2012;26(3):752–7.
16. Salt C, Morris PJ, Wilson D, et al. Association between life span and body condition in neutered client-owned dogs. J Vet Intern Med 2019;33(1):89–99.
17. German AJ, Blackwell E, Evans M, et al. Overweight dogs exercise less frequently and for shorter periods: results of a large online survey of dog owners from the UK. J Nutr Sci 2017;6:e11.
18. Adams VJ, Watson P, Carmichael S, et al. Exceptional longevity and potential determinants of successful ageing in a cohort of 39 Labrador retrievers: results of a prospective longitudinal study. Acta Vet Scand 2016;58(1):29.
19. Esco MR, Fedewa MV, Cicone ZS, et al. Field-based performance tests are related to body fat percentage and fat-free mass, but not body mass index, in youth soccer players. Sports Basel Switz 2018;6(4):105.
20. Yam PS, Naughton G, Butowski CF, et al. Inaccurate assessment of canine body condition score, bodyweight, and pet food labels: a potential cause of inaccurate feeding. Vet Sci 2017;4(2):30.
21. Mawby DI, Bartges JW, d'Avignon A, et al. Comparison of various methods for estimating body fat in dogs. J Am Anim Hosp Assoc 2004;40(2):109–14.
22. Witzel AL, Kirk CA, Henry GA, et al. Use of a novel morphometric method and body fat index system for estimation of body composition in overweight and obese dogs. J Am Vet Med Assoc 2014;244(11):1279–84.
23. Laflamme D. Development and validation of a body condition score system for dogs. Canine Pract 1997;22(4):10–5.
24. Gant P, Holden SL, Biourge V, et al. Can you estimate body composition in dogs from photographs? BMC Vet Res 2016;12(1):18.
25. Silva AM. Structural and functional body components in athletic health and performance phenotypes. Eur J Clin Nutr 2019;73(2):215–24.
26. Stephens JM, Halson SL, Miller J, et al. Effect of body composition on physiological responses to cold-water immersion and the recovery of exercise performance. Int J Sports Physiol Perform 2018;13(3):382–9.
27. McLeod M, Breen L, Hamilton DL, et al. Live strong and prosper: the importance of skeletal muscle strength for healthy ageing. Biogerontology 2016;17:497–510.
28. Yang N-P, Hsu N-W, Lin C-H, et al. Relationship between muscle strength and fall episodes among the elderly: the Yilan study, Taiwan. BMC Geriatr 2018;18:90.
29. Orr RM, Robinson J, Hasanki K, et al. The relationship between strength measures and task performance in specialist police. 2019. Available at: https://research.bond.edu.au/en/publications/the-relationship-between-strength-measures-and-task-performance-i. Accessed September 17, 2020.
30. Freeman LM, Michel KE, Zanghi BM, et al. Evaluation of the use of muscle condition score and ultrasonographic measurements for assessment of muscle mass in dogs. Am J Vet Res 2019;80(6):595–600.
31. Freeman LM, Sutherland-Smith J, Prantil LR, et al. Quantitative assessment of muscle in dogs using a vertebral epaxial muscle score. Can J Vet Res 2017; 81(4):255–60.
32. Orr RM, Robinson J, Hasanki K, et al. The relationship between strength measures and task performance in specialist tactical police. J Strength Cond Res 2020. https://doi.org/10.1519/JSC.0000000000003511.
33. Mertens PA, Unshelm J. Effects of group and individual housing on the behavior of kennelled dogs in animal shelters. Anthrozoös 1996;9(1):40–51.
34. Taylor K, Mills D. The effect of the kennel environment on canine welfare: a critical review of experimental studies. Anim Welf 2007;13.

35. Young RJ. Environmental enrichment for Captive Animals. Blackwell Science; 2003.
36. Gfrerer N, Taborsky M, Würbel H. Benefits of intraspecific social exposure in adult Swiss military dogs. Appl Anim Behav Sci 2018;201:54–60.
37. Emery NJ, Clayton NS, Frith CD. Introduction. Social intelligence: from brain to culture. Philos Trans R Soc B Biol Sci 2007;362(1480):485–8.
38. Hubrecht RC. A comparison of social and environmental enrichment methods for laboratory housed dogs. Appl Anim Behav Sci 1993;37(4):345–61.
39. Tarou LR, Bashaw MJ. Maximizing the effectiveness of environmental enrichment: suggestions from the experimental analysis of behavior. Appl Anim Behav Sci 2007;102(3):189–204.
40. Wells DL. Sensory stimulation as environmental enrichment for captive animals: a review. Appl Anim Behav Sci 2009;118(1–2):1–11.
41. Kogan LR, Schoenfeld-Tacher R, Simon AA. Behavioral effects of auditory stimulation on kenneled dogs. J Vet Behav 2012;7(5):268–75.
42. Kollock RO, Games KE, Wilson AE, et al. Vehicle exposure and spinal musculature fatigue in military warfighters: a meta-analysis. J Athl Train 2016;51(11): 981–90.
43. Kazemi R, Haidarimoghadam R, Motamedzadeh M, et al. Effects of shift work on cognitive performance, sleep quality, and sleepiness among petrochemical control room operators. J Circadian Rhythms 2016;14:1.
44. Ganesan S, Magee M, Stone JE, et al. The impact of shift work on sleep, alertness and performance in healthcare workers. Sci Rep 2019;9:4635.
45. Zion N, Shochat T. Cognitive functioning of female nurses during the night shift: the impact of age, clock time, time awake and subjective sleepiness. Chronobiol Int 2018;35(11):1595–607.
46. Chinoy ED, Harris MP, Kim MJ, et al. Scheduled evening sleep and enhanced lighting improve adaptation to night shift work in older adults. Occup Environ Med 2016;73(12):869–76.
47. Caldwell JA, Caldwell JL, Thompson LA, et al. Fatigue and its management in the workplace. Neurosci Biobehav Rev 2019;96:272–89.
48. Jenkins EK, Lee-Fowler TM, Angle TC, et al. Effects of oral administration of metronidazole and doxycycline on olfactory capabilities of explosives detection dogs. Am J Vet Res 2016;77(8):906–12.
49. Carioto L. Miller's anatomy of the dog, 4th edition. Can Vet J 2016;57(4):381.
50. Dycus DL, Levine D, Marcellin-Little DJ. Physical rehabilitation for the management of canine hip dysplasia. Vet Clin North Am Small Anim Pract 2017;47(4): 823–50.
51. Millis DL, Levine D. Canine rehabilitation and physical therapy. 2nd edition 2013. https://doi.org/10.1016/C2009-0-52108-3.
52. Zink MC, Van Dyke JB. Canine sports medicine and rehabilitation. Incorporated: John Wiley & Sons; 2011. Available at: http://ebookcentral.proquest.com/lib/upenn-ebooks/detail.action?docID=1132530. Accessed May 8, 2020.
53. Ludwig O, Kelm J, Hammes A, et al. Neuromuscular performance of balance and posture control in childhood and adolescence. Heliyon 2020;6(7):e04541.
54. Viton JM, Mesure S, Bensoussan L, et al. Analyse de la posture et du mouvement et médecine du sport. Ann Réadapt Médecine Phys 2004;47(6):258–62.
55. Howell DR, Hanson E, Sugimoto D, et al. Assessment of the Postural Stability of Female and Male Athletes. Clin J Sport Med 2017;27(5):444–9.

56. Zink MC, Van Dyke JB. Canine sports medicine and rehabilitation. John Wiley & Sons, Incorporated; 2013. Available at: http://ebookcentral.proquest.com/lib/upenn-ebooks/detail.action?docID=1132530. Accessed September 17, 2020.

57. Farr BD, Ramos MT, Otto CM. The penn vet working dog center fit to work program: a formalized method for assessing and developing foundational canine physical fitness. Front Vet Sci 2020;7:470.

58. Elliott RP. Dogsteps: a new look. Fox Chapel Publishing; 2014.

59. Brown CM, Bonnie D. Dog locomotion and gait analysis. 1986. Available at: http://books.google.com/books?id=aC9WAAAAYAAJ. Accessed September 15, 2021.

60. Walter RM, Carrier DR. Rapid acceleration in dogs: ground forces and body posture dynamics. J Exp Biol 2009;212(12):1930–9.

61. Martín-Serra A, Figueirido B, Palmqvist P. A three-dimensional analysis of the morphological evolution and locomotor behaviour of the carnivoran hind limb. BMC Evol Biol 2014;14(1):129.

62. Deban SM, Schilling N, Carrier DR. Activity of extrinsic limb muscles in dogs at walk, trot and gallop. J Exp Biol 2012;215(2):287–300.

63. Baltzer WI, Owen R, Bridges J. Survey of handlers of 158 police dogs in New Zealand: functional assessment and canine orthopedic index. Front Vet Sci 2019;6:85.

64. Otto CM, Cobb ML, Wilsson E. Editorial: working dogs: form and function. Front Vet Sci 2019;6:351.

65. Worth AJ, Cave NJ. A veterinary perspective on preventing injuries and other problems that shorten the life of working dogs. Rev Sci Tech Int 2018;37(1):161–9.

66. Gamble KB, Jones JC, Biddlecome A, et al. Qualitative and quantitative computed tomographic characteristics of the lumbosacral spine in German shepherd military working dogs with versus without lumbosacral pain. J Vet Behav 2020;38:38–55.

67. Sabanci SS, Ocal MK. Categorization of the pelvic limb standing posture in nine breeds of dogs. Anat Histol Embryol 2018;47(1):58–63.

68. Adrian CP, Haussler KK, Kawcak C, et al. The role of muscle activation in cruciate disease. Vet Surg 2013;42(7):765–73.

69. Caspersen CJ, Powell KE, Christenson GM. Physical activity, exercise, and physical fitness: definitions and distinctions for health-related research. Public Health Rep 1985;100(2):126–31.

70. Cain B, Jones JC, Holásková I, et al. Feasibility for measuring transverse area ratios and asymmetry of lumbosacral region paraspinal muscles in working dogs using computed tomography. Front Vet Sci 2016;3:34.

Hunting Dogs

Marcella Ridgway, VMD, MS, DACVIM (SAIM)

KEYWORDS

- Sporting breeds • Upland game • Bird dogs • Sport dogs • Zoonoses
- Scent hounds • Gun dogs

KEY POINTS

- Hunting dog breeds vary in their occupational specialties and breed traits; pertinent information to be familiar with includes nuances of each breed, general dangers encountered while hunting specific prey, and specific microclimate threats based on work environment.
- Working-level hunting breed dogs have high energy, and intense demeanor, and, will work despite severe illness or pain, thereby masking clues that they are ailing or the nature of the problem.
- Through sustained or repeated contact with other animal species and their habitats, these dogs may be affected by infectious diseases, including parasitic infections, not commonly seen in dogs.
- Proper conditioning, gear functionality, identification, nutrition, and hydration are important for safety and optimal hunting performance.

INTRODUCTION

Hunting dogs are used to locate, chase, and/or retrieve other animals, typically individual wild animals. Unlike most other canine occupations, hunting is done predominantly by dogs of breeds developed over centuries to millennia specifically for that purpose. Hunting breeds have been selected with specific skills optimized for a successful hunt. There are breeds for locating quarry (eg, pointer), flushing out birds and waterfowl (eg, spaniels), retrieving birds and waterfowl (eg, retrievers), or trailing game (eg, hounds). Hunting breed dogs generally have high energy, and intense demeanor and, will work despite severe illness or pain, thereby masking clues that they are ailing or the nature of the problem. Veterinarians providing care for working hunting dogs should familiarize themselves with the nuances of the particular breed, general dangers encountered while hunting, specific microclimate threats, as well as characteristics unique to that individual dog. Monitoring and intervention by the handler are critical to keep dogs from literally working themselves to death, and veterinarians should take an active role in training handlers in addressing common problems.

Hunting dogs typically work outdoors in rural to wilderness environments with continuous exposure to other domestic animals and wildlife, infectious disease

---

University of Illinois College of Veterinary Medicine, 1008 West Hazelwood Drive, Urbana, IL 61802, USA
E-mail address: ridgway@illinois.edu

Vet Clin Small Anim 51 (2021) 877–890
https://doi.org/10.1016/j.cvsm.2021.04.006
0195-5616/21/© 2021 Elsevier Inc. All rights reserved.

reservoirs and vectors, rugged terrain, and weather extremes. Many dogs live outdoors even when not working, further increasing exposure. Through sustained or repeated contact with other animal species and their habitats, these dogs may be affected by infectious diseases, including parasitic infections, not commonly seen in dogs. The general principles for preventive care and health considerations for working dogs presented in the article "Preventative Health Care for Working Dogs" by Marcella Ridgway this issue, apply to hunting dogs. Specific health concerns of hunting dogs are addressed here.

WORKING HUNTING DOGS

Hunting occurs worldwide for purposes of food acquisition, control of wildlife populations, elimination of pest animals, and sport. Humans have likely used dogs to assist them in hunting for 8000 to 9000 years.[1] Since then, dogs have developed tremendous phenotypic variation through selective breeding for defined physical and behavioral characteristics. A study of hunting dogs showed evidence of strong selection for genes associated with muscular, neurologic, and cardiovascular functions and, surprisingly, with auditory function deficiency (congenital deafness, accelerated hearing loss with loud noise exposure): positive selection for genes associated with hearing problems may have occurred because this resulted in a reduced startle response to sudden loud noises.[2] Hunting encompasses a variety of specific tasks depending on the type of animal being hunted and type of assistance desired by the handler. Individual hunting dog breeds are therefore often further specialized, especially behaviorally, in the type of work for which they were developed, including chasing, holding at bay, pointing, retrieving, flushing, or following the blood trail of a wounded animal. The genetic basis of pointing behavior has been investigated[3] but the genetics supporting most specialized hunting breed traits are unknown. Most hunting tasks involve protracted periods of endurance activity with intermittent short periods of sprinting and usually require excellent olfactory function. Physical performance and olfaction are affected by hydration status, nutrition, certain supplements and medications, and presence of disease (see the article, "Special Senses," in this issue).

SPECIAL HEALTH CONSIDERATIONS IN HUNTING DOGS
General

General recommendations for health assessment and maintenance presented in the article, "Preventative Health Care for Working Dogs," in this issue, should be applied for hunting dogs. Hematological and biochemical normal ranges can vary considerably across different breeds.[4–10] Exercise as well can affect these values. Levels of acute phase proteins (haptoglobin, serum amyloid A, and C-reactive protein), often used as biomarkers of pathologic conditions, increase with hunting exercise and rapidly normalize afterward. Increases in these parameters in exercising hunting dogs should not be misinterpreted as indicating underlying disease conditions.[11,12] Routine infectious disease screening appropriate for all regions in which the dogs work is vital in light of heightened exposure through working in natural areas, proximity to wildlife reservoirs, and often being kenneled outdoors year-round. Aggressive control of ticks and other insect vectors is imperative and simultaneous use of multiple preventive products is often necessary.

Hydration and Nutrition

Few publications have specifically addressed the water and nutritional needs of hunting dogs,[13–17] but generally energy and water requirements increase proportional to the total amount of work done and are increased in hot or, especially, cold conditions. When hunting every day, as on multiple-day hunting trips, dogs may have excessive weight loss even when fed 3 to 4 times daily: calorie-dense diets formulated for sporting dogs offer the best chance of maintaining condition (see the article, "Nutrition in Working Dogs," in this issue). Hypoglycemia is rare in otherwise healthy adult dogs but, with intense or prolonged exercise, hunting dogs may experience exertional hypoglycemia manifested by altered mentation, weakness, trembling, ataxia, seizures, and/or collapse and death. Veterinarians should confirm that handlers know about the condition, preventive measures (proper conditioning of the dog, feeding a calorie-dense diet, intermittent calorie [carbohydrate] supplementation during prolonged exercise) and how to respond in the field with cessation of activity, providing a rapidly available oral carbohydrate source (Karo or other syrup, Nutri-Cal, sugar-containing beverage, jam/jelly, honey) followed by feeding and continued rest. Olfaction can be affected by factors such as dehydration and nutrient content of the diet (see the article, "Special Senses," in this issue). Some hunting dog handlers claim that heartworm preventives reduce dogs' scenting ability, but the effect, if any, of these products on olfaction has not been evaluated. Even so, their benefit in preventing heartworm infection in this predisposed dog population predominates.

Conditioning

Proper conditioning is important for safety and optimal performance. However, many hunting dogs are seasonally active depending on their designated hunting season and lose conditioning in the off-season. Overweight condition and obesity may develop in inactive dogs; Labrador and golden retrievers and beagles are especially susceptible. Handlers should be advised to maintain year-round condition and weight management and to build the dog's conditioning appropriately in advance of hunting season to achieve best hunting performance and help prevent musculoskeletal injury, exertional hypoglycemia, exertional rhabdomyolysis, and heat stroke.[18]

Safety

Visibility and individual identification are critical concerns for hunting dogs, which often work at distance from their handler following unpredictable paths after their quarry: they are at risk of becoming lost or of encountering other hunters, landowners, and vehicle operators who need to quickly recognize the unexpected presence of a dog and identify it as owned. Dogs should be individually identified by a permanent identification method (microchip, tattoo) that cannot become detached in rough terrain and should also wear a readily visible form of identification (collar and tags). Hunting dogs typically work in flat strap collars. Many hunters prefer a central O-ring safety collar: the central ring is intended to allow the collar to flex if snagged, allowing the dog to escape (**Fig. 1**). Identification is often incorporated into the collar as a riveted nameplate or lettering on the collar material itself rather than free-hanging tags, which are more likely to snag or be lost. Specifically designed protective equipment is available commercially through hunting outfitters. Ear, head, leg, chest, and tail protectors and protective vests limit abrasions, punctures, and lacerations of vulnerable body regions by heavy brush, thorns, and wire. Heavier protective vests help prevent injury from prey (hogs) or snakebite. Hog dog collars are wide and constructed of heavy material to protect vulnerable neck structures from tusk injury. Dog boots help maintain warmth and protect feet from injury by rocks, burrs, brush, and debris. Topical products such as Tuff-Foot, Pad Heal, and Mushers Secret paw wax help protect from injury from sand, road salt, hot or cold surfaces, formation of interdigital snow or ice balls, and chemical injury and counter dryness and cracking of foot

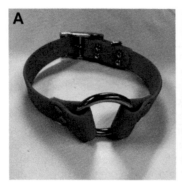 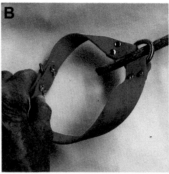

Fig. 1. (A) Central O-ring safety collar. Leash ring sits flat against dog's neck so is less likely to snag than common D-ring collar. (B) If the ring does snag, the center ring construction allows the collar to flex so that the dog can slip free.

pads. Neoprene vests provide insulation to maintain warmth in cold weather as well as protect against external injury. Because neoprene repels water, these vests do not become waterlogged and heavy when dogs swim, and some feature an additional foam flotation layer to help prevent fatigue while swimming. Many hunting dog handlers use electronic collars to allow communication with the dog at distance. Dog tracking collars and dog bells for collars or vests help handlers track the dog's location. Hunting dog equipment is usually available in high-visibility colors, helpful for visually tracking the dog and visibility to other hunters and traffic. Dog-worn equipment should be fitted snuggly to reduce the chance of snagging and trapping the dog in vegetation or tight spaces or becoming entangled with the prey species. Some hunting kennels routinely remove all dewclaws to prevent injury from hooking vegetation when dogs work in heavy thatch.

Disease Considerations

Studies of the nature and relative frequency of hunting dog ailments are limited. A postmortem study of 52 hounds culled from 10 Irish hunting kennels identified renal changes in 48%, including glomerulonephritis in 33%, but few dogs with obvious infectious or other systemic disease; most had been culled for behavioral or performance problems.[19] Identifying disease and disease transmission in hunting dogs is important not only for the dogs' health but also as a means of surveillance (the dog as a sentinel) of infectious disease prevalence in environments shared by other potentially susceptible domestic and wildlife species and humans.[20–22] Dogs may facilitate transmission of diseases that are vector borne[23] or have a wildlife reservoir (rabies, leptospirosis) to humans. The risk of transmission of specific diseases depends on the type of prey and the specific environments in which the dog hunts; for example, dogs retrieving migratory waterfowl and avian influenza[24] (**Fig. 2**). Hunting dogs are a potential source of disease (canine distemper, canine parvovirus, dirofilariasis, *Brucella canis*, *Sarcoptes scabiei*, *Neospora caninum*) spilling from a domestic animal source to wildlife, especially in remote communities. This danger is a particular threat in wild canids. Hunting dogs may further affect wildlife when the presence of dogs alters habitat use by other species.

Trauma

Hunting dogs work off leash and are at risk for dog-vehicle collisions. They may sustain dermal, eye, ear, or foot injury and infection from heavy brush, burrs, embedded

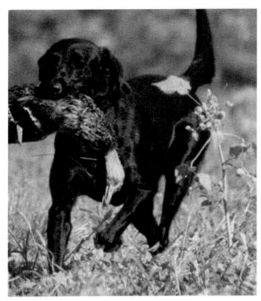

Fig. 2. Labrador retriever with duck. Hunting dogs may contribute to significant geographic spread of infectious disease not only through traveling widely to hunting locations but potentially even more widely through direct contact with migratory species.

seeds, thorns, grass awns (foxtails), wire, and other human debris. Migrating plant material or other foreign bodies may incite inflammation and introduce pathogenic organisms into other tissues and cause disease in essentially any organ: pyothorax is a classic example[25] but other conditions, such as foreign body hepatitis with focal peritonitis[19] and sublumbar myositis presented as back pain, are reported.[26] Snagging on collars, tags, other gear, or the dog's dewclaws may also promote injury by brush or thatch. Dogs may be injured by the prey species (hogs, raccoons) or by animals they encounter incidentally (other dogs) while hunting. Intent on their prey, hunting dogs may be injured by running into trees, fences, or other hazards and are susceptible to falls from cliffs, stream banks, structures, and other heights. Gunshot injury warrants particular attention because hunting dogs are at risk of accidental or intentional (unhappy landowner) gunshot wounding. Despite an obvious increased exposure, hunting dogs do not predominate in reports of gunshot injury in dogs,[27,28] suggesting that intentional wounding is most common. Gunshot dogs may present anywhere along a spectrum from acute life-threatening injury to incidental finding of embedded metal projectiles from a past incident. Prognosis varies widely and depends on the tissues affected, the severity of the wounding, and consequent blood loss or organ dysfunction, with thoracic wounds associated with higher fatality.[27] In addition to direct wounding, further harm may occur by corrosion of chronically embedded steel pellets and consequent inflammation.[29] Hunting dogs may be accidental victims of traps set for other species. Traps may cause significant tissue injury (foot-hold/leg-hold traps) or death (body-gripping traps), detain the dog to be injured by other animals or the trapper, or subject them to dehydration and exposure to elements if traps are infrequently tended. Trapping is a regulated activity but laws vary by country and state. Hunting dog handlers should be familiar with what traps are in use and how to release the traps (various instructional videos are available online). Dogs are often working at speed and focused on their prey so are susceptible to falls when hunting near steep banks or cliffs. Dogs leaping into water to retrieve may suffer impalement on submerged woody vegetation.

Toxins

Hunting dogs may encounter poisons intentionally placed to kill pests. Lethal M-44s (spring-loaded canisters that release cyanide), strychnine, compound 1080, antifreeze, or xylitol, as well as illicit other poisons (ie, methomyl, aldicarb), used to eliminate coyotes and other pests may poison nontarget animals, including dogs. Lead intoxication may occur in dogs that are fed game shot with lead-based ammunition.[30] Transient gastrointestinal and behavioral signs have been attributed to ingestion of oral rabies vaccine baits by dogs.[31]

Infectious disease

Hunting dogs have an increased risk of exposure to infectious disease related to increased likelihood of direct or indirect contact with wildlife reservoirs, exposure to insect vectors, or the practice of feeding them raw tissues of quarry species or allowing access to areas where game is field dressed and entrails can be ingested. Heartworm infection is more common in unprotected hunting dogs than in pet dogs,[32] and, in hunting dogs on heartworm preventives, failure of prophylaxis may occur because of problems of emerging resistance; individual differences in drug absorption or metabolism; or, most commonly, faulty administration. Prophylaxis failure in hunting dogs is associated with greater number of hours spent outdoors at dawn, dusk, and at night (when mosquitoes are most active).[33] Hunting dogs may be transported widely to hunt regions other than the home environment: handlers must be made aware of regional differences in transmission seasons (longer seasons in warmer regions) and apparent parasite resistance to macrocyclic lactone preventive medications. Many hunting dog handlers have significant misunderstanding of heartworm transmission and the use and effectiveness of preventives and could benefit from educational resources provided through their veterinarians.[34] Infection with *Pythium insidiosum* is of special concern in dogs working in bodies of water. In the United States, pythiosis occurs most commonly in the southern states and California and may manifest as cutaneous or gastrointestinal disease. Humans are also susceptible to environmental exposure but the infection is not zoonotic. Hunters are at risk for tularemia (*Francisella tularensis*), which can be severe to fatal, caused by bites from infected ticks or contact with infected animals, especially rabbits and hares.[35] Exposed dogs seroconvert to *Francisella* but rarely become ill; exposed dogs, although asymptomatic, can transmit infection to humans.[36,37] Leptospirosis is another bacterial disease for which hunting dogs have increased risk,[38] especially to certain serovars (grippotyphosa).[39] With leptospirosis, illness occurs more frequently in dogs than in humans. Infected dogs can be a source of human infection. Hunting dogs and hunters may be exposed to plague (*Yersinia pestis*) when hunting in enzootic areas. Dogs are often subclinically affected but may still be a source of animal-human transmission.[40,41] Other bacterial diseases of public health significance have been reported as isolated findings (bovine tuberculosis in working foxhounds in the United Kingdom)[42–44] or studies of hunting dogs with no nonhunting dog data for comparison.[45] Many studies document a high exposure rate to tick-borne diseases (ehrlichiosis, anaplasmosis, borreliosis, babesiosis, hepatozoonosis, bartonellosis, coxiellosis) in hunting dogs worldwide. Coinfection with multiple vector-borne disease agents is common, although the pattern of coinfecting pathogens varies by region corresponding with the geographic distribution of tick vectors.[46] Hunting dogs may also increase human exposure to tick-borne pathogens by carrying unattached ticks into the proximity of handlers.[23,46] Dogs may acquire *Hepatozoon americanum* infection by swallowing an infected tick while self-grooming or ingestion of infected ticks on a prey species or tissues of a prey species containing *H americanum* cystozoites.[47,48] Leishmaniasis is a zoonotic disease for which dogs are the principal domestic reservoir host. In the United States, infection is endemic in hunting dogs, with 8.9% to 53% (average, 20.2%–26.7%) of hunting hounds testing positive for the organism,[49,50] which parallels 20% to 26% seropositivity rates in other endemic areas of Brazil, Tunisia, and Italy.[49,51] In the United States, infection with *Leishmania* is maintained by vertical transmission rather than vector (sand fly) transmission.[49] Infected dogs pose a public health risk as well as being source of infection of wild canids.[51] Infection in dogs is often asymptomatic, but co-infection with tick-borne disease increases the likelihood of progression to clinical leishmaniasis in hunting dogs.[52] Canine *Leishmania* vaccines are available in Europe and Brazil but none are licensed in the United States. Infection with *Trypanosoma cruzi* (American trypanosomiasis or Chagas disease) is more common in hunting dogs, which move between domestic and natural areas and thus may participate in both the domestic and sylvatic cycles of transmission.[53,54] In addition to vector-mediated transmission (Reduviidae), infection with *T cruzi* may be transmitted by vertical transmission, blood transfusion, or exposure to infected tissues. *Toxoplasma gondii*, *N caninum*, and *Cryptosporidium* spp are other protozoan pathogens found with increased frequency in hunting dogs[55–58]: dogs may transmit infection to other species, including humans. Intestinal parasites in hunting dogs, like other infections, are important not only from the standpoint of individual health of the dog but also for the potential for hunting dogs to disseminate infective ova over large areas. In moving across natural, rural, and residential areas and through consumption of uncooked carcasses, hunting dogs have a heightened potential for exposure to parasitic agents,[59–63] and ongoing conscientious endoparasite control measures are warranted. *Echinococcus* spp, with reservoirs in wild canids and for which dogs serve as a definitive host, is of particular concern because of the potential for this zoonotic cestode to cause devastating disease in humans.[61,64–67] Other parasitic infections found more frequently in hunting dogs include *Capillaria plica*[68,69] and *Spirocerca lupi*.[70] Leeches of various species are present in diverse microenvironments and may parasitize dogs: oral parasitism is most commonly reported but other areas of attachment, usually unhaired surfaces (nasal mucosa, interdigital skin, ventral abdomen, prepuce), are possible.[71] Because of prolonged periods spent outdoors and work in diverse, sometimes remote, environments, hunting dogs may be affected by sporadic or unusual infections, such as severe disease reported in a group of hunting dogs with trombiculid mite infestation.[72]

Dogs used to hunt feral pigs and wild boar, or hog dogs, are at particular risk of injury and exposure to infectious diseases not encountered by most hunting dogs. Hog dogs include bay dogs, which specialize in locating and chasing the hog, and catch dogs, which physically grip and hold the hog until the hunter arrives. Hog dogs often wear special protective gear to reduce injury from the dangerous tusks of their prey. Lacerations are very common and injuries may include tearing of ears and tails, stabbing wounds, contusions, body cavity perforation, evisceration, and fractures. Wound frequency is highest for the abdomen, head and neck, and rear limbs, but any body region can be affected. Pseudorabies (Suid herpesvirus 1 or Aujeszky disease) is often fatal in dogs and is of particular concern in pig-hunting dogs.[73–77] Pseudorabies has been eradicated from domestic pigs in the United States but the disease is endemic in US feral swine populations. Dogs are exposed by direct or indirect contact with infected swine. Pigs are a reservoir for *Brucella suis*, which can cause discospondylitis and back pain, lameness, and/or reproductive tract disease in dogs. Dogs can be infected through pig-hunting activities or eating raw meat from feral pigs. Infected dogs can transmit infection to other animals and to humans.[78,79] *Paragonimus westermani* infection is reported in Japanese boar-hunting dogs associated with feeding of raw boar meat.[80–82] Pig-hunting dogs have been shown to have a high seropositivity to *T gondii*,[83] *Trichinella* spp,[20] and eastern, western, and Venezuelan encephalitis viruses.[84]

Other disease concerns

Exertional rhabdomyolysis is a syndrome of acute muscle necrosis following intense prolonged exercise, especially when it extends across consecutive days. Associated myoglobinuria may cause acute renal failure. The condition is most common in racing sled dogs and hunting dogs, particularly when the exercise exceeds the dog's level of conditioning. Coonhound paralysis is an acute polyradiculoneuritis causing ascending flaccid paralysis in dogs, which may occur 7 to 14 days following a raccoon bite: immune-mediated demyelination is suspected but the underlying mechanism is unknown. Tick paralysis is an ascending paralysis caused by a neurotoxin secreted from the salivary glands of feeding female ticks. Tick bites by Lone Star and other tick species have been associated with subsequent development of food allergy, particularly to red meats and mammal products, in humans and animals, including dogs. This condition is referred to as alpha-Gal syndrome in reference to the sugar molecule alpha-Gal (galactose-alpha-1,3-galactose). Alpha-Gal is found in tick saliva and in mammalian products, including red meats, and is thought to be the substance toward which the affected person or animal becomes sensitized. The condition occurs worldwide with different associated tick species. Acute caudal myopathy, or limber tail, is a transient flaccid paralysis of a dog's tail, usually following an episode of overuse, strain, or other injury of tail muscles (swimming, exposure to cold wet weather, prolonged cage confinement, overexertion, and poor conditioning). The whole tail may be affected or the proximal tail may retain tone, show dorsal piloerection, and may be painful on manipulation. Limber tail occurs most commonly in sporting breeds, especially retrievers, pointers, setters, and hounds, and typically resolves spontaneously in a few hours, days, or weeks.[85] Infraspinatus muscle injury and subsequent infraspinatus fibrosis/contracture[86] is seen most commonly in highly active dogs, especially bird dogs, and presents as a forelimb lameness and restricted extension of the shoulder. Surgical treatment is indicated. Special risks for water dogs include drowning from becoming snagged or from exhaustion while swimming. Thermal injury may affect any hunting dog traveling into a hot or cold environment with insufficient acclimation. Dogs hunting in cold weather may develop hypothermia or frostbite even while physically active, especially if they become wet. Areas of the body with thin to no hair (nipples, scrotum, ventrum) and extremities (ears, tail, toes) are most susceptible to frostbite: lesions may not be readily apparent initially until tissue necrosis ensues. Water dogs may be especially vulnerable to hypothermia from periods of inactivity waiting in blinds in cold weather, especially after becoming wet, and from swimming in cold waters. Hunting dogs are also at risk for heat stress and heat stroke, particularly if they are not well conditioned or travel to a warmer environment to hunt or trial. Hunting dog pulmonary edema, a syndrome of acute onset of dyspnea during or following hunting (active chase) activity, has been described in Swedish hunting dogs. Affected dogs have pulmonary edema without underlying heart disease and a mechanism of neurogenic pulmonary edema resulting from high catecholamine levels from the stress and excitement of the hunt has been proposed.[87,88]

CLINICS CARE POINTS

- Handler monitoring and intervention are critical to keep dogs from overworking, which can result in significant distress and even death. Veterinarians should take an active role in training handlers on identifying and addressing health problems.

- Hunting dogs have an increased risk of exposure to infectious disease related to increased likelihood of direct or indirect contact with wildlife reservoirs, exposure to insect vectors, or the practice of feeding them raw tissues of quarry species or allowing access to areas where game is field dressed and entrails can be ingested.

- Routine infectious disease screening appropriate for all regions in which the dogs work is vital in light of heightened exposure through working in natural areas, proximity to wildlife reservoirs, and often being kenneled outdoors year round. Aggressive control of ticks and other insect vectors is imperative and simultaneous use of multiple preventive products is often necessary.

- Veterinarians should confirm that handlers know about hypoglycemia, preventive measures (proper conditioning of the dog, feeding a calorie-dense diet, intermittent calorie [carbohydrate] supplementation during prolonged exercise), and how to respond in the field.

- Hunting dogs are also at risk for heat stress and heat stroke, particularly if they are not well conditioned or travel to a warmer environment to hunt or trial.

- Hunting dogs may be transported widely to hunt regions other than their home environment: veterinarians must be made aware of travel and exposure history.

DISCLOSURE

There are no conflicts of interests to disclose.

REFERENCES

1. Grimm D. Oldest images of dogs show hunting, leashes. Science 2017; 358(6365):854.
2. Kim J, Williams FJ, Dreger DL, et al. Genetic selection of athletic success in sport-hunting dogs. Proc Natl Acad Sci U S A 2018;115(30):E1712–21.
3. Akkad DA, Gerding WM, Gasser RB, et al. Homozygosity mapping and sequencing identify two genes that might contribute to pointing behavior in hunting dogs. Canine Genet Epidemiol 2015;2(5). https://doi.org/10.1186/s40575-015-0018-5.
4. Miglio A, Gavazza A, Siepi D, et al. Hematological and biochemical reference intervals for 5 adult hunting dog breeds using a blood donor database. Animals (Basel) 2020;10(7):1212–31.
5. Harper EJ, Hackett RM, Wilkinson J, et al. Age-related variations in hematologic and plasma biochemical test results in Beagles and Labrador Retrievers. J Am Vet Med Assoc 2003;223(10):1436–42.
6. Matwichuk CL, Taylor S, Shmon CL, et al. Changes in rectal temperature and hematologic, biochemical, blood gas, and acid-base values in healthy Labrador Retrievers before and after strenuous exercise. Am J Vet Res 1999;60(1):88–92.
7. Sharkey L, Gjevre K, Hegstad-Davies R, et al. Breed-associated variability in serum biochemical analytes in four large-breed dogs. Vet Clin Pathol 2009; 38(3):375–80.
8. Bourgès-Abella NH, Gury TD, Geffré A, et al. Reference intervals, intraindividual and interindividual variability, and reference change values for hematologic variables in laboratory beagles. J Am Assoc Lab Anim Sci 2015;54(1):17–24.

9. Chang YM, Hadox E, Szladovits B, et al. Serum biochemical phenotypes in the domestic dog. PLoS One 2016;11(2):e0149650.

10. Lawrence J, Chang YM, Szladovits B, et al. Breed-specific hematological phenotypes in the dog: a natural resource for the genetic dissection of hematological parameters in a mammalian species. PLoS One 2013;8(11):e81288.

11. Rovira S, Munoz A, Bento M. Effect of exercise on physiological, blood and endocrine parameters in search and rescue-trained dogs. Vet Med 2008;53:333–46.

12. Casella S, Fazio F, Russo C, et al. Acute phase proteins response in hunting dogs. J Vet Diagn Invest 2013;25(5):577–80.

13. Davenport GM, Kelley RL, Altom EK, et al. Effect of diet on hunting performance of English pointers. Vet Ther 2001;2(1):10–23.

14. Ahlstrom O, Skrede A, Speakman J, et al. Energy expenditure and water turnover in hunting dogs: a pilot study. J Nutr 2006;136:2063S–5S.

15. Ahlstrom O, Redman P, Speakman J. Energy expenditure and water turnover in hunting dogs in winter conditions. Br J Nutr 2011;106:S158–61.

16. Davidson MG, Geoly FJ, Gilger BC, et al. Retinal degeneration associated with vitamin E deficiency in hunting dogs. J Am Vet Med Assoc 1998;213(5):645–51.

17. Stephens-Brown L, Davis M. Water requirements of canine athletes during multiday exercise. J Vet Intern Med 2018;32:1149–54.

18. Marcellin-Little DJ, Levin D, Taylor R. Rehabilitation and conditioning of sporting dogs. Vet Clin North Am 2005;35:1427–39.

19. Jahns H, Callanan JJ, McElroy MC, et al. Post-mortem findings in Irish culled hounds. J Comp Pathol 2011;145(1):59–67.

20. Gomez-Morales MA, Selmi M, Ludovisi A, et al. Hunting dogs as sentinel animals for monitoring infections with Trichinella spp. in wildlife. Parasit Vectors 2016;9: 154–65.

21. Gabriele-Rivet V, Brookes VJ, Arsenault J, et al. Hunting practices in northern Australia and their implication for disease transmission between community dogs and wild dogs. Aust Vet J 2019;97(8):268–76.

22. Montagnaro S, Piantedosi D, Ciarcia R, et al. Serological evidence of mosquitoborne flaviviruses circulation in hunting dogs in Campania Region, Italy. Vector Borne Zoonotic Dis 2019;19(2):142–7.

23. Toepp AJ, Willardson K, Larson M, et al. Frequent exposure to many hunting dogs significantly increases tick exposure. Vector Borne Zoonotic Dis 2018;18(10): 519–23.

24. Lane C, Tamru C, Nganwa D, et al. A quantitative risk assessment for the likelihood of introduction of highly pathogenic avian influenza virus strain H5N1 into I.S. hunter retriever dogs. Avian Dis 2010;54(1 suppl):699–706.

25. Frendin J. Pyogranulomatous pleuritic with empyema in hunting dogs. Zetralbl Veterinarmed A 1997;44(3):167–78.

26. Frendin J, Funkqust B, Hansson K, et al. Diagnostic imaging of foreign body reactions in dogs with diffuse back pain. J Small Anim Pract 1999;40:278–85.

27. Capak H, Bottegaro NB, Manojlovic A, et al. Review of 166 gunshot injury cases in dogs. Top Compan Anim Med 2016;31:146–51.

28. Olsen LE, Streeter EM, DeCook RR. Review of gunshot injuries in cats and dogs and utility of a triage scoring system to predict short-term outcome: 37 cases (2003-2008). J Am Vet Med Assoc 2014;245(8):923–9.

29. Bartels KE, Stair EL, Cohen RE. Corrosion potential of steel bird shot in dogs. J Am Vet Med Assoc 1991;199(7):856–63.

30. Hogasen HR, Ornsrud R, Knutsen HK, et al. Lead intoxication in dogs: risk assessment of feeding dogs trimmings of lead-shot game. BMC Vet Res 2016; 12:152–60.

31. Nokireki T, Nevalainen M, Sihvonen L, et al. Adverse reactions from consumption of oral rabies vaccine baits in dogs in Finland. Acta Vet Scand 2016;58(1):53.

32. Orr B, Ma G, Koh WL, et al. Pig-hunting dogs are an at-risk population for canine heartworm (*Dirofilaria immitis*) infection in eastern Australia. Parasit Vectors 2020; 13(1):69.

33. Rohrbach BW, Odoi A, Patton S. Risk factors associated with failure of heartworm prophylaxis among members of a national hunting dog club. J Am Vet Med Assoc 2011;238(9):1150–8.

34. Rohrbach BW, Lutzy A, Patton S. Attributes, knowledge, beliefs, and behaviors relating to prevention of heartworm in dogs among members of a national hunting dog club. Vet Parasitol 2011;176:324–32.

35. Jacob D, Barduhn A, Tappe D, et al. Outbreak of tularemia in a group of hunters in Germany in 2018 – kinetics of antibody and cytokine responses. Microorganisms 2020;8(11):1645–59.

36. Nordstoga A, Handeland K, Johansen TB, et al. Tularaemia in Norwegian dogs. Vet Microbiol 2014;173:318–22.

37. Kwit NA, Schwartz A, Kugeler KJ, et al. Human tularaemia associated with exposure to domestic dogs-United States, 2006–2016. Zoonoses Public Health 2019; 66:417–21.

38. Lee HS, Guptill L, Johnson AJ, et al. Signalment changes in canine leptospirosis between 1970 and 2009. J Vet Intern Med 2014;28:294–9.

39. Adesiyun AA, Hull-Jackson C, Mootoo N, et al. Sero-epidemiology of canine leptospirosis in Trinidad: serovars, implications for vaccination and public health. J Vet Med 2006;53:91–9.

40. Cleri DJ, Vernaleo JR, Lombardi LJ, et al. Plague pneumonia disease caused by *Yersinia pestis*. Semin Respir Infect 1997;12(1):12–23.

41. Nichols MC, Ettestad PJ, Vin Hatton ES, et al. *Yersinia pestis* in dogs: 62 cases (2003-2011). J Am Vet Med Assoc 2014;244(10):1176–81.

42. Are hunting dogs spreading bovine TB? Vet Rec 2017;180(24):583.

43. Eastwood B, Menache A, Dalzell F, et al. Spreading of bovine TB by hunting hounds. Vet Rec 2018;183:327–8.

44. Phipps E, McPhedran K, Edwards D, et al. Bovine tuberculosis in working foxhounds: lessons learned from a complex public health investigation. Epidemiol Infect 2018;9:1–6.

45. Mustapha M, Bukar-Kolo YM, Geidam YA, et al. Phenotypic and genotypic detection of methicillin-resistant *Staphylococcus aureus* in hunting dogs in Maiduguri metropolitan, Borno State, Nigeria. Vet World 2016;9(5):501–6.

46. Mahachi K, Kontowicz E, Anderson B, et al. Predominant risk factors for tick-borne co-infections in hunting dogs from the USA. Parasit Vectors 2020;13: 247–60.

47. Johnson EM, Panciera RJ, Allen KA, et al. Alternate pathway of infection with *Hepatozoon americanum* and the epidemiologic importance of predation. J Vet Intern Med 2009;23:1315–8.

48. Mitkova B, Hrazdilova, Steinbauer V, et al. Autochthonous *Hepatozoon* infection in hunting dogs and foxes from the Czech Republic. Parasitol Res 2016;115(11): 4167–71.

49. Toepp AJ, Schaut RG, Scott BD, et al. *Leishmania* incidence and prevalence in U.S. hunting hounds maintained via vertical transmission. Vet Parasitol 2017; 10:75–81.

50. Vida B, Toepp A, Schaut RG, et al. Immunologic progression of canine leishmaniosis following vertical transmission in United States dogs. Vet Immunol Immunopathol 2016;169:34–8.

51. Piantedosi D, Veneziano V, Di Muccio T, et al. Epidemiological survey on *Leishmania* infection in red foxes (*Vulpes vulpes*) and hunting dogs sharing the same rural area in Southern Italy. Acta Parasitol 2016;61(4):769–75.

52. Toepp AJ, Montiero GRG, Coutinho JFV, et al. Comorbid infections induce progression of visceral leishmaniasis. Parasit Vectors 2019;12:54–66.

53. Bradley KK, Bergman DK, Woods JP, et al. Prevalence of American trypanosomiasis (Chagas disease) among dogs in Oklahoma. JAVMA 2000;12:1853–7.

54. Roegner AF, Daniels ME, Smith WA, et al. *Giardia* infection and *Trypanosoma cruzi* exposure in dogs in the Bosawas Biosphere Reserve, Nicaragua. EcoHealth 2019;16:512–22.

55. Cano-Terriza D, Puig-Riba M, Jimenez-Ruiz S, et al. Risk factors of *Toxoplasma gondii* infection in hunting, pet and watchdogs from southern Spain and northern Africa. Parasitol Int 2016;65:363–6.

56. Machacova T, Bartova E, Sedlak K, et al. Seroprevalence and risk factors of infections with *Neospora caninum* and *Toxoplasma gondii* in hunting dogs from Campania region, southern Italy. Folia Parasitol (Praha) 2016;63:2016, 012.

57. Chukwu VE, Daniels OO, Olorunfemi JC, et al. *Cryptosporidium* oocysts: prevalence in dogs in Abujam Federal Capital Territory, Nigeria. Ann Parasit 2019; 65(4):321–7.

58. Collantes-Fernandez E, Gomez-Bautista M, Miro G, et al. Seroprevalence and risk factors associated with *Neospora caninum* infection in different dog populations in Spain. Vet Parasitol 2008;152:148–51.

59. Ortuno A, Scorza V, Castella J, et al. Prevalence of intestinal parasites in shelter and hunting dogs in Catalonia, Northeastern Spain. Vet J 2014;199:465–7.

60. Pullola T, Vierimaa J, Saari S, et al. Canine intestinal helminths in Finland: prevalence, risk factors and endoparasite control practices. Vet Parasitol 2006; 140(3–4):321–6.

61. Stallbaumer M. The prevalence and epidemiology of cestodes in dogs in Clwyd, Wales. II. Hunting dogs. Ann Trop Med Parasitol 1987;81(1):43–7.

62. Al-Sabi MNS, Kapel CMO, Johansson A, et al. A coprological investigation of gastrointestinal and cardiopulmonary parasites in hunting dogs in Denmark. Vet Parasitol 2013;196(3–4):366–72.

63. Lesniak I, Franz M, Heckmann I, et al. Surrogate hosts: hunting dogs and recolonizing grey wolves share their endoparasites. Int J Parasitol Parasites Wildl 2017; 6(3):278–86.

64. Maas M, Dam-Deisz WDC, van Roon AM, et al. Significant increase of *Echinococcus multilocularis* prevalence in foxes, but no increased predicted risk for humans. Vet Parasitol 2014;202:167–72.

65. Oksanen A, Lavikainen A. Echinococcus canadensis transmission in the North. Vet Parasitol 2015;213(3–4):182–6.

66. Wetscher M, Hacklander K, Faber V, et al. Hunting poses only a low risk for alveolar echinococcosis. Front Public Health 2019;7:7.

67. Grech-Angelini S, Richmonne C, de Garam CP, et al. Identification and molecular characterization of *Echinococcus canadensis* G6/7 in dogs from Corsica, France. Parasitol Res 2019;118(4):1313–9.

68. Bork-Mimm S, Rinder H. High prevalence of *Capillaria plica* infections in red foxes (*Vulpes vulpes*) in Southern Germany. Parasitol Res 2011;108(4):1063–7.

69. Callegari D, Kramer L, Cantoni AM, et al. Canine bladderworm (*Capillaria plica*) infection associated with glomerular amyloidosis. Vet Parasitol 2010;168(3–4): 338–41.

70. Mylonakis ME, Koutinas AF, Liapi MV, et al. A comparison of the prevalence of *Spirocerca lupi* in three groups of dogs with different life and hunting styles. J Helminthol 2001;75:359–61.

71. Alshehabat MA. Sublingual vein infestation with leech *Limnatis nilotica* in a hunting dog. Ann Parasitol 2016;62(4):359–61.

72. Apesteguia MA, Portell JBA, Kassab NH, et al. Severe trombiculiasis in hunting dogs infested with *Neotrombicula inopinata* (Acari: Trombiculidae). J Med Entomol 2019;56(5):1389–94.

73. Cramer SD, Campbell GA, Njaa BL, et al. Pseudorabies virus infection in Oklahoma hunting dogs. J Vet Diagn Invest 2011;23(5):915–23.

74. Pederson K, Turnage CT, Gaston WD, et al. Pseudorabies detected in hunting dogs in Alabama an Arkansas after close contact with feral swine (*Sus scrofa*). BMC Vet Res 2018;14:388–95.

75. Cano-Terriza D, Martinez R, Moreno A, et al. Survey of Aujeszky's disease virus in hunting dogs from Spain. Ecohealth 2019;16(2):351–5.

76. Engelhart S, Schneider S, Buder A, et al. MRI in a dog with confirmed pseudorabies infection. Tierarztl Prax Ausg K Kleintiere Heimtiere 2019;47(4):272–81.

77. Steinrig A, Revilla-Fernandez S, Kolodziejek J, et al. Detection and molecular characterization of Suid herpesvirus type 1 in Austrian wild boar and hunting dogs. Vet Microbiol 2012;157(3–4):276–84.

78. Mor SM, Wiethoelter AK, Lee A, et al. Emergence of *Brucella suis* in dogs in New South Wales, Australia: clinical findings and implications for zoonotic transmission. BMC Vet Res 2016;12:199–208.

79. James DR, Golovsky G, Thornton JM, et al. Clinical management of *Brucella suis* infection in dogs and implications for public health. Aust Vet J 2017;95(1–2): 19–25.

80. Kirino Y, Nakano N, Hagio M, et al. Infection of a group of boar-hunting dogs with *Paragonimus westermani* in Miyazaki Prefecture, Japan. Vet Parasitol 2008; 158(4):376–9.

81. Kirino Y, Nakano N, Doanh PN, et al. A seroepidemiological survey for paragonimiosis among boar-hunting dogs in central and southern Kyushu, Japan. Vet Parasitol 2009;161(3–4):335–8.

82. Irie T, Yamaguchi Y, Doanh PN, et al. Infection with *Paragonimus westermani* of boar-hunting dogs in Western Japan maintained via artificial feeding with wild boar meat by hunters. J Vet Med Sci 2017;79(8):1419–25.

83. Machado FP, Kmetiuk LB, Teider-Juniior PI, et al. Seroprevalence of anti-*Toxoplasma gondii* antibodies in wild boars (*Sus scrofa*), hunting dogs and hunters of Brazil. PLoS One 2019;14(10):e0223474.

84. Kmetiuk LB, de Sousa Hunold Lara MdCC, Villalobos EMC, et al. Serosurvey of Eastern, Western, and Venezuelan Equine Encephalitis viruses in wild boars (*Sus scrofa*), hunting dogs, and hunters of Brazil. Vector Borne Zoonotic Dis 2002. https://doi.org/10.1089/vbz.2019.2596.

85. Steiss J, Braund K, Wright J, et al. Coccygeal muscle injury in English pointers (Limber Tail). J Vet Intern Med 1999;13:540–8.

86. Devor M, Serby R. Fibrotic contracture of the canine infraspinatus muscle: pathophysiology and prevention by early surgical intervention. Vet Comp Orthop Traumatol 2006;19:20 117–121.

87. Ehenvall A, Hansson K, Sateri H, et al. Pulmonary oedema in Swedish hunting dogs. J Small Anim Pract 2003;44:209–17.

88. Egenvall A, Swenson L, Andersson K. Inheritance and determinants of pulmonary oedema in Swedish hunting dogs. Vet Rec 2004;155(5):144–8.

Breeding Program Management

Pamela S. Haney, MS[a],*, Robyn R. Wilborn, DVM, MS, DACT[b]

KEYWORDS

- Breeding colony • Canine breeding management • Breeding stock selection
- Estimated breeding value • K9 • Canine • Working dog

KEY POINTS

- Acquire knowledge regarding breed-specific health conditions and conduct-appropriate medical testing to select foundational breeding stock.
- Establish desired colony phenotypes. Develop a standardized evaluation process for breeding stock and progeny that produces valid, reliable data in the form of numeric scores.
- Replacement breeding stock and outside stud dogs should be held to the same medical and behavioral standards as foundational breeding stock.
- Establish a structured puppy development plan with activities tailored to the 4 developmental stages.
- Capture and organize population data in a useable and accurate format. It is suggested to avoid comments stored as free text as the source of objective information in databases.

INTRODUCTION

Currently, there is an increasing need for specialized working dogs that exceeds the supply available.[1] Working dogs may operate in government, private industry, or service organizations.[2] Working dogs typically consist of large-breed sporting, herding, hound, or working breeds.[3] The main goal of producing purpose-bred working dogs is to make genetic progress to enhance their capabilities. Breeders should strive to improve health and behavioral characteristics in their colony while also balancing clearly defined and attainable production goals. Breeders should educate themselves on the basics of canine genetics and understand that collecting and maintaining accurate records is vitally important for making genetic progress. Pedigree depth should also be established for making guided mating selections to achieve production goals.

The authors declare that the research was conducted in the absence of any commercial or financial relationships that could be construed as a potential conflict of interest.
^a Canine Performance Sciences Program, College of Veterinary Medicine, Auburn University, 104 Greene Hall, Auburn, AL 36849, USA; ^b Department of Clinical Sciences, College of Veterinary Medicine, Auburn University, 1220 Wire Road, Auburn, AL 36849, USA
* Corresponding author.
E-mail address: wiltpam@auburn.edu

Breeders should be knowledgeable about the genetic problems that affect their specific breed. Breeding stock should be medically and behaviorally screened. Knowing there is risk involved with breeding animals, breeders should select mating pairs based on multiple criteria. Breeding a few good-quality litters is easier than dozens of litters,[4] so breeders should grow their population gradually. It is impossible to guarantee that every single puppy will be successful, but gradual growth will allow colony advancement. Breeders should not expect to be clear of all defects after one generation because breeding that "perfect" dog will take several years, likely decades, and many generations, but should realize forward progress should be made with each generation (**Figs. 1–3**).

This article is designed to review active breeding colony management methods of a working dog population and use Auburn University College of Veterinary Medicine's Canine Performance Sciences (AUCPS) Breeding Program (Auburn, AL, USA) as a reference. The ultimate goal of the AUCPS colony is to advance the practices of selective breeding, reproductive health, and cognitive-behavioral development practices of working dogs to scientifically improve and understand how to produce the most elite dogs. AUCPS has always been focused on quality over quantity and has chosen not to compromise on breeding stock selection. The Auburn Dog dynamically represents the vision and values of Auburn University to improve the lives of the people of Alabama, the nation, and the world by enhancing safety, security, and animal health.

COLONY SIZE AND BREED

Breeders should select a breed to produce and then determine if their colony will be self-sustaining or part of a breeding cooperative based on the number of litters they plan to produce each year. Populations that produce 20 to 25 litters of a single breed per year can self-sustain a closed population for at least 15 to 20 years.[4] AUCPS is a medium-sized production colony in its 20th year of production that has produced a total of 140 litters of purpose-bred working dogs. Annually, AUCPS produces an average of 7 litters from a breeding stock ratio of 10 dams to 10 studs. The colony consists of Labrador retrievers and Labrador retriever × German wire-haired pointer

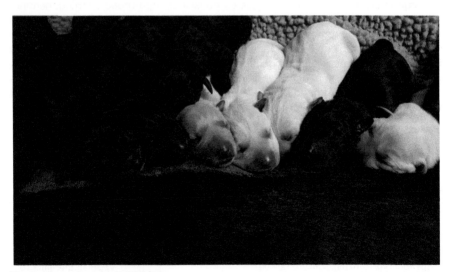

Fig. 1. Three-day-old AUCPS litter.

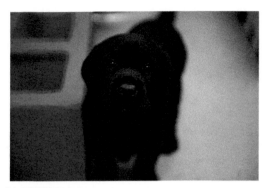

Fig. 2. Five-week-old AUCPS puppy.

crossbred dogs. Comprehending the size, scope, and focus of the AUCPS program will help breeders understand some of the parameters and decision-making factors that are discussed in this article.

PROTOCOLS AND RECORD KEEPING

It is critically important for breeders to document information about their colony and establish program expectations and goals from the beginning. It is key to outline how the following items will be measured and recorded: breeding protocols, behavioral measures, record-keeping systems, and criteria for obtaining breeding stock.[5] Breeders should capture and organize population data in a useable and accurate format.

Record keeping and pedigree depth will allow breeders to better understand and analyze their population. Electronic records are best, as they allow for easier analysis of population data. Avoid the use of comments stored as free text as the source of objective information in population databases. Pedigree depth will help breeders make educated decisions regarding their population. Using breed databases like the Orthopedic Foundation for Animals (OFA), USA[6,7] allows breeders to use pedigree

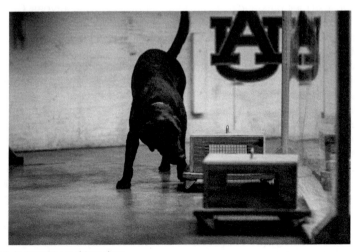

Fig. 3. Adult AUCPS working dog.

information to reduce the incidence of genetic disease, or participating in breeding co-operatives like the International Working Dog Registry,[1] that organizes pedigree and phenotype data on a large number of dogs, will allow breeders to maximize the pedigree depth and historical knowledge of populations to make better informed decisions.

BREEDING STOCK SELECTION

Selection of high-quality breeding stock is crucial to producing high-quality offspring. Breeders should have a methodological approach for selecting breeding stock and should conduct medical and behavioral evaluations on said breeding stock before mating dogs. Screening the entire population to establish complete pedigree data is a best practice for making informed decisions, but screening all breeding stock must occur before mating. It is necessary to acquire knowledge regarding breed-specific health conditions and conduct-appropriate medical testing to select breeding stock.

Health Evaluations

Breeders should establish strict medical requirements for selecting foundational and replacement breeding stock, and they should be especially knowledgeable about the genetic problems that affect their specific breed. Breeding stock should be medically sound, meaning they should be normal/clear of all health defects. Breeders should only select breeding stock that meets those standards in order to reduce the incidence of inherited disease. The Canine Health Information Center (CHIC) is a centralized canine health database jointly sponsored by the American Kennel Club Canine Health Foundation, USA, and the OFA that provides a list of breed-specific health screening tests (www.ofa.org). Breeders can use the breed-specific information listed on the CHIC Web site as a minimum standard of screening tests they should complete before choosing to mate their dogs. This Web site also has helpful links for how testing can be accomplished and even includes submission forms to facilitate the process.

Depending on the ability to breed away from health defects in some breeding populations, it is sometimes necessary to retain a dog that may have a certain health defect because of their outstanding behavioral/performance phenotypes. Genetic diseases with a reliable screening test and a simple recessive pattern of inheritance can be managed effectively within a breeding population by ensuring that carrier dogs are never mated together. Examples of these types of diseases are exercise-induced collapse, centronuclear myopathy, and progressive retinal atrophy. If a genetic carrier exists in the colony, the goal should be to only select progeny with normal/clear results, thus moving toward a more medically sound population.

For radiographic evaluation scores, breeders should have strict requirements that are nonnegotiable for selection of breeding stock. Working dogs that are otherwise successful will not be procured, or will be rejected for service, if they have any radiographic evidence of hip, elbow, shoulder, or stifle joint osteoarthritis or transitional vertebrae.[3,8] Breeding stock should have radiographic evaluations before producing offspring. Breeding colonies that perform radiographic evaluations and researchers have shown that hip and elbow dysplasia are heritable in various working breeds and have heritability scores ranging from 0.18 to 0.76 and 0.31 to 0.77, respectively.[9–18] Several methods are available for obtaining hip dysplasia scoring/assessments. The main radiographic approaches are operated by the OFA in the United States, the British Veterinary Association Kennel Club in the United Kingdom and

Australasia, and the Fédération Cynologique Internationale in Europe.[19] A main cause of hip dysplasia is the presence of excessive hip joint laxity, which causes changes in the acetabulum,[20] and breeders have found the addition of the PennHIP evaluation to be extremely useful in detecting these changes in a more discriminating manner. The PennHIP evaluation measures passive hip joint laxity from radiographic views of the pelvis under stress (ie, compression and distraction views with the use of a distraction bar).[21]

PennHIP distraction index (DI) can be effectively used to make accurate evidence-based potential breeder selection decisions (**Fig. 4**). At least 2 working dog colonies have demonstrated that the PennHIP evaluation has more effectively reduced the prevalence of hip dysplasia in breeding populations, and they recommend colonies use PennHIP evaluations as a selective breeding tool.[10,18,22]

All AUCPS breeding stock must pass all standard medical evaluations before admittance into the breeding colony (**Table 1**). All breeding stock have routine hip joint radiographic evaluations. Radiographs are not conducted if females are in estrus, in accordance with OFA and PennHIP guidelines. AUCPS breeding stock must have a PennHIP DI $\leq$0.30 and an OFA score of "excellent" or "good." Dogs with "excellent" or "good" OFA scores and slightly greater than 0.30 DI have been infrequently permitted as breeding stock because of their other outstanding behavioral phenotypes. AUCPS breeding stock must have normal elbows, shoulders, stifles, and lumbar spine. Ideally, all breeding stock iss normal/clear on all breed-specific genetic tests. Other AUCPS examinations include OFA eye examinations, cardiac examinations, *Brucella canis* screenings, and breeding soundness examinations. Males should be screened for *B canis* twice annually, or before mating if testing is not current.

Proactively using the expertise of a board-certified theriogenologist will aid in the selection and screening of breeding stock. Theriogenologists specialize in veterinary reproduction. Find a veterinary reproduction specialist through the American College of Theriogenologists Web page (www.theriogenology.org). If there is no specialist convenient to your area, the Society for Theriogenology provides resources of veterinary professionals with a special interest in reproduction (www.therio.org).

Behavioral Evaluations

Breeders should define desired phenotypic traits specific to their breed's working task[23] and create a standard evaluation process so that all dogs in the colony may matriculate through the program during development. Breeders should develop a standardized evaluation process that produces valid, reliable data in the form of numeric scores. All dogs produced in the colony should, if possible, complete behavioral evaluations so data can be logged for use in calculating estimated breeding values (EBVs) and mating pair selection decisions. EBVs are statistical predictions of relative genetic worth of individual dogs and can help breeders select dogs with greater potential for producing successful offspring.

Several organizations have developed evaluation measures that provide valid and reliable behavior tests specific to working dog roles, which are valuable tools for screening dogs for selection.[24–26] Detection dog colonies use behavioral evaluations that consist of performance, trainability, and environmental domains.[26] The Swedish Armed Forces (Sweden) use temperament testing to evaluate prospective military working dogs, which consists of both subjective and objective behavioral ratings. The subjective component evaluates global behavior of the subject and is based on overall perception of dog's aggregate behavioral disposition, whereas the objective component is based on observed behaviors in a particular test situation and then are objectively scored.[27] Although beyond the scope of this article, in-depth

10/30/2020   Report Viewer

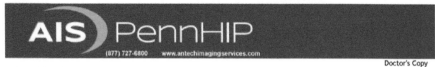

Doctor's Copy

PennHIP Report

Referring Veterinarian: Dr Robert Cole	Clinic Name: Auburn University
Email: rcc0025@auburn.edu	Clinic Address: 1500 Wire Rd College of Veterinary Medicine
	Auburn, AL 36849
	Phone: (334) 844-5045
	Fax:(334) 844-6417

Patient Information

Client: AUBURN, AUBURN	Tattoo Num:
Patient Name: ARIEL6	Patient ID:
Reg. Name:	Registration Num:
PennHIP Num:	Microchip Num:
Species: Canine	Breed: LABRADOR RETRIEVER
Date of Birth: 14 Mar 2019	Age: 11 mon
Sex: Female	Weight: 57.3 lbs/26 kgs
Date of Study: 12 Feb 2020	Date Submitted: 12 Feb 2020
Date of Report: 14 Feb 2020	

Findings

Distraction Index (DI): Right DI = 0.20, Left DI = 0.22.

Osteoarthritis (OA): **No radiographic evidence of OA for either hip.**

Cavitation/Other Findings: No cavitation present.

Interpretation

Distraction Index (DI): The laxity ranking is based on the hip with the greater laxity (larger DI). In this case the DI used is 0.22.

OA Risk Category: The DI is less than or equal to 0.30. This patient is at minimal risk for hip OA.

Distraction Index Chart:

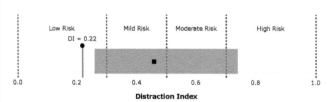

BREED STATISTICS: This interpretation is based on a cross-section of 36151 canine patients of the LABRADOR RETRIEVER breed in the AIS PennHIP database. The gray strip represents the central 90% range of DIs (0.26 - 0.74) for the breed. The breed average DI is 0.46 (solid square). The patient DI is the solid circle (0.22).

SUMMARY: The degree of laxity (DI = 0.22) ranks the hip within the tightest 5% of DIs for the breed. This amount of hip laxity places the hip at a minimal risk to develop hip OA. **No radiographic evidence of OA for either hip.**

INTERPRETATION AND RECOMMENDATIONS: No OA/Minimal Risk: Unlikely to show radiographic evidence of hip OA; even more unlikely to develop clinical signs of hip dysplasia. **Recommendations:** Normal to strenuous activity is permitted. Keep lean: try to maintain BCS at 5/9 for a longer and healthier life. **Breeding Recommendations:** Please Consult the PennHIP Manual.

COMMENTS:

None

Fig. 4. Sample PennHIP report for an AUCPS dog.

Table 1
Auburn University College of Veterinary Medicine's Canine Performance Sciences standard medical testing

Radiology Examinations	Genetic Testing	Other Examinations
Hip dysplasia examination (OFA and PennHIP)	EIC (exercise-induced collapse) genetic test	Brucellosis evaluation
Elbow dysplasia examination	Centronuclear myopathy (CNM) genetic test	Eye examination by a board-certified ophthalmologist (ACVO)
Shoulder dysplasia examination	Progressive rod cone disease-progressive retinal atrophy (PRCD-PRA) genetic test	Advanced cardiac examination
Stifle examination	Retinal dysplasia/oculoskeletal dysplasia 1 genetic test	Stud dogs: breeding soundness examination by a board-certified theriogenologist (ACT)
Lumbar spine (transitional vertebrae) examination		

behavioral characteristics for explosive detection dogs have been well characterized and outlined in other articles.[28]

Assistance dog evaluations at Canine Companions for Independence (Santa Rosa, CA, USA) consist of the Canine Behavioral Assessment and Research Questionnaire (C-BARQ), which focuses on the frequency and severity of problematic behaviors, and a standardized temperament assessment called the In-For-Training (IFT) test. The C-BARQ has been validated in guide and pet dogs and takes about 15 minutes to complete and consists of 100 items that give a glimpse into the dog's behavioral profile. Assessment begins at 8 weeks of age and is conducted at set time points until the dog enters professional training (approximately 18 months of age). The IFT is a standardized temperament test that is conducted when the dog enters professional training. The IFT tests the dog in 6 normal working-life scenarios that are stimulating enough to potentially trigger problem behaviors.[25]

AUCPS has a standard development and training program with set times for behavioral evaluations (**Table 2**). AUCPS performs puppy evaluations at 5 time points throughout the puppy's first year of life and an additional evaluation once a dog is selected as a breeder, but before mating (**Fig. 5**).

Medical screening data and behavioral evaluation data should be included in population databases to calculate EBVs and make informed mating pair selections. EBVs do not yield an absolute genetic value, but provide a rating for each dog based on

Table 2
Auburn University College of Veterinary Medicine's Canine Performance Sciences behavioral evaluation timepoints with ages

Evaluation Timepoint	7-wk Evaluation	3-mo Evaluation	5-mo Evaluation	10-mo Evaluation	12-mo Final Evaluation	Additional Breeder Evaluation
Age of puppy at evaluation	7 wk old (49 d)	12 wk old (84 d)	22 wk old (154 d)	44 wk old (308 d)	52 wk old (365 d)	65 wk old (456 d)

CPS Breeding Program 3 Month Assessment										
Dog		USDA#			DOB	/	/		Age	
Assessor					Date of Assessment	/	/			

LOCATION 1

Performance

	Severe	Moderate	Mild	Very Mild	Absent	Not Exposed	Issues (circle issue(s) only)		Comments		
Reward Possession	1	2	3	4	5		Selective--> yes				
Arousal-Pre-work (workability)	1	2	3	4	5		Reward Persistence	1	2	3	4	5
Sensitivity to object contact	1	2	3	4	5		tight spaces (corners)				
							obstacles	overhead			
Novel Objects (1)	1	2	3	4	5		activated	aggressive	flight	inhibited	
Elevation	1	2	3	4	5		activated	aggressive	flight	inhibited	
Stairs (1) solid	1	2	3	4	5		up	down			
							activated	aggressive	flight	inhibited	
Anxious in unfamiliar locations	1	2	3	4	5						
Noise Sensitivity (1)	1	2	3	4	5		high stimulus	low stimulus			
							activated	aggressive	flight	inhibited	
Hunt	1	2	3	4	5		Handler Engagement	1	2	3	4	5
Task Engagement	1	2	3	4	5		Arousal-Work	1	2	3	4	5
Distraction-->	auditory	visual	people	animal		Air Scenting	1	2	3	4	5

Environmental

	Severe	Moderate	Mild	Very Mild	Absent	Not Exposed	Issues (mark only if an issue)			
Visual Startle (1)	1	2	3	4	5		activated	aggressive	flight	inhibited
Visual Startle (2)	1	2	3	4	5		activated	aggressive	flight	inhibited
Acoustic Startle (1)	1	2	3	4	5		activated	aggressive	flight	inhibited
Acoustic Startle (2)	1	2	3	4	5		activated	aggressive	flight	inhibited
Animated Objects (1)	1	2	3	4	5		activated	aggressive	flight	inhibited
Animated Objects (2)	1	2	3	4	5		activated	aggressive	flight	inhibited

LOCATION 2

Environmental

	Severe	Moderate	Mild	Very Mild	Absent	Not Exposed	Issues (mark only if an issue)			
Traffic	1	2	3	4	5		activated	aggressive	flight	inhibited
People	1	2	3	4	5		single	crowds		
							odd position	children		
							activated	aggressive	flight	inhibited
Stairs (2) solid	1	2	3	4	5		up	down		
							activated	aggressive	flight	inhibited
Anxious in unfamiliar locations	1	2	3	4	5					
Noise Sensitivity (2)	1	2	3	4	5		high stimulus	low stimulus		
							activated	aggressive	flight	inhibited
Surfaces	1	2	3	4	5		slippery floors	grated floors		
							activated	aggressive	flight	inhibited
Novel Objects (2)	1	2	3	4	5		activated	aggressive	flight	inhibited

Overall Comments

Tractability	1		2		3		4		5

Fig. 5. AUCPS 3-month behavioral evaluation.

objective scoring criteria. The Seeing Eye, Inc (Morristown, NJ, USA), a guide-dog foundation, has used EBVs to make replacement breeder selections and have observed genetic improvement in both health and behavioral traits.[29] The use of EBVs could increase the accuracy of identifying potential breeders at an earlier age.[18]

REPLACEMENT BREEDING STOCK

Replacement breeding stock should be held to the same medical and behavioral standards as foundational breeding stock. It is recommended to replace breeding stock from within the colony whenever possible, as the addition of outside stock may bring in undesirable traits.[4] In the AUCPS colony, female breeding stock is typically replaced from within the population, whereas studs are replaced from both within and outside the population.

OUTSIDE COLONY STUD DOG USE

When incorporating an outside stud dog into a closed colony, it is important to perform the same comprehensive medical and behavioral evaluations that were conducted on foundation breeding stock. If possible, breeders should medically and behaviorally screen the outside stud's parents, siblings, and offspring to establish pedigree depth. Evaluating dogs with another colony/agency that has similar working dog characteristics is the best place to start,[5] which highlights the importance of collaboration between like-minded breeding organizations. Outside stud dogs should only be introduced into the colony if the breeder is trying to create genetic diversity within the colony, as outside genetics may bring in undesirable traits.[4]

PUPPY DEVELOPMENT PLAN

Even dogs with the best genetics will not achieve their full potential without a proper development plan. Development plans should consist of environmental exposure and job-specific performance training. Puppies go through 4 periods of development during puppyhood: neonatal, transitional, socialization, and juvenile.[30] Development programs should take into account these 4 unique phases and develop training plans that will successfully progress the puppy through each stage.

Some programs raise puppies in homes with foster families (ie, puppy raisers or puppy walkers), in prison systems with inmates, or in kennel facilities. At The Seeing Eye, puppies are weaned from their mothers around 7 weeks of age and placed in puppy raiser homes. Puppies progress through a structured development plan with their volunteer family until 14 to 18 months of age[5] and then return for medical evaluation and begin a 4-month plus training period where they learn to work as guides for blind people.[18] Puppies from the National Guide Dog School of Scandicci (Florence, Italy) are whelped in a home environment, weaned at 8 weeks, and live with puppy walker families until 12 months of age. Their puppies are given as much environmental stimuli as possible while living with a puppy walker family.[31] Puppies in the Swedish Armed Forces Breeding Program are weaned at 8 weeks of age and are also raised in puppy raiser homes. Their puppy raisers are asked to conduct ordinary house training and obedience training and then return dogs to the Swedish Armed Forces program at 15 to 18 months of age for formal behavioral evaluation.[27]

In the AUCPS colony, puppies are group-housed in the nursery with their littermates and dam until they are 7 weeks old. This period of puppy development includes individual and group development through the introduction of new sounds and sights, reward value building, and obstacle navigations to enhance motor skills and

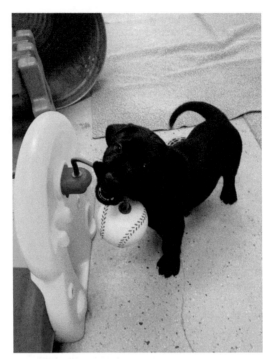

Fig. 6. AUCPS puppy development training at 7 weeks.

problem-solving abilities (**Fig. 6**). The puppies then move to intermediate puppy development from 7 weeks to 6 months of age. During this time, extensive social, environmental, and performance conditioning occurs in the local city and surrounding areas (**Fig. 7**). Puppies are housed in indoor/outdoor kennels, first pair-housed until 13 weeks and then single-housed the remainder of the time. Puppies experience successive approximation of age-appropriate development and exposures, progressing from simple to complex, using positive reinforcement to cultivate a strong working foundation (**Fig. 8**). Intermediate puppy development continues when the puppies are placed in participating prisons for further socialization and development by specially trained inmates from 6 to 10 months of age. Inmates participating in the AUCPS dog program

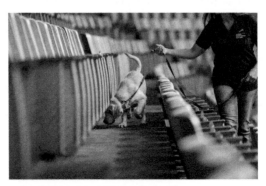

Fig. 7. AUCPS puppy development training at 3 months.

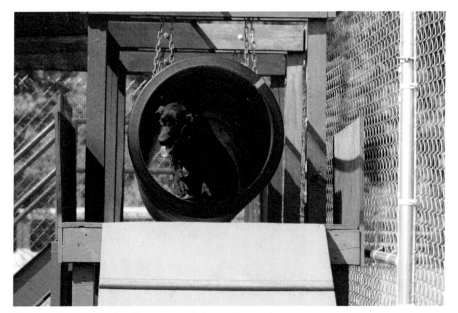

Fig. 8. AUCPS puppy development training at 5 months.

are enrolled in a 1150-hour AUCPS-developed Performance Canine Care and Development course taught in the prisons by trained program managers. The prison program engages dogs in activities like basic odor discrimination games and exposes dogs to tighter living quarters simulating operational work in crowds of people. The

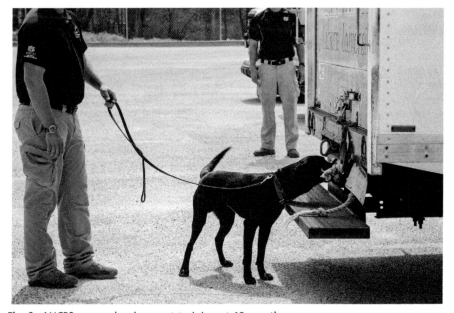

Fig. 9. AUCPS puppy development training at 10 months.

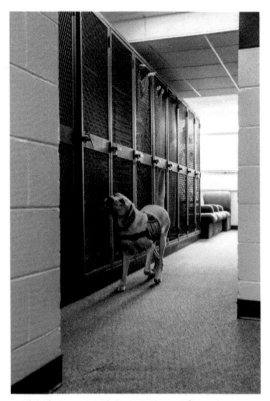

Fig. 10. AUCPS puppy development training at 12 months.

last phase of puppy development commences upon return from the prison program to Auburn at 10 months and continues until the puppies are 12 months and older (**Fig. 9**). During the last phase of development, dogs undergo evaluations for detection performance (**Fig. 10**), physical fitness, environmental soundness, and medical soundness. Final placement of the AUCPS dogs occurs through sale as explosive detection dogs, other types of working dogs, retained for AUCPS breeding or research activities, or, infrequently, offered for adoption. Dogs offered for adoption typically do not possess the necessary behavior repertoire needed for detection work or in-house detection research activities, and/or they are not medically sound (eg, a dog that has transitional vertebrae).

SUMMARY

Breeding colony goals and objectives should be established at the beginning, as well as strict standards for both medical and behavioral screening. Once established, breeders should strive to adhere to these criteria for any dog selected for breeding stock. Quality of the breeding stock should always take precedence, thus creating fewer regrets within a program. Data management is key in a successful program and must be in a clear, objective, and useable format. Breeders should educate themselves in capturing and accurately interpreting the program data in order to use the data effectively. When based on solid medical and behavioral data, breeding decisions become clear, and genetic progress is achieved more readily with each generation.

CLINICS CARE POINTS

- PennHIP distraction index can be effectively used to make accurate evidence-based potential breeder selection decisions.
- Proactively using the expertise of a board-certified theriogenologist will aid in the selection and screening of breeding stock.
- Medical screening data and behavioral evaluation data should be included in population databases to calculate estimated breeding values and make informed mating pair selections.

ACKNOWLEDGMENT

Funding for AUCPS Breeding Program Research was provided by the Auburn University College of Veterinary Medicine Canine Performance Sciences' Help Raise-a-Hero Fund and CPS Donors Walt and Ginger Woltosz, the Alan Kalter and Chris Lezotte Annual Fund for Excellence in Canine Health, Reproduction, and Husbandry, the James M. Hoskins Endowment, and the Diane Carter Memorial Fund.

REFERENCES

1. Leighton EA, Hare E, Thomas S, et al. A solution for the shortage of detection dogs: a detector dog center of excellence and a cooperative breeding program. Front Vet Sci 2018;5:284.
2. Cobb M, Branson N, McGreevy P, et al. The advent of canine performance science: offering a sustainable future for working dogs. Behav Process 2015;110:96–104.
3. Moore GE, Burkman KD, Carter MN, et al. Causes of death or reasons for euthanasia in military working dogs: 927 cases (1993–1996). J Am Vet Med Assoc 2001;219(2):209–14.
4. Leighton EA. Secrets for producing high-quality working dogs. J Vet Behav Clin Appl Res 2009;6(4):212–5.
5. Leighton E, Holle D, Roberts D. The Seeing Eye breeding program: results obtained and lessons learned. Paper presented at: international working dog breeding conference, San Antonio, TX, 10À12 September 2001.
6. Keller GG, Dziuk E, Bell JS. How the Orthopedic Foundation for Animals (OFA) is tackling inherited disorders in the USA: using hip and elbow dysplasia as examples. Vet J 2011;189(2):197–202.
7. Keller GG. The use of health databases and selective breeding: a guide for dog and cat breeders and owners. Columbia (MO): Orthopedic Foundation for Animals; 2018.
8. Worth A, Sandford M, Gibson B, et al. Causes of loss or retirement from active duty for New Zealand police German shepherd dogs. Anim Welf 2013;22(2):166–73.
9. Hou Y, Wang Y, Lu X, et al. Monitoring hip and elbow dysplasia achieved modest genetic improvement of 74 dog breeds over 40 years in USA. PloS One 2013; 8(10):e76390.
10. Haney PS, Lazarowski L, Wang X, et al. Effectiveness of PennHIP and Orthopedic Foundation for Animals measurements of hip joint quality for breeding selection to reduce hip dysplasia in a population of purpose-bred detection dogs. J Am Vet Med Assoc 2020;257(3):299–304.
11. Oberbauer A, Keller G, Famula T. Long-term genetic selection reduced prevalence of hip and elbow dysplasia in 60 dog breeds. PLoS One 2017;12(2): e0172918.

12. Wilson BJ, Nicholas FW, James JW, et al. Heritability and phenotypic variation of canine hip dysplasia radiographic traits in a cohort of Australian German shepherd dogs. PLoS One 2012;7(6):e39620.

13. Mäki K, Liinamo A, Ojala M. Estimates of genetic parameters for hip and elbow dysplasia in Finnish Rottweilers. J Anim Sci 2000;78(5):1141–8.

14. Leighton EA, Linn JM, Willham RL, et al. A genetic study of canine hip dysplasia. Am J Vet Res 1977;38(2):241.

15. Swenson L, Audell L, Hedhammar A. Prevalence and inheritance of and selection for elbow arthrosis in Bernese mountain dogs and Rottweilers in Sweden and benefit: cost analysis of a screening and control program. J Am Vet Med Assoc 1997;210(2):215–21.

16. Guthrie S, Pidduck H. Heritability of elbow osteochondrosis within a closed population of dogs. J Small Anim Pract 1990;31(2):93–6.

17. Studdert V, Lavelle R, Beilharz R, et al. Clinical features and heritability of osteochondrosis of the elbow in Labrador retrievers. J Small Anim Pract 1991;32(11):557–63.

18. Leighton EA, Holle D, Biery DN, et al. Genetic improvement of hip-extended scores in 3 breeds of guide dogs using estimated breeding values: notable progress but more improvement is needed. PLoS One 2019;14(2):e0212544.

19. Flückiger M. Scoring radiographs for canine hip dysplasia-the big three organisations in the world. Eur J Companion Anim Pract 2007;17(2):135–40.

20. Henrigson B, Norberg I, Olssons SE. On the etiology and pathogenesis of hip dysplasia: a comparative review. J Small Anim Pract 1966;7(11):673–88.

21. Lust G, Williams A, Burton-Wurster N, et al. Joint laxity and its association with hip dysplasia in Labrador retrievers. Am J Vet Res 1993;54(12):1990–9.

22. Leighton EA. Genetics of canine hip dysplasia. J Am Vet Med Assoc 1997;210(10):1474–9.

23. Beilharz R. Evolutionary aspects on breeding of working dogs. Behav Biol dogs 2007;166.

24. Harvey ND, Craigon PJ, Sommerville R, et al. Test-retest reliability and predictive validity of a juvenile guide dog behavior test. J Vet Behav 2016;11:65–76.

25. Bray EE, Levy KM, Kennedy BS, et al. Predictive models of assistance dog training outcomes using the canine behavioral assessment and research questionnaire and a standardized temperament evaluation. Front Vet Sci 2019;6:49.

26. Lazarowski L, Haney PS, Brock J, et al. Investigation of the behavioral characteristics of dogs purpose-bred and prepared to perform Vapor Wake® detection of person-borne explosives. Front Vet Sci 2018;5:50.

27. Wilsson E, Sinn DL. Are there differences between behavioral measurement methods? A comparison of the predictive validity of two ratings methods in a working dog program. Appl Anim Behav Sci 2012;141(3–4):158–72.

28. Lazarowski L, Waggoner L, Krichbaum S, et al. Selecting dogs for explosives detection: behavioral characteristics. Front Vet Sci 2020;7(597).

29. Leighton EA. How to use estimated breeding values to genetically improve dog guides. Paper presented at: Presented at a Meeting of the "Original Group 2003.

30. Scott JP, Fuller JL. Genetics and the social behavior of the dog, vol. 570. University of Chicago Press; 2012.

31. Cecchi F, Vezzosi T, Branchi G, et al. Inbreeding and health problems prevalence in a colony of guide dogs: a cohort of 40 Labrador retrievers. Acta Agr Scan 2020;69(3):183–8.

Production and Reproductive Management

Robyn R. Wilborn, DVM, MS[a],*, Pamela S. Haney, MS[b]

KEYWORDS

- Breeding colony • Breeding management • Whelping • Fertility • k9 • Canine
- Working dog

KEY POINTS

- Proactively work with a specialist in veterinary reproduction to help maximize reproductive success and efficient use of resources.
- Determine whether the colony will be self-sustaining or part of a breeding cooperative based on the number of litters produced each year.
- Establish mating protocols based on ovulation timing for fresh, cool-shipped, and frozen semen types.
- Establish whelping protocols and decision points for intervening outlined before parturition for free whelping, assisted free whelping, and cesarean sections.

INTRODUCTION

In working dog programs, reproductive management with veterinary intervention can maximize success. Although large programs may employ their own veterinary team, small to medium-sized programs typically use a local veterinary clinic for their canine medical needs. This article goes into more detail regarding the role of the veterinary team in supporting small to medium-sized canine reproduction programs. Although this veterinary care does come at a cost, which needs to be budgeted, it also greatly improves reproductive efficiency and maximizes use of valuable genetic resources. In turn, this leads to fewer medical washouts from improved health screenings as well as a higher percentage of pups weaned and placed into successful careers.

This article reviews active breeding colony management methods of working dog populations and uses the Auburn University College of Veterinary Medicine's Canine Performance Sciences (AUCPS) Breeding Program (Auburn, AL) as a reference (**Fig. 1**). For a full description of the AUCPS program, see the chapter in this issue entitled "Breeding Program Management" by Haney and Wilborn.

Conflict of interest: The authors declare that this research was conducted in the absence of any commercial or financial relationships that could be construed as a potential conflict of interest.
[a] Department of Clinical Sciences, College of Veterinary Medicine, Auburn University, 1220 Wire Road, Auburn, AL 36849, USA; [b] Canine Performance Sciences Program, College of Veterinary Medicine, Auburn University, 104 Greene Hall, Auburn, AL 36849, USA
* Corresponding author.
E-mail address: wilborn@auburn.edu

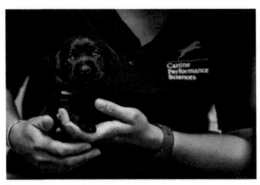

Fig. 1. AUCPS breeding colony puppy.

BREEDING MANAGEMENT
Veterinary Intervention for Reproduction

When it comes to the logistics of reproduction, veterinary intervention can help maximize success. Established breeders should first examine records from the program to determine the areas of greatest need (eg, prebreeding health screenings, pregnancy rates, or neonatal losses) and then partner with a veterinary clinic that routinely works with breeders and understands breeding program goals.

Board-certified theriogenologists, specialists in veterinary reproduction, can help maximize reproductive success. Theriogenologists in a certain geographic area are easily located by visiting the Web site for the credentialing organization, the American College of Theriogenologists (www.theriogenology.org). If there is no specialist convenient to your area, visit the Web site for the Society for Theriogenology (SFT) to find a veterinary clinic with a focus on reproduction (www.therio.org). The SFT is an organization of veterinary professionals with a special interest in reproduction. Although not board certified, these veterinarians are dedicated to reproduction and frequently attend meetings and seminars to further their reproductive knowledge and skills. The SFT has more than 1800 members in the United States alone, so finding a veterinarian through this organization is a viable option in most locations in the United States.

Colony Size and Statistics

Breeders should determine whether their colony will be self-sustaining or part of a breeding cooperative based on the number of litters they plan to produce each year. Large populations that produce 20 to 25 litters of a single breed per year can self-sustain a closed colony population for at least 15 to 20 years.[1] Colonies that produce fewer than 10 litters per year should consider joining a breeding cooperative.

In most colonies, sires produce more offspring than dams. Thus, to maintain genetic diversity, breeders should limit the number of litters produced by an individual sire or dam to keep the level of inbreeding to no more than 1% or 2% per generation. This limitation can often be accomplished in medium-sized breeding colonies by allowing a dam to produce 3 or 4 litters and a sire to produce no more than 4 to 8 litters, depending on the effective population size of the colony.[2,3]

Effective population size is the population genetic parameter that determines the effectiveness of selection relative to random genetic drift (Ne).[4] It measures the average number of individuals who contributed to the next generation. Because of genetic drift, a smaller Ne results in a stronger genetic drift. In an inbred closed colony population, it can be said that effective population size measures the decrease of genetic diversity of the population being studied.[5] Kennel Club–registered United Kingdom Labrador retrievers from 2002 to 2008 had an effective population size range of 54.5 to 82.3, when the entire pedigree was used and when individuals with inbreeding coefficients equal to 0 were removed, respectively.[6]

AUCPS, a medium-sized colony, has produced a total of 140 litters of purpose-bred working dogs with an average of 7 litters annually from available breeding stock ratio of 10 dams to 10 studs. The colony consists of Labrador retrievers and Labrador retriever X German wirehaired pointer crossbred dogs. AUCPS dams are typically bred on the first heat cycle that occurs after 12 months of age, then on each subsequent cycle until they have reached 3 litters. A dam may produce a fourth litter if her previous litters are highly successful and representative of the desired phenotype and medical standards of the population. Stud dogs typically sire an average of 2 to 4 litters before retirement from the breeding program. Average litter size in the AUCPS population is 6.81 ± 2.63 puppies born per litter and 6.41 ± 2.69 puppies weaned per litter (n = 140 litters). See **Table 1** for further statistics about the AUCPS colony.

The Seeing Eye, (Morristown, NJ), a guide dog foundation, is in its 91st year of production and currently produces German shepherds, Labrador retrievers, golden retrievers, and Labrador X golden retriever crossbred dogs. As a large closed colony, they whelp around 20 to 25 litters per year per breed. Dogs in their population are typically selected for breeding at 22 to 24 months of age. Stud dogs are limited to 8 to 10 matings and females, once selected, are bred on each heat cycle until they reach 4 years of age.[2] Litter sizes in The Seeing Eye's Labrador retriever population average 6.72 ± 2.30 puppies born per litter and 6.39 ± 2.41 puppies weaned per litter (n = 618 litters), and German shepherd dogs average 6.38 ± 2.47 puppies born per litter and 6.21 ± 2.51 puppies weaned per litter (n = 703 litters).[7]

Guiding Eyes for the Blind (Yorktown Heights, NY), a guide dog foundation, is also a large closed colony that produces Labrador retrievers and German shepherds. They perform 65 breedings per year, which result in 61 whelped litters per year with an average Labrador retriever litter size of 7.9 puppies born and 7.2 puppies weaned.[8]

The Swedish Armed Forces originally created a closed breeding colony of German shepherds with 70 to 80 females and 15 males, recruiting replacement breeders from

Table 1
Auburn University College of Veterinary Medicine's Canine Performance Sciences breeding colony population statistics reported as averages and standard deviations

Dam Service Life	2.69 ± 1.55 litters n = 140 litters	Litter Inbreeding Coefficient	1.7% ± 2.8% n = 140 litters
Age Of First Estrus	15.37 ± 4.81 mo n = 27 dams	Litters Per Year	7.00 ± 2.15 litters n = 20 y
Interestrus Interval	7.37 ± 1.58 mo n = 25 dams	Pups Per Year	47.70 ± 15.61 pups n = 20 y
Sire Service Life	2.13 ± 2.48 litters n = 140 litters	Puppies Born Per Litter	6.81 ± 2.63 pups n = 140 litters
Outside Stud Dogs	Average 2 mating contracts annually	Puppies Weaned Per Litter	6.41 ± 2.69 pups n = 140 litters
—	—	Pup Weaning Age	6 wk
—	—	Labrador Retriever Pups Produced	866 pups
—	—	Crossbred Pups Produced	88 pups

within the population, and producing around 200 to 300 puppies per year.[9,10] Dams whelped an average 3.36 litters, with an average of 8 puppies born per litter in German shepherd dogs. Labrador retriever dams whelped an average 2.95 litters, with an average of 7.5 puppies born per litter.[11]

Selecting Mating Pairs

Breeding stock should have the highest-quality medical and behavioral standards, and mating pairs should be selected with the goal of improving population genetics. Breeders should know the behavioral characteristics to propagate or eliminate in the colony. The overall goal when selecting mating pairs is to avoid matings that could produce disease-affected puppies. Estimated breeding values (EBVs) are a good resource to calculate a dog's genetic risk for developing specific characteristics.[12] EBVs are statistical predictions of relative genetic worth of individual dogs and can help breeders select dogs with greater potential for producing successful offspring. In the AUCPS colony, once all medical requirements are satisfied, mating selections are based on lower inbreeding coefficients of the expected litter, management of other genetic traits, and behavioral phenotypes.

Inbreeding is the degree to which 2 individuals are related to each other through 1 or more common ancestors. Inbreeding coefficient values increase the closer the relationship of the mating pairs. Inbreeding coefficients that are maintained at a low rate allow an increase in genetic variability.[3,13] The AUCPS colony has maintained an inbreeding coefficient around 1.6%. The Seeing Eye, which is a closed colony, has reported average inbreeding coefficients of 26.2% in German shepherds and 22% in in Labrador retrievers.[2] Ideally, breeding colonies would maintain low inbreeding coefficients to keep the level of inbreeding to no more than 1% or 2% per generation.[1]

Breeders should also establish a protocol for whether or not to repeat mating pairs. Although tempting, the repeating of mating pairs fails to make genetic progress; it simply keeps the status quo. AUCPS does not repeat mating pairs, because the primary aim is quality rather than quantity for the program. Breeders that choose to repeat matings should do so with caution, because each repeat litter may present unique issues compared with the previous litter.

Reproductive Techniques

Most breeding colonies use a combination of reproductive techniques, including both natural mating and artificial insemination (AI). AI can include vaginal AI, surgical AI, and transcervical insemination (TCI). The type of insemination method chosen depends on the availability of the stud dog, the type of semen used (fresh, chilled, or frozen), and the quality of the semen sample. AUCPS has several high-quality stud dogs readily available, thus most breedings use a combination of live cover, vaginal AI, and TCI using fresh semen. When stud dogs outside of the AUCPS colony are used for breeding, chilled semen is shipped via overnight delivery and is deposited using the TCI technique.

The TCI technique requires specialized equipment and uses a rigid endoscope to visualize the cervix and thread a small catheter through the cervix and into the uterus, depositing the semen as far cranially as possible and maximizing conception rates and litter sizes (**Fig. 2**). The vaginal AI and TCI techniques are often compared in scientific literature as well as anecdotal reports from breeding programs. In all of these comparisons, TCI yields a higher conception rate and litter size compared with traditional vaginal AI.[14] In the AUCPS colony, adding at least 1 TCI of fresh semen to each

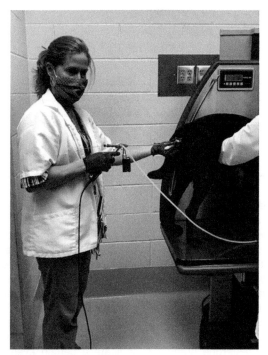

Fig. 2. TCI procedure on an AUCPS bitch.

breeding cycle yielded an increase of 3 puppies per litter compared with cycles where TCI was not performed (unpublished data; AUCPS 2019).

Failure to establish pregnancy or small litter sizes are both detrimental in a canine production program, leading to a high expenditure of resources and time for a very small gain. Moving beyond the reproductive techniques used for breeding, the 2 major challenges that have the biggest impact on fertility in any canine breeding colony are (1) insemination at the improper time, and (2) poor semen quality, both of which are easily managed.

Cycle Management

Insemination at the improper time is a major cause of infertility and subfertility in canine breeding programs.[15–17] For many years, programs relied on vaginal cytology evaluation and/or behavioral receptivity of the female as indications for when to breed. With the increased knowledge and availability of progesterone testing, the measurement of this hormone has become the most reliable method for prediction of the peak fertile window in canine breeding management.[18,19]

For AUCPS, cycle management begins 5 to 7 days after the onset of vulvar swelling or bloody vaginal discharge. Vaginal cytology is measured 2 to 3 times per week until 80% to 100% cornification of vaginal epithelial cells is noted, indicating the transition from proestrus to estrus. At this point, serum samples are taken daily and divided into 2 aliquots from each date. The serum samples are submitted for progesterone testing every 2 to 3 days, with the samples from the remaining days stored in the freezer for later luteinizing hormone (LH) testing (**Table 2**).

Table 2
Auburn University College of Veterinary Medicine's Canine Performance Sciences progesterone values for clinical decisions

Progesterone Value (ng/mL)	Indication
<1.0	Before LH surge
~2.0	LH surge
5–10	Ovulation (typically occurs 2 d after LH surge)
>10	Ovulation complete

Once a progesterone value of ~2.0 ng/mL is identified, the frozen serum samples are then thawed 1 at a time and subjected to a rapid (patient-side) LH test, which indicates a subjective result (positive, negative, or indeterminate) in order to confirm that the LH surge occurred on the day suspected. For the purposes of planning the breeding, peak fertile days are typically days 2 to 4 following ovulation (with ovulation indicated as day 0). This timing is unlike any other species, because the dog ovulates primary oocytes that are not yet capable of fertilization at time of ovulation; canine oocytes require an additional 48 hours following ovulation before fertilization can occur.

It should be emphasized that progesterone testing must be interpreted as a physiologic trend indicating the days of LH surge and ovulation rather than depending on 1 individual progesterone number to indicate a certain event. Also, note that each laboratory may have a slightly different range of values, and the interpretation may need to be adjusted accordingly. This point cannot be overemphasized, especially for those programs that may be new to breeding management.

It is recommended to minimize stress during estrus and gestation to maximize litter success. An increase in cortisol may interfere with the LH surge and jeopardize ovulation. Environmental factors may also increase the chances of spontaneous abortion.[20] It is not recommended to change kennel environments or transport the bitch during this time if it can be avoided.[21] This advice is especially important in high-anxiety temperaments.

Semen Evaluation

The second major cause of infertility and subfertility in a breeding colony is poor semen quality. In programs where AI is used, semen quality is frequently monitored each time a stud dog is collected for insemination or shipping of semen. However, in programs where live cover mating is used, changes in semen quality can remain undetected until females fail to become pregnant and investigation is warranted. Missed cycles are extremely costly in a production program, thus it is always a sound investment to perform a semen evaluation 1 to 2 times per year on males used for live cover matings to ensure that quality parameters are not declining.

A complete semen evaluation is a simple procedure by a reproductive veterinarian. A complete analysis measures 3 parameters: motility (total and progressive motility), morphology (how many of the sperm cells are shaped normally), and concentration (sometimes referred to as sperm count). Once these parameters have been measured, a total number of progressively motile, morphologically normal spermatozoa can be calculated to determine whether quality is adequate. Ideal quality is a progressive motility of 70% or greater and a normal morphology of 60% or greater.[14] Total sperm number varies with the size of the dog and the size of the testicles, with larger breeds able to produce a greater total sperm number than small to medium breeds. The generally accepted breeding dose is a minimum of 150 million progressively motile spermatozoa.[14] AUCPS has established guidelines for outside colony–contracted stud dogs that requires chilled semen shipments to include a minimum of 150 million progressively motile spermatozoa per shipment for a total of 2 shipments per breeding cycle in order to meet the requirement for the contract and disbursement of the breeding portion of the stud fee.

If semen quality parameters decline in an outstanding male, other factors can be adjusted to overcome this setback. For example, rather than continuing to use the stud dog for live cover mating, he could instead be collected and the fresh semen used for a TCI in order to give the poor-quality semen the best chance of establishing a pregnancy.

Brucellosis Testing

Brucella canis is a routine screening test and should always be part of the initial breeding management visit, no matter the health status or breeding history of the female. Male dogs in a kennel situation should be tested annually regardless of their breeding status. Stud dogs should be tested twice yearly if actively used for breeding or shipping of semen.

Reproductive implications from canine brucellosis include abortions in females and orchitis in males. Discospondylitis (acute inflammatory spinal disease) or ophthalmic disease can also occur in either gender as a result of infection, and dogs that have been spayed or neutered can also be infected and shed the disease. Dogs that have never been mated before can contract and shed canine brucellosis. Although often thought to be just a reproductive disease spread through mating and shipped semen, canine brucellosis is also shed in the urine, saliva, and nasal secretions of infected dogs. Most infected dogs show no clinical signs of disease, thus the disease spreads quickly through a kennel in a very short time frame because it is highly contagious from dog to dog through casual contact.[22] Brucellosis is also zoonotic and poses a human health risk to workers within a canine program.

In the AUCPS colony, females are tested at the beginning of each estrus cycle and stud dogs are tested before each mating unless a recent (<6 months) negative test is confirmed and no other matings have occurred in that time frame.

Mating Protocols

Many different mating protocols are used successfully, indicating that there is not necessarily a right/wrong method but slightly different opinions based on both scientific research and anecdotal experience. Breeders should examine the protocols that have been successful for other programs and then combine this with the options or limitations within their program to find a system that maximizes litter success. Guiding Eyes for the Blind mates dogs most often on day 3 or 4 and 5 or 6 after LH surge (initial increase in serum progesterone levels of 1.5 and 2 ng/mL), and this protocol yields an average of 7.9 puppies per litter in Labrador retrievers within their colony.[8] The Seeing Eye mates dogs on days 3 and 5 following LH surge by either live coverage or AI using fresh semen, yielding an average of 6.72 ± 2.30 puppies born per Labrador retriever litter.[7] AUCPS standardized a breeding protocol in 2018 where the sire and dam are mated for 3 days in a row starting 2 days after ovulation, using a combination of TCI and live coverage or vaginal AI with fresh semen, recently yielding an average of 7.47 ± 2.65 puppies per litter (**Fig. 3**).

Since 2018 in the AUCPS colony, dams have been bred using only fresh and chilled semen with the standardized protocol, which has resulted in a 100% conception rate

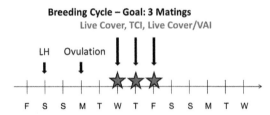

Fig. 3. AUCPS standardized breeding protocol. VAI, vaginal artificial insemination.

and an observed increase from 6 to 7 puppies per litter compared with historical un-standardized mating protocols (**Table 3**).

Estimating Due Dates

Gestation is best estimated by using progesterone concentrations to determine the day of LH surge and ovulation. Parturition normally occurs 65 days (±1 day) from LH surge and 63 days (±1 day) from ovulation, with ovulation usually occurring 48 hours after the LH surge.[23] Guiding Eyes for the Blind bases due dates on 65 days after initial increase in serum progesterone level, whereas AUCPS estimates 63 days ± 1 day from LH surge because of logged colony parturition data (which include declining progesterone values as parturition nears, nesting behavior, and first signs of stage II labor).

Other methods for estimating due dates include gestational aging measurements taken via ultrasonography at the time of pregnancy diagnosis.[23] Although this method is effective, it also has much greater variability and is not recommended as the sole predictor of due dates. However, gestational aging measurements taken at the time of pregnancy diagnosis can be a good method to help confirm due dates that have already been calculated based on progesterone data indicating LH surge and ovulation.

Pregnancy Diagnosis

Ultrasonography is considered the most reliable method to confirm canine pregnancy (**Fig. 4**). Ultrasonography is an excellent tool to confirm pregnancy status, confirm viability of the pregnancy through visualization of fetal heartbeats, and estimate litter size. AUCPS dams receive pregnancy confirmation ultrasonography examinations 30 days after ovulation. Guiding Eyes for the Blind verifies pregnancy and approximates litter size 33 days after initial increase in progesterone level.[8]

Ultrasonography is a useful technique to estimate litter size. In the event of a very small litter (1–2 puppies), this information is crucial in the planning process because

Table 3 Auburn University College of Veterinary Medicine's Canine Performance Sciences prenatal survival litter size					
Number of Litters	Conception Rate (%)	Semen Type Used	Litter Size (Mean)	Litter Size (Median)	Litter Size (Range)
19	100	Fresh or cool shipped	7.47 ± 2.65 pups	7.5 pups	2–12 pups

Unpublished data from AUCPS breeding colony April 2018 to August 2020.

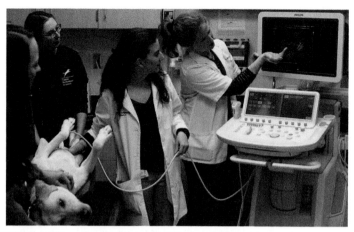

Fig. 4. AUCPS dam ultrasonography at day 30 of gestation.

this could indicate the need for an elective cesarean section (C-section) versus a natural free whelping. It is well documented that medium to large breed dams carrying very small litters often fail to initiate the process of parturition, leading to prolonged gestation and death of the puppies if not recognized in a timely manner. Because the AUCPS colony is almost exclusively Labrador retrievers, elective C-sections are always performed for litters of 1 to 2 puppy in order to minimize neonatal losses.

Other popular methods for pregnancy diagnosis include radiography (discussed in detail later) and serum levels of relaxin in the dam. Relaxin is produced by the canine placenta and is therefore a very specific pregnancy hormone. Testing is quick and easy but does have some drawbacks. Increased relaxin levels indicate the presence of placental tissue but do not confirm the viability of the current pregnancy. In addition, in the event of a very small litter (eg, singleton), it is possible to have a negative relaxin result, in which case the pregnancy would go undetected.

Radiographs

AUCPS dams receive abdominal radiographs approximately 10 days before expected due date for the purposes of confirming puppy count (**Fig. 5**). This radiograph is a simple management tool that pays big dividends, especially in colonies where most dams whelp naturally. It is crucial for the whelping staff to know how many puppies are expected so that they can confirm that the dam has finished the birthing process. Although radiographs can be performed anytime following the mineralization of fetal skeletons (gestational day 45), it is recommended to wait until the last 7 to 10 days of gestation, when puppies are easily visualized and are also at their mature size.

For best radiographic results, dams should be fasted for 4 to 6 hours before radiographs to facilitate an empty stomach and should also be allowed several opportunities to defecate before radiographs. A stomach distended with food or a colon full of fecal material can often lead to difficulty in confirming the number of fetal skeletons present, especially with very large litters.

WHELPING PROCEDURES

Colonies should have established whelping protocols and decision points for intervening outlined before parturition. Progesterone timing performed during estrus management produces a more exact estimated due date for puppies. At AUCPS, 3 days

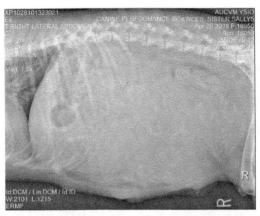

Fig. 5. AUCPS dam abdominal radiograph at day 54 of gestation confirming the presence of 8 pups. Stomach is empty, but note the presence of feces in the colon. The full colon is not problematic in this dam, but could make visualization difficult with a larger litter.

before a dam's estimated due date, blood draws to monitor progesterone levels, ultrasonography scans to check for fetal heat rates and maturation, and maternal behaviors are closely monitored. Guiding Eyes for the Blind dams follow similar processes and begin progesterone level tracking starting 2 to 3 days before the estimated due date. They have found that, if progesterone levels are 2 ng/mL, the dam typically whelps within 24 to 36 hours; if progesterone levels are 1 ng/mL, she typically whelps within 18 to 24 hours; and if progesterone levels are less than 1 ng/mL, whelping has begun or will begin within 18 hours.[8]

Free Whelping

Free whelping is the natural process by which a dam delivers her puppies. At Guiding Eyes for the Blind, normal parturition is monitored via video monitors by staff nearby a whelping suite. Guiding Eyes for the Blind has established decision points for allowing the dog to free whelp with or without assistance.[8] At AUCPS, dams are either free-whelped assisted or have an elective C-section (**Figs. 6** and **7**).

In AUCPS current population protocols, dams are monitored via video monitors by staff nearby and are typically free-whelped assisted for their first litter and have elective C-sections for subsequent litters. Both forms have been regularly conducted at AUCPS. Our comparison of puppy survivability from past free-whelped assisted versus

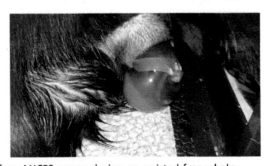

Fig. 6. Delivery of an AUCPS puppy during an assisted free whelp.

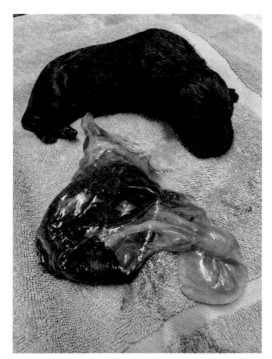

Fig. 7. AUCPS assisted free-whelped puppy with placenta attached.

C-section litters suggests that both can be used with good results (**Table 4**). A factor for AUCPS in making whelping decision is the anticipated availability of resources to conduct video surveillance to ensure dam well-being in the prewhelping phase, and also available trained personnel to assist with the free whelping (**Fig. 8**). Free whelping the first litter also allows staff to observe maternal behaviors during the parturition process.

| Table 4 | | | |
Auburn University College of Veterinary Medicine's Canine Performance Sciences free whelping versus cesarean section whelping statistics			
Elective C-section Delivery Time	47 ± 11 min n = 17 litters	C-section Puppy Survivability	87% n = 28 litters
Free-whelping Delivery Time	237 ± 66 min n = 12 litters	Free-whelping Puppy Survivability	96% n = 23 litters

Emergency Cesarean Section

Dystocia is the inability of the dam to expel a fetus during parturition.[24] If dystocia occurs, the dam has visible mild or intermittent labor contractions for more than 2 hours without progressing to hard labor, or hard, almost continuous contractions have been occurring for more than 30 minutes without the appearance of the puppy at the vulva. An additional parameter that is often overlooked is the appearance of dark green vaginal discharge that is not followed by delivery of a puppy within 30 minutes. This type of discharge indicates placental separation and resulting hypoxia for the neonate. Dystocia and other types of fetal distress typically result in emergency C-sections.

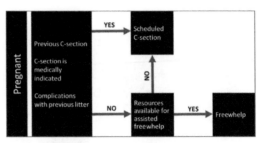

Fig. 8. AUCPS protocol for selecting dam whelping procedure.

Other signs of fetal distress include fetal heart rates of less than 200 beats per minute (bpm) via ultrasonography. When fetal heart rates are consistently at 170 bpm or less, steps are taken to proceed to C-section immediately. Guiding Eyes for the Blind perform a C-section if labor fails to initiate by day 66 from the progesterone initial increase date measured during estrus or within 24 to 36 hours after the progesterone level decreases to less than 2 ng/mL.[8]

In order to understand more reasons for dystocia, Guiding Eyes for the Blind examined factors other than uterine inertia and malpositioned fetuses that resulted in C-sections in purpose-bred Labrador retrievers. They analyzed 667 litters and found that lighter dams with heavier puppies were more likely to require an emergency C-section.[8] The Seeing Eye found that dog adult weight and height were highly heritable at 0.44 and 0.46, respectively.[25] Therefore, it is recommended to consider using EBVs to track the maternal and paternal effects of puppy size and to consider the size of females when selecting breeding stock. It has been recommended that females substantially less than the average population weight and height should not be selected as breeders.[8]

Elective Cesarean Section

As mentioned earlier, AUCPS plans elective C-sections on many dams. Dams are monitored via physical examination, ultrasonography, and progesterone values starting 2 to 3 days before expected due date. Progesterone values are monitored at the same time each morning until the value is less than 2.0 ng/mL. Although there is a predictable increase in progesterone level when the dam is in estrus, there is no predictability in the rate at which progesterone level declines at the end of pregnancy. However, once progesterone decreases to less than 2.0 ng/mL, the dam initiates labor in 12 to 36 hours. This marker is useful for the timing of elective C-sections but can also be a useful marker to establish when the dam will initiate labor in the case of natural free whelping.

On ultrasonography, fetal kidneys are well defined after day 57 with a consistent ratio of renal parenchyma to renal pelvis. Fetal intestines are the last organ to mature, so great emphasis is placed on this portion of the ultrasonography examination as visualization of the intestinal lumen is confirmed, followed by peristalsis as parturition nears.[23] Fetal heart rates are also monitored at these visits, with normal fetal heart rates greater than 200 bpm. Heart rates consistently less than 170 bpm may indicate fetal distress.

In addition to these measures, AUCPS dams are monitored daily for behaviors such as nesting, lack of appetite, and body temperature, which usually declines to less than 37.2°C (99° F) when progesterone level declines before whelping. Video footage is reviewed each morning from the night before in order to gauge restlessness or nesting behaviors.

Table 5
Common practices regarding volume and route of administration of serum or plasma to neonates when colostrum is unavailable

	Volume of Plasma to be Given	Route of Administration	Notes
Puppies	4.5 mL/kg	PO if <12 h SQ if >12 h	Can be given at once; no more than 5 mL/site if SQ
Kittens	15 mL total	PO if <12 h SQ if >12 h	Given in 5-mL boluses at birth, 12 h and 24 h

Abbreviations: PO, by mouth; SQ, subcutaneously.

Neonatal care

A complete discussion of neonatal care is beyond the scope of this article, but a few key management points should be emphasized. Providing adequate warmth and nutrition in the first 5 to 7 days of life cannot be overemphasized, especially when training nursery staff. Steady weight gain is the single best indicator of neonatal health and well-being, and puppies should be weighed twice daily for the first week of life, providing supplemental tube or bottle feeding of milk replacer when needed.

Adequate colostrum intake from healthy, well-vaccinated dams provides the best immunity for neonates. When colostrum is unavailable because of loss of the dam or lack of milk production, plasma from another well-vaccinated colony adult can be used as an alternative (**Table 5**). Plasma is administered orally if within the first 12 hours of birth and subcutaneously thereafter. However, the immunoglobulin G levels provided by colostrum are superior to plasma.

A complete review of newborn assessment and recommendations can be found in the VCNA chapter by Wilborn entitled Small Animal Neonatal Health.[26]

SUMMARY

Breeders should determine whether their colony will be self-sustaining or part of a breeding cooperative based on the number of litters produced each year. Once all medical requirements are satisfied, mating selections should be based on EBVs, lower inbreeding coefficients of the expected litter, management of other genetic traits, and behavioral phenotypes. Breeders should work with a veterinary reproduction specialist to help maximize reproductive success. Ovulation timing using a combination of progesterone and LH testing is the most reliable method for prediction of the peak fertile window in canine breeding management. Poor semen quality parameters can compromise pregnancy rates and litter sizes, which can be detrimental to a canine production program. Gestation is best estimated by using progesterone concentrations to determine the day of LH surge and ovulation. Establish whelping protocols and decision points for intervention before parturition for free whelping, assisted free whelping, and C-sections.

CLINICS CARE POINTS

- Two major challenges that have the biggest impact on fertility in any canine breeding colony are (1) insemination at the improper time, and (2) poor semen quality, both of which are easily managed.

- It is recommended to minimize stress during estrus and gestation to maximize litter success. An increase in cortisol level may interfere with the LH surge and jeopardize ovulation.[21] It is not recommended to change kennel environments or transport the bitch during this time if it can be avoided.

- Adjustments can be made to overcome a decline in semen quality parameters for outstanding studs with continued desire for genetics. For example, the stud dog could be collected and the fresh semen used for a TCI in order to give the poor-quality semen the best chance of establishing a pregnancy rather than live cover.

- Popular methods for pregnancy diagnosis include ultrasonography, radiography, and serum levels of relaxin in the dam. Relaxin testing is quick and easy, but does have some drawbacks.

- For the best puppy count radiographic results, dams should be fasted for 4 to 6 hours before radiographs to facilitate an empty stomach and should also be allowed several opportunities to defecate before radiographs.

- It is recommended to consider using EBVs to track the maternal and paternal effects of puppy size and to consider the size of females when selecting breeding stock. It has been recommended that females substantially less than the average population weight and height should not be selected as breeders.[8]

ACKNOWLEDGMENT

Funding for AUCPS Breeding Program Research was provided by the Auburn University College of Veterinary Medicine Canine Performance Sciences' Help Raise-a-Hero Fund and CPS Donors Walt and Ginger Woltosz, the Alan Kalter and Chris Lezotte Annual Fund for Excellence in Canine Health, Reproduction, and Husbandry, the James M. Hoskins Endowment, and the Diane Carter Memorial Fund.

REFERENCES

1. Leighton EA. Secrets for producing high-quality working dogs. J Vet Behav Clin Appl Res 2009;6(4):212–5.
2. Cole J, Franke D, Leighton E. Population structure of a colony of dog guides. J Anim Sci 2004;82(10):2906–12.
3. Mäki K, Groen A, Liinamo A-E, et al. Population structure, inbreeding trend and their association with hip and elbow dysplasia in dogs. Anim Sci 2001;73(2): 217–28.
4. Charlesworth B. Effective population size and patterns of molecular evolution and variation. Nat Rev Genet 2009;10(3):195–205.
5. Leroy G, Mary-Huard T, Verrier E, et al. Methods to estimate effective population size using pedigree data: Examples in dog, sheep, cattle and horse. Genet Sel Evol 2013;45(1):1.
6. Wiener P, Sánchez-Molano E, Clements DN, et al. Genomic data illuminates demography, genetic structure and selection of a popular dog breed. BMC Genomics 2017;18(1):1–13.
7. Hare E, Leighton EA. Estimation of heritability of litter size in Labrador Retrievers and German Shepherd dogs. J Vet Behav 2006;1(2):62–6.
8. Dolf G, Gaillard C, Russenberger J, et al. Factors contributing to the decision to perform a cesarean section in Labrador retrievers. BMC Vet Res 2018;14(1):57.
9. Foyer P. Early experience, maternal care and behavioural test design: effects on the temperament of military working dogs. Linkoping (Sweden): Linköping University Electronic Press; 2015.

10. Wilsson E, Sinn DL. Are there differences between behavioral measurement methods? A comparison of the predictive validity of two ratings methods in a working dog program. Appl Anim Behav Sci 2012;141(3–4):158–72.

11. Van der Waaij E, Wilsson E, Strandberg E. Genetic analysis of results of a Swedish behavior test on German Shepherd Dogs and Labrador Retrievers. J Anim Sci 2008;86(11):2853–61.

12. Leighton EA. How To Use Estimated Breeding Values to Genetically Improve Dog Guides. Paper presented at: Presented at a Meeting of the "Original Group2003.

13. Sonesson A. Minimization of rate of inbreeding for small populations with overlapping generations. Genet Res 2001;77(3):285–92.

14. Mason SJ. Current review of artificial insemination in dogs. Vet Clin Small Anim Pract 2018;48(4):567–80.

15. Freshman JL. Clinical approach to infertility in the cycling bitch. Vet Clin North Am Small Anim Pract 1991;21(3):427–35.

16. Goodman M. Ovulation timing: Concepts and controversies. Vet Clin Small Anim Pract 2001;31(2):219–35.

17. Moxon R, Batty H, Irons G, et al. Periovulatory changes in the endoscopic appearance of the reproductive tract and teasing behavior in the bitch. Theriogenology 2012;78(9):1907–16.

18. Concannon P, Hansel W, Mcentee K. Changes in LH, progesterone and sexual behavior associated with preovulatory luteinization in the bitch. Biol Reprod 1977;17(4):604–13.

19. Concannon P, McCann J, Temple M. Biology and endocrinology of ovulation, pregnancy and parturition in the dog. J Reprod Fertil Suppl 1989;39:3.

20. Holyoak GR, Makloski C, Morgan GL. In: Lorenz MD, Neer TM, DeMars P, editors. Abortion, abnormal estrous cycle, and infertility. Third Edition; Wiley Blackwell; Small Anim Med Diagn 2013;337–57.

21. Wilborn RR, Maxwell HS. Clinical approaches to infertility in the bitch. Vet Clin Small Anim Pract 2012;42(3):457–68.

22. Kauffman LK, Petersen CA. Canine brucellosis: old foe and reemerging scourge. Vet Clin Small Anim Pract 2019;49(4):763–79.

23. Lopate C. Gestational aging and determination of parturition date in the bitch and queen using ultrasonography and radiography. Vet Clin Small Anim Pract 2018; 48(4):617–38.

24. Purohit G, Gaur M. Dystocia and its management in the bitch and queen: a review. J Canine Develop Res 2004;4:90–100.

25. Helmink S, Rodriguez-Zas S, Shanks R, et al. Estimated genetic parameters for growth traits of German shepherd dog and Labrador retriever dog guides. J Anim Sci 2001;79(6):1450–6.

26. Wilborn RR. Small animal neonatal health. Vet Clin Small Anim Pract 2018;48(4): 683–99.

Development and Training for Working Dogs

Lucia Lazarowski, PhD*, Melissa Singletary, DVM, PhD, Bart Rogers,
Paul Waggoner, PhD

KEYWORDS

- Dog training • Puppy development • Socialization • Canine • K9

KEY POINTS

- Behavioral problems are one of the most commonly reported causes of working dog attrition.
- Early life experiences and environments can greatly impact the future suitability of a working dog.
- Different types of training practices differ in their effectiveness and impacts on working dog welfare.

INTRODUCTION

Individual differences in behavior lead to wide variability in a dog's suitability for working roles, and are greater determinants of success than physical characteristics.[1] A large proportion of working dog candidates fail to successfully complete training and matriculate into operational roles for behavioral reasons,[2] and behavioral problems which are also reported as the most common reason for early release of dogs deployed in the field.[3] Aside from genetic influences, the behavioral repertoire necessary for a working dog to succeed in a given role is largely molded by two important aspects of their preparation: 1) environmental influences and specific experiences during early development; and 2) specialized training to perform the tasks required for the role. Thus, an understanding of how aspects of development and training can affect a working dog's performance is critical for practitioners to evaluate and treat behavioral concerns in working dogs. This article provides an overview of the critical aspects of puppy development that can influence future behavior, which are largely generalizable across all types of working dogs, and reviews important features of training that can influence a dog's ability to learn and perform its designated task.

Canine Performance Sciences, 104 Greene Hall, Auburn, AL 36849, USA
* Corresponding author.
E-mail address: lzl0017@auburn.edu

Vet Clin Small Anim 51 (2021) 921–931
https://doi.org/10.1016/j.cvsm.2021.04.009
0195-5616/21/© 2021 Elsevier Inc. All rights reserved.
vetsmall.theclinics.com

DEVELOPMENT

Environmental influences during development can have a greater and longer-lasting impact on adult behavior than those occurring at later stages,[4] such as the development of fear and anxiety,[5] aggression,[6–8] hyperactivity,[9] and learning disabilities.[10–12] In working dogs, specific experiences during early puppyhood and indirect factors associated with the environment across the first year of life have been shown to influence trainability and suitability for work.[11,13–19] For example, prospective guide dog puppies were more likely to be successful if raised by more experienced volunteer puppy raisers, were raised in homes without children, and with other resident dogs.[15,16] The impact of such experiences may be latent and manifest when triggered by exposure to some environmental stressor later in their career. Therefore, preparing dogs for future working roles begins with laying the foundation during early developmental periods, and problems presented later in life are better understood given the context of the dog's developmental history.

The Socialization Period

The socialization period runs from roughly 2 to 3 weeks until 12 to 14 weeks and is considered a critical period of development during which puppies are particularly susceptible to environmental influences, including an increased readiness to approach and accept interactions with humans and other nonsocial stimuli, with lasting effects on adult behavior.[4] Early socialization for working dog puppies often involves exercises to prepare puppies for their future roles. Examples include acclimation to wearing a harness handle for guide dog puppies,[20] exposure to sounds of sirens and other ambient noises for police dog puppies,[13,14] and habituation to kennels and crates likely to be used for transport and housing.[19,21,22] Because of limitations in exposure opportunities when puppies' immune systems are still vulnerable, exposure to audiovisual representations of different objects and environments are effective alternatives.[23] Because one cannot predict every scenario a working dog may encounter in the future, the socialization period is an opportune time to habituate puppies to the concept of novelty, which is likely to generalize to novel experiences in the future.[24]

A hypersensitivity period occurs around 8 weeks of age where effects of even a single exposure to a frightening stimulus are particularly traumatizing,[25] indicating the close of the socialization period. However, significant differences in timing of this period have been reported between breeds.[26,27] For example, German shepherds demonstrated greater levels of fear during a 5-week physical examination compared with Labrador retrievers raised at the same facility, suggesting that the German shepherds had begun to reach the close of their socialization period earlier than their Labrador counterparts.[27] These breed differences can have important implications for working dog facilities housing both of these breeds, two of the most common among working dogs, where differences in the timing of the onset of fear can differentially impact the different breeds reared in the same environment.[27] Therefore, standardized socialization protocols may not be appropriate given differences in sensitivity to stimuli at different stages of development.

The timing of puppies' peak vulnerability to fearful experiences also tends to coincide with the time puppies typically leave the nursery and are moved to kennels or volunteer puppy-raiser homes, the stress of which could be impactful on future behavior.[4] However, waiting to make the transition toward the end of the period could mean a missed opportunity for socialization to the type of environment puppies are likely to experience for the remainder of their lives, because it is recommended that puppies are introduced to the types of situations they will experience as adults before 8 and no later than

12 weeks for effective acclimation and socialization to occur.[28] However, separating working dog puppies from their mother at 6 weeks can lead to negative effects on physical health and separation-related stress, indicating the risk of removing puppies too early.[29] Although early recommendations suggested 6 to 8 weeks as the best time to remove a puppy from its litter,[28] more recent data suggest 7 to 9 weeks as the period of time resulting in the lowest likelihood of developing behavior problems.[4] Stress of the transition is mitigated by gradually weaning puppies and habituating them to brief separations rather than abrupt removal and drastic change in environment.[4,21]

Early Life Stress

Early life stress can have irreversible effects on behavioral development because of the influence of high levels of glucocorticoids on the development of the central nervous system.[4,30] It is therefore critical that significant stressors, such as social isolation, confinement, prolonged separation from the mother and litter, early weaning, transport, and exposure to loud noises (eg kennel environments) are avoided during early, and even prenatal, development.[24] Nevertheless, mild to moderate stress can have an inoculation effect important for the development of the central nervous system, hypothalamic-pituitary-adrenal axis, and stress resilience critical for dogs working in dynamic and highly variable environments..[4,30,31] Effects of stress inoculation on working dog performance have been illustrated through extensive neonatal handling,[32,33] mental and physical challenges,[34] and style of maternal care.[35,36]

TRAINING

Although early development plays a critical role in laying the foundation for future working dog success, working dogs also need to be trained to perform the specific tasks that are required for their jobs. Different types of training and factors related to training can have important effects on dogs' performance. In the following sections, The use of the term "handler" refers to the primary individuals working with the dog (eg, law enforcement) or for whom the dog performs its tasks (eg, guide dogs).

Types of Training

Methods used for training working dogs largely rely on the principles of operant conditioning,[37] using rewards and punishers to modify behavior. Positive reinforcement involves increasing the future likelihood of a behavior occurring by arranging a behavior-consequence contingency in which the behavior produces a stimulus (colloquially, a reward). For example, if a dog is given a treat for sitting on command, the behavior of sitting on command is likely to increase. Negative reinforcement also increases future occurrences of behavior, but does so by removing a stimulus, typically one that is aversive, contingent on the behavior occurring. Negative reinforcement typically involves the dog learning to perform a behavior that escapes or avoids the stimulus. For example, using leash pressure or pushing the dog's rear end to force into a sit position and releasing the pressure once the dog sits may reinforce compliance of the sit behavior by removal of the pressure. It is important to consider that reinforcers are defined by their effect on behavior and not by the stimulus itself. For example, food may not function as an effective reinforcer to an animal that is not hungry. Scolding a dog for misbehaving can function as a reinforcer if the dog finds the attention reinforcing, and the dog continues to perform the behavior to gain attention.

In contrast to reinforcement, punishment involves decreasing the frequency or future likelihood of the behavior occurring. Like reinforcement, punishment can involve delivering a stimulus contingent on a behavior occurring, or removing a stimulus contingent on a behavior occurring. The terms positive and negative often lead to confusion based on the assumption that positive refers to good and negative refers to bad; conceptualizing operant conditioning by mathematical operations may be more comprehensible, where "positive" refers to the addition of a stimulus and "negative" refers to its subtraction. Punishment can function by adding a stimulus that causes a decrease in a behavior (positive punishment), typically an aversive stimulus, or by removing a stimulus that causes its decrease (negative punishment), typically something the dog desires. Negative punishment is often implemented as time-out (removal of access to all sources of reinforcement), or as a response cost (behavior results in a loss of a specific and current reinforcer). Troisi and colleagues[37] provide examples of reinforcement and punishment related to dog training.

Operant behavior can often be a function of opposing forces of punishment and reinforcement working together. A dog that receives collar pressure when pulling on the leash may learn not to pull (positive punishment, because the pressure resulted in the decrease of the pulling behavior), and/or may learn to walk appropriately to avoid the collar pressure (negative reinforcement, because removing or avoiding the pressure resulted in the increase of appropriate walking behavior). As one can see, these scenarios often differ only by a matter of semantics and most behaviors are two-sided, where decreasing one behavior naturally increases its counterpart. Furthermore, for negative reinforcement to be effective (ie, for the animal to learn to avoid or escape an aversive stimulus), the stimulus must have first been used as a punisher. Although many dog trainers refer to the four processes of operant conditioning as the "four quadrants," it may be more constructive to recognize the processes as whether or not they involve aversive control. For example, in positive punishment and negative reinforcement, behavior results from experiencing or avoiding an aversive stimulus. However, in positive reinforcement and negative punishment, behavior results from gaining or losing access to reinforcers and are often referred to as "force-free" training by modern dog trainers. Although losing access to a reinforcer may be thought of as an aversive experience, it is considered more humane and effective than the application of an aversive stimulus.

Effects of Training on Performance and Welfare

Importantly, different types of training vary in their effectiveness and impact on dogs' well-being. Traditionally, working dog training has relied on the use of punitive methods, shown to be associated with poorer operational performance and compromised welfare.[38,39] Accordingly, modern working dog training has largely shifted away from the use of aversives.[24] The use of compulsion-based training may be a function of the dog's role, such as protection dogs trained for bite-work that are resistant to releasing their grip.[39] However, Haverbeke and coworkers[40] found that training sessions that included positive dog-handler interactions led to better performance for military working dogs (MWDs), and recommend avoiding the use of aversive methods by conducting more frequent and reward-based training to improve obedience and the dog-handler relationship. For example, the authors suggested training dogs to perform behaviors more compatible with the desired outcomes, such as releasing a bite in exchange for a different "decoy" target.[40]

Although obedience training has generally been found to have positive behavioral effects, the amount and type of obedience training used depends on the nature of the dog's task. For example, guide dogs are responsible for safely navigating their handler around obstacles in their environment. Although they require a high level of obedience in appropriate leash-walking, ignoring distractions, and responding to commands, they are also taught "intelligent disobedience" where they should disobey potentially unsafe cues given by their handler, such as a command to cross the street in oncoming traffic.[41] Similarly, explosives-detection dogs are taught "obedience to odor" where the dog should follow the scent trail to a target even if given conflicting commands from the handler.[42] If the dog has had a significant amount of obedience training, especially using compulsory methods, the dog may be hesitant to "disobey" the handler's command.[43] Furthermore, dogs trained for roles requiring a high degree of independence are generally not taught typical obedience to avoid the dog becoming too dependent on the handler or overly sensitive to human cues.

Factors that Affect Training and Performance

Arousal

Psychological or physiologic arousal is associated with an increased responsiveness to the environment resulting from a general activation of the cerebral cortex,[44] and can have a substantial impact on working dog performance regardless of whether the underlying emotional state is positive (ie, excitement) or negative (ie, distress). Levels of arousal can reflect the current state of the individual because of acute changes in the environment, and more constant trait-level features.[37] Different types of working dogs vary in their baseline levels of arousal as a result of selection for specific temperament profiles suitable for different working roles.[45] For example, MWDs and detection dogs are typically selected for higher energy levels and strong motivational drives to enable working over long periods of time and in harsh conditions with infrequent reinforcement,[38,46,47] whereas assistance and guide dogs tend to exhibit much calmer and docile temperaments more compatible with assimilation into anthropocentric environments.[20,45,48,49]

The relationship between arousal and performance is expressed as a bell-shaped curve, known as the Yerkes-Dodson law, where performance improves as arousal increases up to a certain point and then declines when arousal becomes too high.[50] For working dogs, effects of increased arousal vary across different types of working dogs as a function of baseline level. For example, Bray and colleagues[45] found that increasing arousal by the experimenter speaking to the dog in a high-pitched, excited voice improved performance on a problem-solving task for assistance dogs, who showed lower baseline levels of arousal, compared with a group of pet dogs exhibiting higher baseline arousal and for which performance was reduced when excited. For working dogs with high baseline levels of arousal, further increases can lead to compromised performance and welfare.[37,51,52] It is therefore important to consider the many potential stressors encountered by working dogs, such as housing conditions, transport, and training methods, and adapt practices to the dogs' level of arousal and excitability.[37] This is of particular importance when considering presentation and expectations during clinical evaluation, such as the use of high-pitched tones typically used with pet dogs and manner of handling. Such techniques include speaking calmly and with a lower tone, using low-stress handling techniques,[53] and encouraging active handler participation as reasonable.

Training frequency

The frequency and schedule of training has been shown to impact the amount of time taken to learn a task. Search and rescue dogs that spent at least 4 hours training per week were more likely to pass their certification test, which is the minimum amount of time for weekly training recommended for working dogs.[43,54] However, the spacing of training sessions may be just as, if not more, important than total amount of time. For example, dogs trained once a week learned a task in fewer total sessions than dogs trained daily,[55] and dogs trained one to two times a week in short sessions learned a task faster than dogs trained for the same total amount of time but on a daily basis or in longer training sessions.[56] This suggests that although less frequent training would mean a more extended period of time to completion, less time and resources would need to be devoted to actual training time.

Postlearning consolidation

The effects of training regimen may be in part caused by increased opportunity for memory consolidation in between sessions, which occurs during sleep and during waking hours in between learning.[56] It is therefore important that training sessions are kept short and dogs are allowed sufficient opportunities to rest. Amount of time spent resting in the kennel during evening hours has been found to be predictive of successful guide dog certification, which the authors suggested may have been caused by better rest leading to a better ability to focus during training in the day time.[57] However, other studies have found that specific activities following training may boost learning and long-term retention, such as a post-training period of play[58,59] or exercise.[60] The working dog has a different lifestyle than the average pet dog, thus it is important to consider the work/rest cycles and schedule demands of the working dogs under veterinary care.

Addressing Training Issues and Behavior Problems

Some behaviors that may be considered undesirable or inappropriate for pet dogs are often not a concern or are even considered desirable behaviors for working dogs, such as hyperactivity and obsession-like motivational drives.[17] Similarly, some behavioral problems common to working dogs, such as a lack of aggression needed in protection dogs, are not problems for pet dogs.[61] Thus, the determination of whether a behavior should be considered problematic should be based on whether it impacts the dogs' ability to perform its task or would endanger its welfare.[61] This consideration is made according to a proposed classification scheme for managing behavioral problems in working dogs, which identifies four categories of behavior problems: (1) difficulty learning a task, which is often related to suitability for the role and thus identified during selection rather than in operations; (2) degradation in the dogs' ability or willingness to perform a learned task (eg, caused by neurodegenerative disease)[62]; (3) secondary problems unrelated to the trained task but that nonetheless impact performance, such as distractibility detracting from the dog performing its job or free access to reinforcers outside of work that can decrease dogs' motivation to work; and (4) husbandry problems, referring to those outside of the working context that compromise the welfare of the dog, its handler, or others, such as the development of abnormal behavior that leads to self-injury.[61]

Fear and anxiety are commonly reported as problems for working dogs[63–65] and typically develop in adulthood,[61] although this is likely an artifact of dogs showing earlier signs being weeded out early during the selection process. When fear responses develop, the dog's environment and routine should be examined to identify stimuli that elicit the fear behavior so that behavior modification protocols can be used.[24] These methods may include systematic desensitization, where the dog is gradually increasingly exposed to the stimulus while extinguishing the conditioned fear response. This should be done by determining the threshold level at which the dog is in the presence of the stimulus but exhibits little to no response. The intensity of or distance to the stimulus is then gradually increased, allowing for the dog's response to subside before moving to the next level. Counterconditioning is another approach that involves pairing the presence of the fear-eliciting stimulus with a desired stimulus, so that the initial effect of the feared stimulus is reversed and becomes associated with positive emotions. Treatment with anxiolytics may be effective in some cases, but potential impacts of psychoactive drugs on performance need to be carefully considered.[61] In the extreme, working dogs may experience either high-level acute or amass low-level chronic exposure to stress-inducing stimuli to the point of exhibiting canine post-traumatic stress disorder, observed in MWDs deployed in combat zones.[61] For serious behavior problems, a board-certified veterinary behaviorist should be consulted.

SUMMARY

Behavioral characteristics are critical to effective working dog performance, and are largely shaped by early development, training, and other environmental influences. In this article we have reviewed the importance of experience and specific training regimens on working dog performance, which should be considered when evaluating behavioral problems in a working dog. When assessing behavioral issues, a holistic and systematic strategy should be used. The working task, conditions in which it occurs, and the dog's past experiences, as best they can be known, should all be considered. Additionally, the working dog's nonworking conditions, which necessarily occupy a more significant balance of their daily lives, needs to be considered. This includes the home or kennel environment, transportation, and attention to the dog's general behavioral and social welfare. Changes/interventions should be made in an iterative fashion to identify the causes and effective solutions to the problems, which may be as discrete as changing an element of a training routine or as diffuse as adding enriching off-duty activities to improve general welfare.

CLINICS CARE POINTS

- High levels of stress during early puppy development can have negative impacts on the behavioral development of a working dog.

- Mild to moderate stress during puppy development can have a stress inoculation effect, building resilience toward stressors critical for working dog suitability.

- The socialization period from approximately 2 to 3 weeks to 12 to 14 weeks is considered a critical period of development during which puppies are particularly susceptible to influences of environmental stimuli.

- Training methods can have differential impacts on performance and welfare.

- Working dogs are commonly selected for their high baseline arousal, which makes low-stress handling techniques and engagement of the handler important to achieving a smooth clinical evaluation.

- Use of distractions, such as frozen treats or stationary treat mazes, when approved by the handler, are an effective tool during clinical evaluation.

- With high baseline arousal, it is important to ensure regular enrichment is provided during off-duty hours to deter development or exacerbation of obsessive-compulsive behaviors.

- Common behavioral modifying medication could have an impact on working dog performance and consultation with a board-certified veterinary behaviorist should be considered.

DISCLOSURE

The authors declare no conflicts of interest.

REFERENCES

1. Graham LT, Gosling SD. Temperament and personality in working dogs. In: Helton WS, editor. Canine ergonomics: the science of working dogs. Boca Raton: CRC Press/Taylor & Francis; 2009. p. 63–81.
2. Sinn DL, Gosling SD, Hilliard S. Personality and performance in military working dogs: reliability and predictive validity of behavioral tests. Appl Anim Behav Sci 2010;127(1–2):51–65.
3. Evans RI, Herbold JR, Bradshaw BS, et al. Causes for discharge of military working dogs from service: 268 cases (2000–2004). J Am Vet Med Assoc 2007; 231(8):1215–20.
4. Serpell JA, Duffy DL, Jagoe JA. Becoming a dog: early experience and the development of behavior. In: Serpell JA, editor. The domestic dog: its evolution, behavior and interactions with people. 2nd edition. Cambridge (MA): Cambridge University Press; 2017. p. 93e117.
5. Tiira K, Lohi H. Early life experiences and exercise associate with canine anxieties. PLoS One 2015;1–16. https://doi.org/10.1371/journal.pone.0141907.
6. Bennett PC, Rohlf VI. Owner-companion dog interactions: relationships between demographic variables, potentially problematic behaviours, training engagement and shared activities. Appl Anim Behav Sci 2007;102(1–2):65–84.
7. Casey RA, Loftus B, Bolster C, et al. Human directed aggression in domestic dogs (Canis familiaris): occurrence in different contexts and risk factors. Appl Anim Behav Sci 2014;152:52–63.
8. Pirrone F, Pierantoni L, Pastorino GQ, et al. Owner-reported aggressive behavior towards familiar people may be a more prominent occurrence in pet shop-traded dogs. J Vet Behav Clin Appl Res 2016;11:13–7.
9. McMillan FD, Serpell JA, Duffy DL, et al. Differences in behavioral characteristics between dogs obtained as puppies from pet stores and those obtained from noncommercial breeders. J Am Vet Med Assoc 2013;242(10):1359–63.
10. Fuller JL. Transitory effects of experiential deprivation upon reversal learning in dogs '. Psychonomic Science 1966;4(7):273-274.
11. Pfaffenberger CJ, Scott JP. The relationship between delayed socialization and trainability in guide dogs. J Genet Psychol 1959;95(1):145–55.
12. Thompson WR, Heron W. The effects of restricting early experience on the problem-solving capacity of dogs. Can J Psychol 1954;8(1):17–31.
13. Chaloupková H, Svobodová I, Vápeník P, et al. Increased resistance to sudden noise by audio stimulation during early ontogeny in German shepherd puppies. Rosenfeld CS. PLoS One 2018;13(5):e0196553.
14. Alves JC, Santos A, Lopes B, et al. Effect of auditory stimulation during early development in puppy testing of future police working dogs. Top Companion Anim Med 2018. https://doi.org/10.1053/j.tcam.2018.08.004.
15. Serpell JA, Duffy DL. Aspects of juvenile and adolescent environment predict aggression and fear in 12-month-old guide dogs. Front Vet Sci 2016;3:1–8.
16. Harvey ND, Craigon PJ, Blythe SA, et al. Social rearing environment influences dog behavioral development. J Vet Behav Clin Appl Res 2016;16:13–21.
17. Foyer P, Bjällerhag N, Wilsson E, et al. Behaviour and experiences of dogs during the first year of life predict the outcome in a later temperament test. Appl Anim Behav Sci 2014;155:93–100.
18. Foyer P, Wilsson E, Wright D, et al. Early experiences modulate stress coping in a population of German shepherd dogs. Appl Anim Behav Sci 2013;146(1–4): 79–87.

19. Vaterlaws-Whiteside H, Hartmann A. Improving puppy behavior using a new standardized socialization program. Appl Anim Behav Sci 2017;197(August): 55–61.

20. Arata S, Momozawa Y, Takeuchi Y, et al. Important behavioral traits for predicting guide dog qualification. J Vet Med Sci 2010;72(5):539–45. Available at: http://www.ncbi.nlm.nih.gov/pubmed/20009419. Accessed September 4, 2016.

21. Lord K. Kennel enrichment. Dog studies program and Lemelson assistive technology. Amherst (MA): Development Center; 2003. https://doi.org/10.13140/RG. 2.2.29510.73289.

22. Rooney NJ, Gaines SA, Bradshaw JWS. Behavioural and glucocorticoid responses of dogs (Canis familiaris) to kennelling: investigating mitigation of stress by prior habituation. Physiol Behav 2007;92(5):847–54.

23. Pluijmakers JJTM, Appleby DL, Bradshaw JWS. Exposure to video images between 3 and 5 weeks of age decreases neophobia in domestic dogs. Appl Anim Behav Sci 2010;126(1–2):51–8.

24. Rooney NJ, Clark CCA, Casey RA. Minimizing fear and anxiety in working dogs: a review. J Vet Behav Clin Appl Res 2016;16:53–64.

25. Fox MW, Stelzner D. The effects of early experience on the development of inter and intraspecies social relationships in the dog. Anim Behav 1967;15(2–3): 377–86.

26. Morrow M, Ottobre J, Ottobre A, et al. Breed-dependent differences in the onset of fear-related avoidance behavior in puppies. J Vet Behav 2015;10(4):286–94.

27. Lord K, Schneider RA, Coppinger R. Evolution of working dogs. In: Serpell JA, editor. The domestic dog: its evolution, behavior, and interactions with people. 2nd edition. Cambridge University Press; 2017. p. 42–66.

28. Scott JP, Fuller JL. Genetics and the social behavior of the dog. Chicago: University of Chicago Press; 1965.

29. Slabbert JM, Rasa OA. The effect of early separation from the mother on pups in bonding to humans and pup health. J S Afr Vet Assoc 1993;64(1):4–8. Available at: http://www.ncbi.nlm.nih.gov/pubmed/7802733. Accessed December 12, 2018.

30. Nagasawa M, Shibata Y, Yonezawa A, et al. The behavioral and endocrinological development of stress response in dogs. Dev Psychobiol 2014;56(4):726–33.

31. Parker KJ, Buckmaster CL, Sundlass K, et al. Maternal mediation, stress inoculation, and the development of neuroendocrine stress resistance in primates. Proc Natl Acad Sci U S A 2006;103(8):3000–5.

32. Gazzano A, Mariti C, Notari L, et al. Effects of early gentling and early environment on emotional development of puppies. Appl Anim Behav Sci 2008; 110(3–4):294–304.

33. Battaglia CL. Periods of early development and the effects of stimulation and social experiences in the canine. J Vet Behav 2009. https://doi.org/10.1016/j.jveb. 2009.03.003.

34. Duffy DL, Serpell JA. Effects of early rearing environment on behavioral development of guide dogs. J Vet Behav 2009;4(6):240–1.

35. Foyer P, Wilsson E, Jensen P. Levels of maternal care in dogs affect adult offspring temperament. Sci Rep 2016;6:19253.

36. Bray EE, Sammel MD, Cheney DL, et al. Effects of maternal investment, temperament, and cognition on guide dog success. Proc Natl Acad Sci U S A 2017; 113(32):9128–33.

37. Troisi CA, Mills DS, Wilkinson A, et al. Behavioral and cognitive factors that affect the success of scent detection dogs. Comp Cogn Behav Rev 2019;14:51–76.

38. Haverbeke A, Laporte B, Depiereux E, et al. Training methods of military dog handlers and their effects on the team's performances. Appl Anim Behav Sci 2008; 113(1–3):110–22.

39. Schilder MBH, Van Der Borg JAM. Training dogs with help of the shock collar: short and long term behavioural effects. Appl Anim Behav Sci 2004;85(3–4): 319–34.

40. Haverbeke A, Messaoudi F, Depiereux E, et al. Efficiency of working dogs undergoing a new Human Familiarization and Training Program. J Vet Behav Clin Appl Res 2010;5(2):112–9.

41. Guide Dogs for the Blind. Available at: https://www.guidedogs.com/meet-gdb/dog-programs/guide-dog-training#:~:text=In. addition to learning how, when there is oncoming traffic).

42. Lazarowski L, Waggoner LP, Krichbaum S, et al. Selecting dogs for explosives detection: behavioral characteristics. Front Vet Sci 2020;7. https://doi.org/10.3389/fvets.2020.00597.

43. Alexander M Ben, Friend T, Haug L. Obedience training effects on search dog performance. Appl Anim Behav Sci 2011;132(3–4):152–9.

44. Strain GM. Consciousness and higher cortical function. In: Dukes HH, Reece WO, editors. Dukes' physiology of domestic animals. 12th edition. Comstock Publishing Associates, Cornell University; 2004. p. 935–51.

45. Bray EE, MacLean EL, Hare BA. Increasing arousal enhances inhibitory control in calm but not excitable dogs. Anim Cogn 2015;18(6):1317–29.

46. Brady K, Cracknell N, Zulch H, et al. Factors associated with long-term success in working police dogs. Appl Anim Behav Sci 2018;207(June):67–72.

47. Hall NJ. Persistence and resistance to extinction in the domestic dog: basic research and applications to canine training. Behav Process. 2017;141:67–74.

48. Fadel FR, Driscoll P, Pilot M, et al. Differences in trait impulsivity indicate diversification of dog breeds into working and show lines. Sci Rep 2016;6:1–10.

49. Svartberg K. Breed-typical behaviour in dogs: historical remnants or recent constructs? Appl Anim Behav Sci 2006;96(3–4):293–313.

50. Yerkes RM, Dodson JD. The relationship of strength of stimulus to rapidity of habit formation. J Comp Neurol Psychol 1908;18:59–482.

51. Gazit I, Terkel J. Explosives detection by sniffer dogs following strenuous physical activity. Appl Anim Behav Sci 2003;81(2):149–61.

52. Cao X, Irwin DM, Liu YH, et al. Balancing selection on CDH2 may be related to the behavioral features of the Belgian malinois. PLoS One 2014;9(10):1–7.

53. Yin SA. Low stress handling, restraint and behavior modification of dogs & cats: techniques for developing patients who love their visits. Davis, CA: CattleDog Pub.; 2009.

54. SWGDOG. SWGDOG SC8- SUBSTANCE DETECTOR DOGS: Explosives Detection. 2007. Available at: https://swgdog.fiu.edu/approved-guidelines/sc8_explosives.pdf. Accessed February 5, 2019.

55. Meyer I, Ladewig J. The relationship between number of training sessions per week and learning in dogs. Appl Anim Behav Sci 2008;111(3–4):311–20.

56. Demant H, Ladewig J, Balsby TJS, et al. The effect of frequency and duration of training sessions on acquisition and long-term memory in dogs. Appl Anim Behav Sci 2011;133(3–4):228–34.

57. Tomkins LM, Thomson PC, McGreevy PD. Behavioral and physiological predictors of guide dog success. J Vet Behav Clin Appl Res 2011;6(3):178–87.

58. Affenzeller N, Palme R, Zulch H. Playful activity post-learning improves training performance in Labrador Retriever dogs (Canis lupus familiaris). Physiol Behav 2017;168:62–73.
59. Affenzeller N. Dog–human play, but not resting post-learning improve re-training performance up to one year after initial task acquisition in labrador retriever dogs: a follow-on study. Animals (Basel) 2020;10(7):1235.
60. Snigdha S, de Rivera C, Milgram NW, et al. Exercise enhances memory consolidation in the aging brain. Front Aging Neurosci 2014;6(FEB):1–14.
61. Burghardt WF. Behavioral considerations in the management of working dogs. Vet Clin Small Anim Pract 2003;33:417–46. Available at: https://pdfs.semanticscholar.org/b9c3/2a54104f0b2afe89102f244abff7e7d04037.pdf. Accessed May 10, 2018.
62. Osella MC, Re G, Odore R, et al. Canine cognitive dysfunction syndrome: prevalence, clinical signs and treatment with a neuroprotective nutraceutical. Appl Anim Behav Sci 2007;105(4):297–310.
63. Goddard ME, Beilharz RG. A factor analysis of fearfulness in potential guide dogs. Appl Anim Behav Sci Belhar 1984;12:253–65.
64. Lazarowski L, Haney P, Brock J, et al. Investigation of the behavioral characteristics of dogs purpose-bred and prepared to perform Vapor Wake® detection of person-borne explosives. Front Vet Sci 2018;5:50.
65. Dollion N, Paulus A, Champagne N, et al. Fear/reactivity in working dogs: an analysis of 37 years of behavioural data from the Mira Foundation's future service dogs. Appl Anim Behav Sci 2019;221:104864.

Military Working Dogs
An Overview of Veterinary Care of These Formidable Assets

Andrew L. McGraw, DVM, MS*, Todd M. Thomas, DVM, MSpVM

KEYWORDS

- Military working dog (MWD) • Degenerative lumbosacral stenosis • Chagas disease
- Mesenteric volvulus • Procurement • Canine • K-9

KEY POINTS

- Preventive care is integral to maintaining the health and operational capability of military working dogs (MWDs).
- Veterinary assessment of candidate working dogs is vital to selection of the most ideal dog to work effectively under a variety of challenging conditions.
- Heat-related injury, degenerative lumbosacral stenosis, cauda equina syndrome, and Chagas disease are just some of the conditions of interest that affect MWDs.

INTRODUCTION

The capability they (military working dogs) bring to the fight cannot be replicated by man or machine. By all measures of performance their yield outperforms any asset we have in our inventory. Our Army (and military) would be remiss if we failed to invest more in this incredibly valuable resource.[1] Gen. David H. Petraeus (USA)

War dogs have, indeed, served the nation well and saved many lives. Dogs continue to serve to protect Americans both in combat zones and in homeland security roles.[2] Gen. Colin Powell (USA)

For those who have served the health care needs of military working dogs (MWDs) throughout their respective careers, quotations from key leaders, such as these, are inspiring; they serve to clarify one of the primary motivations behind caring for these amazing animals. Quite simply, the operational effectiveness of MWDs translates into saved lives. Indirectly, veterinary caregivers play a key role in preserving the lives of the US countrymen and countrywomen as well as US allies by ensuring the

Auburn Veterinary Specialists–Gulf Shores, Auburn University Educational Complex, 21541 Coastal Gateway Boulevard (County Road 8), Gulf Shores, AL 36542, USA
* Corresponding author.
E-mail address: mcgraal@auburn.edu

Vet Clin Small Anim 51 (2021) 933–944
https://doi.org/10.1016/j.cvsm.2021.04.010
vetsmall.theclinics.com
0195-5616/21/© 2021 Elsevier Inc. All rights reserved.

readiness and fitness of supported MWDs. It is critical to ensure that the life, health, and abilities of MWDs are optimized throughout their careers.

Dogs have been employed by military forces since antiquity. They have served in a variety of roles that capitalized on their stamina, speed, power, and olfactory prowess. Those same attributes make them effective tools even today. Broad categories of use include explosives detection and nonexplosives detection. Explosives detector dogs serve this function in a variety of forms: on lead or off lead, voice, radio, or hand/arm signals, utilized by military police, engineers, or special operations personnel. Nonexplosives detector dogs conventionally serve a patrol function: tracking enemy combatants, biting and apprehending hostile forces, and searching for drugs and other contraband. Today's conventional MWD is a dual-certified canine who serves in a patrol capability as well as in either an explosives or narcotics detection capability. Given the various methods of utilization of MWDs, musculoskeletal integrity and endurance, and visual and audiological acuity as well as olfactory function, all must perform adequately to allow MWDs to serve effectively.

PROCUREMENT

MWDs are procured for service through 1 of 3 means: overseas commercial vendors, United States–based commercial vendors, or via the Department of Defense (DOD) Military Working Dog Breeding Program at Lackland Air Force Base (AFB), Texas. US Army veterinary personnel serve a key function in screening candidate working dogs for service. Once these candidate dogs pass an operational screening assessment by DOD trainers and evaluators to ensure that they possess the temperament and fortitude to perform in the face of a variety of stimuli, they then are presented for their veterinary examination and assessment.

A complete physical examination is performed to ensure overall physical health of the candidate working dog. A wide variety of breeds are considered, but the German shepherd, Belgian Malinois, and Dutch shepherd are preferred. Dogs should be no less than 12 months and no greater than 36 months of age upon presentation. Emphasis on the oral cavity is given to ensure there is no malocclusion or dental disease that would hinder a dog's ability to prehend or bite an aggressor (see Stephen Juriga and Karin Bilyard's article, "Working Dog Dentistry," in this issue). Poor body condition, external parasitism, evidence of atopic dermatitis, otitis externa, heart murmur, lymphadenopathy, retinal abnormalities or blindness, and poor conformation are just some of the more common physical examination findings that result in rejection of the dog for service.

The cornerstone of the veterinary examination is a radiological evaluation consisting of flexed lateral projections of both elbows, ventrodorsal hip-extended projection of the coxofemoral joints, and a lateral projection of the lumbar spine to include T13 to the caudal aspect of the sacrum. Observing ossification of all relevant bony structures assures minimal age requirements are met. Any evidence of osteoarthritis, dysplasia, osteomyelitis, osteochondrosis, or transitional vertebra results in a recommendation to not purchase the dog. Dogs with transitional vertebra are not recommended for purchase because this congenital abnormality, common in German shepherd dogs,[3,4] has been associated with development of cauda equina disease,[4] a historically significant disease cited[5] as the cause of death or euthanasia in 15.6% of MWDs in 1 retrospective study.

Hematology, biochemistry, and heartworm disease screening are key components in further evaluating the health status of the candidate working dog. Complete blood cell count and biochemistry analysis to include electrolytes, urinalysis, and heartworm antigen testing are performed in order to ensure there is no underlying hepatopathy, renal disease, or heartworm infection that could shorten the working life span of an MWD or result in unavailability for service during the rigors of training and/or deployment. An abbreviated analysis may be performed under more austere, remote screening conditions utilizing handheld analyzers. Bitches serving in the DOD Breeding Program as well as their offspring receive PennHip and Canine Eye Registry Foundation ophthalmologic examinations in order to ensure that those with heritable diseases that would disqualify breeding stock from service are identified and removed from the breeding pool.

INITIAL MEDICAL PROCESSING

Dogs that pass the operational and veterinary screening assessment and examination are medically processed in order to prepare them for future service as MWDs. Core vaccines administered to all MWDs include immunization against rabies virus, canine distemper virus, canine adenovirus type 2, and canine parvovirus, consistent with most recently published guidelines.[6] Leptospirosis (quadrivalent vaccine) is administered as a noncore vaccine. All MWDs are immunized on a triennial frequency with core vaccines and annually with leptospirosis given that vaccine's advertised duration of immunity. An exception to this scheme is considered for routinely or imminently deploying dogs that may need more frequent boosters based on country import requirements. The challenge of refraining from vaccinating more than clinically necessary with concurrently meeting the myriad country import requirements is significant; each MWD's frequency of immunization is assessed on a case-by-case basis by the attending veterinarian and the kennel master (active-duty service member responsible for the care, training, and deployability of assigned MWDs). Other noncore vaccines, such as canine influenza, *Borrelia burgdorferi*, and so forth, generally are not administered to MWDs. Regional medical threat differences, changes in lifestyle and living conditions, emergence of an epizootic disease, and other factors, however, allow for the fact that some dogs may require noncore vaccinations as the attending veterinarian and supporting veterinary clinical specialist deem necessary. These exceptions are approved by the supporting veterinary clinical specialist after informing the director of the DOD Military Working Dog Veterinary Service (DODMWDVS).

GASTROPEXY, TATTOOING, AND STERILIZATION

After procurement, further processing involves general anesthesia. In addition to microchip implantation, MWDs also are tattooed in their left ear to provide visible, permanent identification. Assigned alphanumeric tattoos are unique to each dog. With the exception of bitches selected for breeding programs, all female dogs undergo an ovariectomy (or ovariohysterectomy when indicated). Although surgeon preference influences the choice of ovariectomy or ovariohysterectomy, efficacy for sterilization and prevention of future reproductive problems is similar.[7] Postoperative pain also is similar. Ovariectomy often results in shorter incisions and surgical time, while avoiding the need for specialized training and equipment needed for laparoscopic or laparoscopic-assisted procedures.[8-10] Male dogs are not castrated routinely; however, those with medical conditions that warrant castration (eg, cryptorchidism or severe scrotal diseases) undergo that procedure as well.

While anesthetized, all dogs undergo a thorough oral examination. Conditions involving oral health may lead to pain, poor appetite, poor health, and weight loss as well as reluctance or inability to bite and hold. Dental radiography is performed when additional information is needed prior to formulating a treatment plan. Dental diseases requiring care (eg, severe calculus, periodontal disease, and fractured teeth) are addressed on an individual basis as required. Common dental procedures may include any combination of dental cleaning and polishing, endodontic (ie, root canals) procedures, and simple or surgical extractions (see Stephen Juriga and Karin Bilyard's article, "Working Dog Dentistry," in this issue).

As published in 2001,[5] gastric dilatation and volvulus (GDV) was once the fifth leading cause of death in MWDs. More importantly, the condition was the most common preventable cause of death. Since that time, a variety of prophylactic gastropexy techniques have been used. The gastropexy program gradually increased over several years, with all dogs in at-risk breeds undergoing the procedure prior to training since approximately 2010. Various surgical techniques have been utilized, including multiple gastropexy techniques via a ventral midline incision, laparoscopic-assisted gastropexy,[11,12] and the right paracostal (paramedian) gastropexy (RPG).[13] Currently, the most commonly performed prophylactic procedure is the RPG. GDV occurs infrequently now and typically involves newly procured dogs awaiting gastropexy or contract working dogs utilized by the DOD.

HEAT-RELATED INJURIES

Of all the potentially preventable diseases that MWDs experience, heat-related injuries (HRIs) are among the most encountered. HRIs encompass a spectrum of disease from mild (heat stress, or exertional hyperthermia), moderate (heat exhaustion), and severe (heat stroke). One retrospective study[14] showed that heat stroke was the second most common reason for discharge in MWDs less than 5 years of age. Numerous variables,[15] such as environmental conditions (ambient temperature and relative humidity), poor acclimation, elevated body condition score (BCS), large body size (>15 kg), and poor fitness, all are significant factors in determining whether or not a working dog sustains an HRI. Additionally, a recent retrospective study[16] revealed what many clinicians have personally experienced: working dogs suffering an HRI are more likely to experience a subsequent HRI. Although the obviously life-threatening condition of heat stroke is the most limiting, with a 50% mortality rate,[17] repeated episodes of heat stress or heat exhaustion may have an adverse impact on the likelihood of operational utilization of an MWD due to a loss of confidence in both the veterinarian's and the kennel master's recommendation to deploy these dogs to environmentally austere environments. See Marcella Ridgway's article, "Preventative Health Care for Working Dogs"; and Lee Palmer's article, "Operational Canine," in this issue, for normal deviations in body temperature of working dogs during periods of work.

The common occurrence of HRI in MWDs demands that handlers employing these animals be trained thoroughly in identifying the signs of HRI and what interventions should be implemented prior to and en route to veterinary care. Although concurrent implementation of cooling measures did not prove a statistically significant survival advantage in dogs suffering from heatstroke in 1 study,[17] handlers are trained to perform these measures as well as to expeditiously transport these animals to veterinary caregivers when indicated. Additionally, given the dynamic caloric demands of working dogs, due to variable conditions, such as workload, environmental conditions, and so forth, monthly monitoring BCS is critical to avoid obesity.

Advising trainers and handlers on the ideal work-rest cycles to govern the employment of MWDs during periods of increased heat and humidity can be challenging. Given this constraint, DOD researchers have developed a Canine Thermal Model[18] that factors the dog's physical measurements (mass and length), current meteorologic data, and accelerometer data to predict a core temperature. The dog's core temperature can be tracked on a smart device and assists personnel in identifying dangerous and sustained periods of exertional hyperthermia as well as ensuring appropriate recovery from elevations in body heat has occurred. This model, in conjunction with the future development of wearable devices by the working dog, can serve to provide more objective data on how to best identify work-rest cycles applicable to various climates and conditions.

A critical point is that the working dog's temperature needs to be correlated with the clinical presentation. A working dog with a rectal temperature of 106°F can be consistent with exertional hyperthermia,[19,20] if it is demonstrating controlled panting, is neurologically normal, and rapidly recovers given appropriate rest, shade, and time. Conversely, a working dog that is obtunded yet normothermic may present a more dire case of HRI if the dog succumbed to heat stroke yet received cooling measures before and en route to veterinary care.

MUSCULOSKELETAL AND NEUROMUSCULAR CONDITIONS

Many musculoskeletal and neuromuscular conditions affect MWDs and may have widely varied etiologies. Various types and degrees of trauma create clinically significant injuries that influence daily operations as well as MWD longevity. Many of the relevant conditions, however, also have both a repetitive, work-related nature, and a degenerative component (either as the inciting cause or subsequent to the injury). Even relatively minor injuries, such as footpad abrasions or lacerations and tail trauma, may affect MWD utilization adversely during treatment (eg, outpatient treatment, surgical repair, or hospitalization). Because common musculoskeletal and neuromuscular conditions may be intertwined, have overlapping clinical signs, or affect the same patient simultaneously, the epidemiology of these conditions is reviewed together.

Both musculoskeletal and neuromuscular conditions frequently lead to veterinary visits and MWD losses.[5,10,21] A similar finding involving orthopedic conditions also was seen in German shepherd police dogs seen at the University of Pennsylvania veterinary hospital.[22] In 1 report of non–combat-related illnesses and injuries in MWDs deployed to Iraq, approximately 14% of veterinary visits involved musculoskeletal and neuromuscular conditions. A majority of musculoskeletal diseases (approximately 47%) were localized to the pelvic limbs, and a majority of vertebral conditions (approximately 76%) were localized to the lumbar region.[10] Appendicular degenerative joint disease (DJD) was the most common cause of death in a previous MWD epidemiologic article, and spinal cord–cauda equina disease was the third most common cause. When combined, these 2 categories represented approximately one-third of MWD deaths during a 4-year period.[5] A later review of causes for discharge of MWDs from service revealed that spinal cord disease, DJD, or a combination of both systems accounted for greater than 50% of discharges of MWDs 5 years of age or older.[10]

Few, if any, publications have described the prevalence of individual musculoskeletal conditions in MWDs. The veterinary and operational impacts of this category are based largely on cumulative data for all conditions. Conditions commonly affecting large breeds and very active, working, sport, or agility dogs also are diagnosed in MWDs in an author's (TMT) experience. These conditions include DJD (specifically coxofemoral and stifle), cranial cruciate ligament (CCL) injures, tendinopathies (frequently due to repetitive motion or overexertion), and other injuries resulting in joint instability (eg, hyperextension, tendon rupture, and collateral ligament injuries). Digit injuries, in particular fractures, are common and require treatment, but long bone fractures are infrequent. Immune-mediated and infectious musculoskeletal conditions generally are rare. Given the decades of archived MWD records, this untapped resource could provide valuable information for a wide variety of conditions.

Although screening radiographs are performed routinely during procurement, and discussed previously, conditions affecting the coxofemoral joints still occur later in life. CCL injuries are a common condition and may occur virtually at any age. Genetics as well as degeneration over time both play important roles in these conditions. Additionally, the consistently strenuous nature of working dog activities is substantial and cannot be overlooked. Tasks that involve frequent, vigorous activity with rapid acceleration, deceleration, and turning sharply also are critical factors in developing clinical disease. Lunging, jumping, or rearing on the pelvic limbs are contributing factors that are influenced by rough terrain, uneven surfaces and obstacles. Stifle injuries, especially partial CCL tears, may go undiagnosed without a thorough sedated orthopedic examination. When combined with the muscle mass, excitement in veterinary facilities, patient temperament, and desire to perform the definitive diagnosis of many orthopedic injuries, but especially CCL injuries, is challenging. Treatment includes surgical repair and rehabilitation. MWDs are treated with tibial plateau leveling osteotomies; however, extracapsular stabilization techniques have been used historically and occasionally still are used for select patients. Return to duty after recovery is expected, but individual MWD factors affecting the likelihood include chronicity, secondary degenerative changes, other orthopedic or neuromuscular conditions, and the MWD's intended use.

Thoracic limb conditions frequently include shoulder tendinopathies and carpal hyperextension injuries. Although not eliminated by screening, elbow conditions, including DJD in older MWDs, are uncommon. Acute, severe shoulder injuries also are uncommon. Most are repetitive in nature and present with a more insidious onset. Most carpal injuries are acute in nature and result from some type of injury while falling or jumping from, or over, elevated surfaces. Medical management, including nonsteroidal anti-inflammatory drugs; controlled, low-impact activity; and rehabilitation are beneficial; however, surgical treatment is necessary in patients that fail to improve. Tendinopathy patients may take considerable time and rehabilitation before improving but return to duty is the expectation. Return to duty is possible, but the prognosis for carpal injuries requiring arthrodesis is highly variable in MWDs.

In the pelvic limb, collateral ligament injuries as well as calcaneal tendon injuries both occur. These injuries tend to be acute and related directly to working, with a much less significant degenerative component. Milder, unrecognized, or untreated conditions can progress. When this occurs, chronic or secondary changes already may be present. Joint luxations occur, but infrequently. Because MWDs rely so heavily on their pelvic limbs to propel them when performing apprehension work, navigating obstacles, and rearing to search elevated areas, injuries to ligamentous structures in the pelvic limbs can be challenging to achieve a favorable outcome.

In addition to a thorough orthopedic examination, diagnostic tools utilized for MWD musculoskeletal conditions include radiographs, computed tomography (CT)/magnetic resonance imaging (MRI), and musculoskeletal ultrasound. A thorough evaluation of the patient is critical in establishing potential for return to duty. The breeds utilized, combined with the strenuous nature of their work, results in many dogs having more than 1 musculoskeletal or neuromuscular condition. These additional conditions are important complicating factors in the decision-making process as treatment options are considered. Whether a patient is a pet or MWD, prognosis and outcome goals are important for any treatment; however, return to duty is an additional factor that must be discussed with all stakeholders.

Neuromuscular conditions most commonly involve the spine. Of particular interest is the lumbar spine, with the lumbosacral spine affected most frequently. Other clinical diseases involving the cervical or thoracic lumbar spine are seen and must be ruled out; however, the frequency is much lower. Conditions like discospondylitis, cervical and thoracolumbar intervertebral disc disease, fibrocartilaginous emboli, neoplasia, and spinal fractures all are seen in MWDs but generally are lumped together with the more common diseases.

Cauda equina syndrome, or degenerative lumbosacral stenosis, is a multifactorial degenerative disorder in which myriad abnormalities affecting the bones, joints, discs, and neurovascular structures occur alone or in combination and may result in neural or vascular compression of the cauda equina. German shepherds, a common MWD breed, are known to be predisposed.[23] During procurement, screening for congenital anatomic abnormalities, such as transitional vertebrae, is important to reducing the risk. Due to the strenuous nature of their work, however, this fails to completely eliminate the condition in MWDs. Clinical signs frequently reported to veterinary personnel include pelvic limb weakness, spinal or pelvic limb pain, lameness, and either the inability or reluctance to perform necessary tasks (eg, standing on the pelvic limbs to search elevated positions and obstacle course work). Although signs may appear acute, because the condition most commonly involves Hansen type II disc disease, many cases are chronic at the time of initial presentation.

In addition to radiography, the diagnostic plan for neuromuscular conditions requires ready access to 3-dimensional imaging modalities (CT, MRI, or both for some individual patients). Because instability is a common factor (both predisposing and progressive sequela) in the condition, imaging in multiple positions (ie, pelvic limbs flexed and extended) often is necessary. Surgical correction is necessary in most clinical cases; however, medical management often is attempted during the diagnostic process and prior to surgical intervention. Mildly affected MWDs may respond to short periods of limited activity, rehabilitation, and multimodal pain management. Additionally, patients deemed poor surgical candidates also may be treated with epidural steroid injections with methylprednisolone acetate.[24] Surgical treatment includes dorsal laminectomy. Additional procedures (eg, discectomy, foraminotomy, and stabilization) vary based on the assessment of individual patients, their clinical signs, and imaging findings. Prognosis for return to normal duty generally is guarded for MWDs, with 1 report of less than 50% returning to normal. As age and severity of clinical signs increase, the prognosis for successful outcome decreases.[25] Surgery combined with aggressive, inpatient rehabilitation, however, shows potential for improving outcomes.[26]

In addition to surgical correction, physical rehabilitation and regenerative medicine strategies are becoming increasingly common in veterinary medicine, and their utility for MWDs appears to have enormous potential. Underwater treadmills, therapeutic ultrasound, extracorporeal shockwave therapy, and guided injections with pharmaceutical or biologic agents are gaining use. Although much of their current reported usefulness involves small numbers of pets or sporting animals, the same techniques show similar promise for MWDs. Definitive care that includes surgery, preoperative, and postoperative rehabilitation all are potential treatment options for MWD musculoskeletal conditions. The sports medicine and rehabilitation service at DODMWDVS provides both inpatient and outpatient on-site care as well as consultations during treatment.

BALLISTIC AND EXPLOSION INJURIES

Significant injuries from gunshot wounds, explosions, and flying debris or shrapnel usually are combat related. Although injuries similar to those of civilian working dogs occur, MWDs almost exclusively are overseas, frequently in remote locations, when they occur. One study[27] evaluating causes of death for MWDs during Operation Iraqi Freedom (OIF) and Operation Enduring Freedom (OEF) showed that injuries caused 77% of deaths, with more than half of the external injuries resulting from gunshots, explosions, or blasts. Another article[28] specifically reviewed gunshot wounds to MWDs during OEF and OIF. Most injuries were from high-caliber, high-velocity weapons, with 50% involving the thorax. Of the 29 injured dogs, 11 (38%) survived. All dogs that survived received care at the point of injury, returned to full duty, and subsequently deployed to combat zones again. For dogs that are unable to return to duty, prognosis for function and good quality of life, along with suitability for adoption, are important considerations for treating trauma patients.

First responders may be the handler or human health care providers (HCPs), such as a combat medic or corpsman. Additionally, medical evacuation for these types of injuries, as well as other emergent conditions, must be planned carefully. Depending on the accessibility of veterinary care, the closest medical asset may be a human hospital. Predeployment, canine-specific, tactical combat casualty care training for dog handlers and HCPs is emphasized for units deploying with or supporting MWDs. Clinical practice guidelines for MWDs for HCP use are available for a variety of emergent conditions affecting MWDs.[29] These guidelines, developed in collaboration with human and veterinary specialists, provide guidance for HCPs on how to intervene on behalf of an injured MWD when veterinary personnel are geographically separate from the injured dog and transport either is unavailable or untenable due to inclement weather and/or the patient needs more immediate resuscitative care.

CANINE CHAGAS DISEASE

American trypanosomiasis is a disease of major importance[30] and concern in MWDs. Lackland AFB, in Bexar County, is identified[31] as 1 of the most heavily endemic counties of canine Chagas disease in the state of Texas. Outdoor kennel facilities are in heavily wooded areas that serve as ideal host and vector habitats. Vector surveillance performed at Medina Training Annex found 52.6% of triatomes were infected with *Trypanosoma cruzi* organisms (detected by polymerase chain reaction [PCR]).[32] Medina Training Annex serves as a quarantine facility for procured MWDs and consistently houses approximately 250 dogs, approximately a quarter of the MWD population on Lackland AFB. Seroprevalence among the fluctuating dog population on the installation typically has been less than 2% for the past decade (Ms Kristine Ritter, personal communication). Public health concerns for veterinary staff, which conceivably could become exposed to infected blood through needlestick, necropsy knife cut, and so forth, pose the primary zoonotic disease risk.

Experience with canine Chagas disease in MWDs over the previous 12 years has revealed much about clinical manifestations of infection as well and the impacts on affected dogs' ability to certify, work, and serve effectively throughout their working life span. All working dogs at Lackland AFB are screened no less than annually for *T cruzi* antibodies utilizing immunofluorescent antibody techniques through the DOD Food Analysis and Diagnostic Laboratory located at Fort Sam Houston, Texas. Utilizing a cutoff of 1:160, animals identified as seropositive receive a cardiovascular evaluation consisting of physical examination, *T cruzi* PCR, 6-lead electrocardiogram, 2-view thoracic radiographs, echocardiographic evaluation, and troponin assay. Of the potential outcomes[30] of infection with *T cruzi* (acute, chronic symptomatic, and chronic asymptomatic), in 1 author's experience (ALM), the chronic asymptomatic form is the typical manifestation of Chagas disease in the MWD; most affected dogs go on to experience uncomplicated work histories. This correlates to findings in humans, which show that most people who may be seropositive for the disease and progress from the acute phase to chronic phase of the disease experience no untoward effects.[33] A small number of MWDs at Lackland AFB participated in a multicenter study[34] evaluating the effectiveness of amiodarone and itraconazole for treating Chagas disease in dogs. Although the study showed favorable results for treated dogs compared with untreated controls, this regimen currently is not recommended for MWDs due to the following concerns: the high financial cost of treating dogs for prolonged periods of time (due to serum drug monitoring as well as the pharmaceuticals themselves), the unacceptable incidence of gastrointestinal and hepatic side effects of treatment, and the questionable long-term benefit of treating seropositive asymptomatic dogs. Future studies are indicated to determine what the ideal treatment and diagnostic tools can be leveraged to better understand this disease.

END OF SERVICE CONSIDERATIONS

In 2000, Congress amended Chapter 153 of title 10, US Code, to read, "The Secretary of Defense may make a military working dog of the Department of Defense available for adoption by a person or entity referred to in subsection (c) at the end of the dog's useful working life or when the dog is otherwise excess to the needs of the Department, unless the dog has been determined to be unsuitable for adoption under subsection (b)."[35] This legislation, also known as Robby's Law, is significant in that it mandates that MWDs that reach the end of their effective service, regardless of being due to medical or training deficiency–related reasons, would be afforded an opportunity for adoption. Prior to this time MWDs that reached their service life span were euthanized.

Determining the outcome of MWDs, which are evaluated for their future ability to serve as MWDs, is called the disposition process. MWDs undergoing the disposition process either are retained for service or declared excess to the needs of the DOD. For animals that are retained by the DOD, the dogs could be retained by the accountable unit, transferred to another unit within the DOD, or utilized as training aids (trained dogs who would be utilized to facilitate training for human service members enrolled in the Handler's Course at Lackland AFB). For those animals declared excess, they could experience 1 of 3 potential outcomes: adoption (either by a former handler or another person qualified to care for a retired MWD), transfer to a civilian law enforcement agency or other federal agency, or euthanasia.

The decision to euthanize an MWD that undergoes the disposition process rests with the commander of the law enforcement unit that is responsible for the dog. Input from the attending veterinarian and the supporting veterinary clinical specialist is considered heavily in the commander's determination and includes the veterinarian's professional opinion regarding the dog's suitability based on observed behaviors, personal interaction, history of provoked or unprovoked bites, and temperament assessment (based on video review of behavior) as well as medical diagnoses/problems. All efforts to make a definitive diagnosis are expended in order to elucidate any medical constraints having an impact on the life of the MWD. This is critical not only for outcome determination but also to indicate in the dog's medical record any health issues a prospective adopter may need to know as well as to assist researchers in learning more about MWD service limitations. Happily, greater than 90% of MWDs that undergo the disposition process currently are placed under a former handler's care as a pet animal.[36]

SUMMARY

MWDs are critically important assets whose athletic skill and amazing inborn physical attributes enable them to provide a level of security to service members that is unmatched. These characteristics in addition to the tremendous bond enjoyed between animal and handler serve to make them among the most valuable teams employed on the battlefield. Ensuring competency in treating common canine conditions as well as the unique medical threats MWDs experience requires that veterinarians familiarize themselves with all facets of caring for these valued patients.

CLINICS CARE POINTS

- Musculoskeletal and neuromuscular conditions affecting the pelvic limbs and spine, respectively, are common causes of veterinary visits and MWD losses.
- Handler and first responder training is related directly to survival after ballistic and blast injuries.
- Although a disease of interest in MWDs, canine Chagas disease affects a minority of MWDs; further studies are needed to evaluate the long-term effects of exposure on seropositive dogs and their ability to serve effectively.
- HRIs are a preventable cause of morbidity in young MWDs. Development of tools to aid handlers in employing these assets in hot and humid weather could reduce these injuries.

DISCLOSURE

The authors have no financial or commercial conflicts of interest to disclose.

REFERENCES

1. Pongo A. Military working dog, human handler bond in Baghdad. Department of Defense News; 2017. Available at: https://www.defense.gov/Explore/News/Article/Article/1097173/military-working-dog-human-handler-bond-in-baghdad/. Accessed August 30, 2020.
2. Cruse SD. Military working dogs: classification and treatment in the U.S. Armed Forces. Anim L 2015;21:249.
3. Damur-Djuric N, Steffen F, Hassig M, et al. Lumbosacral transitional vertebrae in dogs: classification, prevalence, and association with sacroiliac morphology. Vet Radiol Ultrasound 2006;47:32–8.
4. Morgan JP, Bahr A, Franti CE, et al. Lumbosacral transitional vertebrae as a predisposing cause of cauda-equina syndrome in German-Shepherd dogs – 161 cases (1987–1990). J Am Vet Med Assoc 1993;202:1877–82.
5. Moore GE, Burkman KD, Carter MN, et al. Causes of death or reasons for euthanasia in military working dogs: 927 cases (1993–1996). J Am Vet Med Assoc 2001;219:209–14.
6. Ford RB, Larson LJ, McClure KD. 2017 AAHA canine vaccination guidelines. J Am Anim Hosp Assoc 2017;53:243–51.

7. Schaefers-Okkens A, Kooistra H, Nickel R. Comparison of long-term effect of ovariectomy versus ovariohysterectomy in bitches. J Reprod Fertil 1997;51: 227–31.

8. Moldal ER, Kjelgaard-Hansen MJ, Peeters ME, et al. C-reactive protein, glucose and iron concentrations are significantly altered in dogs undergoing open ovariohysterectomy or ovariectomy. Acta Vet Scand 2018;60(1):32.

9. Pereira MAA, Gonçalves LA, Evangelista MC, et al. Postoperative pain and short-term complications after two elective sterilization techniques: ovariohysterectomy or ovariectomy in cats. BMC Vet Res 2018;14:335.

10. Peeters ME, Kirpensteijn J. Comparison of surgical variables and short-term postoperative complications in healthy dogs undergoing ovariohysterectomy or ovariectomy. J Am Vet Med Assoc 2011;238:189–94.

11. Rawlings CA, Foutz TL, Mahaffey MB, et al. A rapid and strong laparoscopic-assisted gastropexy in dogs. Am J Vet Res 2001;62:871.

12. Rawlings CA, Mahaffey MB, Bement S, et al. Prospective evaluation of laparoscopic-assisted gastropexy in dogs susceptible to gastric dilatation. J Am Vet Med Assoc 2002;1576:221.

13. Steelman-Szymeczek SM, Stebbins ME, Hardie EM. Clinical evaluation of a right-sided prophylactic gastropexy via a grid approach. J Am Anim Hosp Assoc 2003;39:397.

14. Evans RI, Herbold JR, Bradshaw BS, et al. Causes for discharge of military work-ing dogs from service: 268 cases (2000-2004). J Am Vet Med Assoc 2007;231: 1215–20.

15. Bruchim Y, Horowitz M, Aroch I. Pathophysiology of heatstroke in dogs-revisited. Temperature 2017;4:356–70.

16. Gogolski SM, O'Brien CO, Lagutchik MS. Retrospective analysis of patient and environmental factors in heat-induced injury events in 103 military working dogs. J Am Vet Med Assoc 2020;256:792–9.

17. Bruchim Y, Klement E, Saragusty J, et al. Heat stroke in dogs: a retrospective study of 54 cases (1999–2004) and analysis of risk factors for death. J Vet Intern Med 2006;20:38–46.

18. O'Brien C, Tharion WJ, Karis AJ, et al. Predicting military working dog core tem-perature during exertional heat strain: validation of a Canine Thermal Model. J Therm Biol 2020;90:1–8.

19. Vogelsang R. Care of the military working dog by medical providers. J Spec Oper Med 2007;7:33–47.

20. Headquarters, Department of the Army. Veterinary care and management of the military working dog (TB MED 298) 2019.

21. Takara MS, Harrell K. Noncombat-related injuries or illnesses incurred by military working dogs in a combat zone. J Am Vet Med Assoc 2014;245:1124–8.

22. Parr JR, Otto CM. Emergency visits and occupational hazards in German Shep-herd police dogs (2008-2010). J Vet Emerg Crit Care (San Antonio) 2013;23: 591–7.

23. Björn P. Meij BP, Bergknut N. Degenerative lumbosacral stenosis. In: Johnston SA, Tobias DM, editors. Pathophysiology of degenerative lumbosacral stenosis, 2nd edition. Veterinary Surgery, vol. 2.

24. Björn P. Meij BP, Bergknut N. Degenerative lumbosacral stenosis. In: Johnston SA, Tobias DM, editors. Medical treatment of degenerative lumbosacral stenosis, 2nd edition. Veterinary Surgery. vol 2.

25. Linn LL, Bartels KE, Rochat MC, et al. Lumbosacral stenosis in 29 military working dogs: epidemiologic findings and outcome after surgical intervention (1990-1999). Vet Surg 2003;32:21–9.
26. Thomas TM, Burlison CD, Henderson A, et al. Influence of rehabilitation on outcomes of military working dogs following dorsal laminectomy. Vet Surg 2018; 47:E61.
27. Miller L, Pacheco GJ, Janak JC, et al. Causes of death in military working dogs during operation Iraqi freedom and operation enduring freedom, 2001-2013. Mil Med 2018;183:9–10.
28. Baker JL, Havas KA, Miller LA, et al. Gunshot wounds in military working dogs in Operation Enduring Freedom and Operation Iraqi Freedom: 29 cases (2003–2009). J Vet Emerg Crit Care 2013;23:47–52.
29. Lagutchik M. Clinical practice guidelines for military working dogs. In: Joint trauma system clinical practice guidelines. 2018. Available at: https://jts. amedd.army.mil/assets/docs/cpgs/Military_Working_Dog_CPGs/MWD_CPG_ 12_Dec_2018_ID16.pdf. Accessed September 13, 2020.
30. Barr SC. Canine Chagas' Disease (American Trypanosomiasis) in North America. Vet Clin Small Anim 2009;39:1055–64.
31. Kjos SA, Snowden KF, Craig TM, et al. Distribution and characterization of canine Chagas disease in Texas. Vet Parasitol 2008;152:249–56.
32. McPhatter L, Lockwood N, Roachell W. Vector surveillance to determine species composition and occurrence of *Trypanosoma cruzi* infection at three military installations in San Antonio, TX. AMEDD J 2012;12–21.
33. Malik LH, Singh GD, Amsterdam EA. The epidemiology, clinical manifestations, and management of Chagas heart disease. Clin Cardiol 2015;38:565–9.
34. Madigan R, Majoy S, Ritter K, et al. Investigation of a combination of amiodarone and itraconazole for treatment of American trypanosomiasis (Chagas disease) in dogs. J Am Vet Med Assoc 2019;255:317–29.
35. House Resolution 5314.
36. Dowling M. The 9 biggest myths about military working dogs. In: Military.com. 2015. Available at: https://www.military.com/undertheradar/2015/02/the-9-biggest-myths-about-military-working-dogs. Accessed September 12, 2020.

Operational Canine

Lee Palmer, DVM, MS, CCRP, EMT-T, NRP, TP-C

KEYWORDS

- Law enforcement • Search and rescue • Canine • K9 TECC • Preveterinary care

KEY POINTS

- Operational K9s (OpK9) encompass a unique population of working dogs that serve as a force multiplier in various civilian law enforcement, force protection, search and rescue, and humanitarian operations.
- Occupational hazards are inherent to an OpK9's high-demanding job. Hazards common to OpK9s include soft tissue and paw pad injuries, environmental illnesses, dehydration, extreme fatigue, dermatologic conditions, gastrointestinal-related issues, and musculoskeletal injuries.
- Operational K9s remain at risk for various toxicologic hazards. Awareness and preplanning are necessary for managing a potential toxicologic exposure. Personal protection is paramount during any suspect or known toxicologic exposure.
- Gastric dilatation and volvulus (GDV) is a life-threatening condition requiring immediate surgical intervention. Prophylactic gastropexy can significantly reduce the incidence of GDV in at-risk breeds.
- Bite wounds constitute a potentially debilitating occupational hazard for people working around OpK9s. Mitigating bite risks warrants handler involvement, understanding canine behaviors and associated body languages, and implementation of low-stress handling and restraint techniques.

INTRODUCTION TO OPERATIONAL CANINES

Working dogs (WDs) encompass a wide array of specially trained canines that serve humanity in various settings and roles.[1,2] Operational K9s (OpK9) encompass the distinct subpopulation of WDs that routinely perform in high-threat or tactical environments, often in the way of life-threatening harm.[3,4] Trained in various disciplines, OpK9s serve local, state, and federal, governmental and nongovernmental law enforcement (LE) and security, force protection, and search-and-rescue (SAR) organizations (see Lucia Lazarowski and colleagues' article, "Development and Training for Working Dogs," in this issue).[1,5–8] Their proven role as a force multiplier in the success

Dr L. Palmer is a Veterinary Clinical Officer assigned to the 20th Special Forces Group, Alabama Army National Guard, Certified Tactical Paramedic, and Lead for the K9 Tactical Emergency Casualty Care Working Group and Veterinary Committee on Trauma, Prehospital Subcommittee. 1883 Quail Hollow, Auburn, AL 36830, USA
E-mail address: Lpalmer2508@gmail.com

Vet Clin Small Anim 51 (2021) 945–960
https://doi.org/10.1016/j.cvsm.2021.04.011
0195-5616/21/© 2021 Elsevier Inc. All rights reserved.

of various missions makes OpK9s an essential component of any team or agency that they serve.

Since the early part of the twenty-first century, the global war on terror along with increasing active shooter and natural disaster events significantly increased the demand for OpK9s in safeguarding society. The ongoing demand for these specialized canines contributes to a growing shortage of high-quality canines to fill these roles.[9,10] Although the absolute number of OpK9s serving in the United States remains unknown, estimates indicate that approximately 50,000 are actively in service.[11,12]

Law Enforcement (Also Known as Police Dog or Police K9), Force Protection, and Security

Operational K9s supporting LE, force protection, and security missions provide many invaluable tasks to include detecting illicit materials (**Box 1**) and electronic storage components, apprehending suspects, protecting officers, and providing safety to the nation and local community.[13,14] Detection, apprehension, and tracking constitute the 3 main disciplines of this group of OpK9s whereby they train for a single purpose (eg, detection or apprehension or tracking), dual-purpose (eg, detection and apprehension, detection and tracking) or multipurpose role (detection, apprehension, and tracking).[1,15,16] Detection canines work at airports, train stations, public events, federal buildings, schools, and ports of entry, searching for the presence of explosives, weapons, illicit drugs, accelerants, or electronic storage components.[13,14,16,17] They aid crime scene and forensic investigations by performing *article searches*, locating items of evidence such as currency, firearms, and other contraband.[18]

Apprehension or *patrol* canines employ as an essential, nonlethal option and deterrence to quickly deescalate a potentially hostile situation.[19,20] Their primary purpose is to locate and subdue suspects by either physical apprehension "*Bite-and-Hold*" or by "*Circle-and-Bark*" or "*Bark-and-Hold*" with no physical contact.[19,20] Apprehension with contact (ie, bite) is not always a necessity as long as the suspect complies with the LE officer's (LEO) directions, does not resist arrest, and poses no further threat to the LEO or public.

German shepherds (GSDs), Belgian Malinois, Dutch shepherds, and Labrador retrievers constitute the stereotypical LE canine breeds; however, various other purebred and mixed-breed canines are successfully used as well. The breed selected often depends on the canine's desired role (patrol vs detection) and the breed's anticipated traits, mainly related to obedience, trainability, drive, and environmental soundness.[1,6] Agencies routinely select Belgian Malinois and GSDs for dual-purpose patrol work because of their combined prey drive, olfactory acuity, and intimidating appearance, while many select bloodhounds predominantly for their tracking ability. The cost to fund 1 OpK9 team for the first year approximates between $75,000 and $125,000.[21,22] This includes price of purchasing and training the canine, handler training and salary, specialized vehicle and associated equipment (eg, heat alarm system, kennel), associated canine training equipment and outerwear, and veterinary and other maintenance (food) costs.

Search and Rescue

SAR canines fulfill a variety of roles and can operate in a vast array of environments.[1] Teams operate either as part of a local, state, or federal LE or emergency management agency (eg, Federal Emergency Management Agency) or as private, volunteers; for the latter, the handler personally owns the canine. SAR canines detect the volatilome of a specific person, specializing in either *live find* to locate a missing living person or

---

Box 1
Common characteristics and disciplines of law enforcement detection canines

General Overview: Odor Detection

Trained to locate and alert to various categories of items[a]:
○ Explosives and explosive materials
○ Narcotics (illicit drugs)
○ Accelerants
○ Electronic components
○ Articles of evidence (currency, firearms, clothing, other)

• "Search areas" commonly trained to work in include the following:
  ○ Open area or perimeter search
  ○ Motor vehicle search
  ○ Building and room search
  ○ Person or crowd search

Explosive Detection Canine:

• Detects and alerts to the presence of explosives and/or explosive materials of both commercial and improvised home-made explosives to include the following:
  ○ 2,4,6-trinitrotoluene (TNT)
  ○ Black powder and black powder substitutes
  ○ Smokeless powders
  ○ Dynamite (nitroglycerin or ethylene glycol dinitrate-based)
  ○ Pentaerythritol tetranitrate (PETN)
  ○ Trinitro-triazacylohexane (RDX)
  ○ Ammonium nitrate
  ○ Improvised explosive or explosive materials (eg, peroxide-based)
  ○ Others

Narcotic detection (also known as drug dog):

• Locates and alerts to the presence of various illicit drugs such as cocaine, methamphetamines, heroin, marijuana, phencyclidine (PCP), lysergic acid diethylamide (LSD), and others.

Accelerant detection (arson dog)[16]:

• Locates and alerts to the presence and location of minute quantities of ignitable liquid accelerants, such as gasoline, diesel, charcoal lighter, lighter fluid, kerosene, and more.

• Supports fire departments, fire marshals, forensic investigators, and other arson task forces engaged in arson investigations.

Electronic storage detection:

• Locates and alerts to the presence electronic devices, such as hard drives, thumb drives, smartphones, and computers that may contain evidence related to a particular case.

[a]Note: Because a canine cannot relay to the handler what type of material they actually found, from both a legal and safety standpoint, a canine is rarely, if ever, trained to detect more than one category of materials; for example, a detection canine is trained to detect either narcotics or explosives, not both.

---

recovery to locate human remains (ie, human remains detection or cadaver dog).[1,23] They operate in large and small areas and in various environments, including urban, wilderness, deserts, water, and avalanche.[1,24–28] Their keen sense of smell allows them to locate persons buried under several feet of rubble, snow, or water, as well as cover several miles of wilderness in a short time. An SAR canine team endures several weeks of intense initial training and dedicates several hours of training per month to maintain proficiency. Obedience, trainability, drive, sociability, and environmental soundness are key traits for an SAR canine. **Table 1** describes the common scenting disciplines of SAR canines.

OCCUPATIONAL HAZARDS AND INJURIES COMMON TO OPERATIONAL K9S

Occupational hazards are inherent to an OpK9's high-demanding job. The hazards vary for each OpK9 and depend on their breed characteristics, trained discipline and job-related activities, and operational environment.[2,8,24–29] Data regarding common line of duty (LOD) injuries and illnesses for nonmilitary OpK9s remain limited; however, extrapolating data collected from military WDs (MWDs) fills some of these critical knowledge gaps. Mey and colleagues[8] showed that age, breed, and occupational certification are associated factors for increased injury risk in MWDs. Older MWDs display a higher injury risk compared with younger dogs; particularly, for musculoskeletal injuries. In 2001, Moore and colleagues[30] identified appendicular degenerative joint disease, neoplasia, spinal cord disease, nonspecific geriatric decline, and gastric dilatation–volvulus (GDV) as the leading causes of euthanasia or death in MWDs. While deployed in combat operations, gunshot wounds (GSW), explosions/blast injuries, and heat-related illnesses constituted the leading causes of

Table 1	
Scenting disciplines of search-and-rescue canines[1]	
Discipline	**Characteristics**
Tracking	• Operates with the handler using a harness and 20- to 30-foot leash. • Follows the actual tracks left by the POI by keeping their nose to the ground on the exact path of the POI. • Tracks by detecting the odor of one of a combination of the following: ○ Specific to the POI; requires use of a *scent article* or any item that came into contact with the POI and contains the distinct odor and VOCs of the POI such as a piece of clothing, bedding, car seat, or other. ○ Odor caused by *environmental (ground) disturbances* (eg, crushed vegetation). Tracking by ground disturbance may cause error as the track becomes older (scent dissipates) and/or if track becomes *contaminated* by other persons or animals that have crossed or walked on the same path. • Limited by the age of the track; the older the track, the lower probability the canine can locate the POI. • Works best without other canine teams in the immediate area.
Trailing	• Operates on or off leash. • Uses a scent article to follow the specific scent of the POI. • Does not need to directly follow the track or path of the POI; rather they can *work* within a few feet of the POI's track. • Do not track using environmental disturbance, therefore, are not affected by a trail *contaminated* by another person or animal as compared with a tracking canine. • Not limited by the age of the track as compared with a tracking only canine. • Works best without other canine teams in the immediate area.
Air scent	• Capable of working effectively off leash over a very large area. • Does not require a scent article or trail to follow. • Sniffs the air to identify human scent, then works into the wind following the *scent cone* to the source. • Capable of working effectively with other canine teams in the area.

Abbreviations: POI, person of interest; VOC, volatile organic compounds.

trauma-related deaths.[31] For MWDs suffering GSWs, wounds to the thorax followed by to the head account for the leading cause of death, whereas those suffering GSWs only to the extremity were most likely to survive.[32] Dermatologic, soft tissue trauma, alimentary, and musculoskeletal issues represent the most prevalent noncombat-related illnesses for MWDs operating in a deployed environment (**Box 2**).[33]

Civilian OpK9s are at risk for many of the same occupational hazards discussed for MWDs. Soft tissue injuries (lacerations and puncture wounds), paw pad injuries, environmental illnesses, dehydration, extreme fatigue, dermatologic conditions, gastrointestinal-related issues (diarrhea, vomiting), and musculoskeletal injuries are common to all disciplines of OpK9s.[5,8,24–28,34] Breeds commonly used as OpK9s are prone to degenerative disorders such as lumbosacral disease, hip dysplasia, cranial cruciate ligament tear, and elbow dysplasia.[5,8,34,35] Combined with the physical tasks and extreme athleticism (agility, endurance, strength, balance, and coordination) required of many OpK9 jobs, their risk for musculoskeletal injuries remains high.[34–36] In a retrospective study, orthopedic injuries along with gastrointestinal disease constituted the 2 most likely reasons GSD police dogs presented on emergency.[5] OpK9s wearing ballistic armor may still suffer major internal injuries from blunt force trauma when shot with a high-velocity projectile.[37] Excessive neck pressure applied repetitively by a collar can lead to cervical injuries and elevations in intraocular

---

Box 2
Most prevalent noncombat-related injuries/illnesses for military working dogs in a combat zone[33]

Dermatologic Disease (25.0%)

- Otitis externa (34.6%)

- Generalized superficial pyoderma (10.7%)

- Atopic dermatitis (9.2%)

- Acute moist dermatitis (8.0%)

Soft tissue trauma (21.0%)

- Foot pad or paw injuries (32.0%)

- Lacerations in locations other than foot pads or paws (16.2%)

- Tail tip trauma (10.9%)

- Dog bite wounds (10.9%)

Alimentary system (17.1%)

- Diarrhea (31.6%)

- Vomiting (20.3%)

- Hematochezia (13.4%)

- Gastrointestinal foreign bodies (7.8%)

Musculoskeletal system (14.3%)

- Hind limbs (47.2%)

- Forelimbs (26.9%)

- Vertebral column and associated musculature (10.9%)

- Tail (5.7%)

pressure.[38–40] Transient hearing deficits occur in OpK9s that have frequent exposure to intense noise, including gunfire, flashbangs, and helicopter operations (Pete "Skip" Scheifele MD, PhD, e-mail communication, January 2020).

Heat-Related Illness

Heat-related illnesses remain a leading cause of *preventable* LOD deaths in OpK9s.[29,31,41] Early recognition followed by appropriate and immediate actions prevents mild *heat stress* from cascading into a severe *heat stroke*. Research is ongoing to evaluate the most effective, field-practical preventive measures, such as optimal hydration strategies, pre- and post-cooling techniques, and core temperature monitoring.[42–49] Although traditional recommendations suggested against the need for electrolyte-enriched fluids for rehydrating canines experiencing heat-related illness, a recent study showed that administration of electrolyte-enriched fluids to canines before performing moderate-intensity exercise in hot, arid climatic conditions helped maintain lower peak core temperatures without causing electrolyte abnormalities.[43] In this study, canines experienced an average peak core temperature or more than 41°C (105.8°F) with only 1 canine displaying signs of mild heat stress; that canine possessed a core temperature of 42.8°C (109°F), recovered uneventfully, and completed the study. Another canine with a peak core temperature of 42.88°C (109.18°F) did not show any behavioral or clinical signs of heat stress. Prior observations show that well-conditioned, acclimated canines may reach peak core temperatures of more than 41.1°C (106°F) while working, yet display no behavioral or clinical signs of heat stress.[45,46] Available data demonstrate that repetitive exposure to moderate to high-intensity exercise in conjunction with acclimation to hot climates may invoke adaptive cellular responses that lower the risk of heat-related events in working canines.[47] Collectively, data support that physical conditioning and acclimation can mitigate heat-related illnesses in OpK9s.[43,47]

Gastric Dilatation–Volvulus/Mesenteric Volvulus

Most medium to large OpK9 breeds remain at high risk for gastric dilatation and volvulus (GDV). The pathogenesis of GDV is multifactorial and remains completely unknown.[50] Although several host and environmental predisposing factors (eg, genetic, gender, age, breed, diet, exercise) are implicated with an increased likelihood for GDV, evidence supporting the relevant importance of these associated risk factors remains inconclusive.[50–57]

Most preventive measures used for reducing the likelihood of GDV are empirical and anecdotal in nature; however, the prophylactic gastropexy possesses a documented decrease in the incidence and lifetime probability of death (up to 29-fold in some breeds) from GDV in at-risk breeds.[51,58–60]

Mesenteric volvulus (MV) and rare occurrences of volvulus/torsion of the ileocecocolic junction and transverse and descending colon are reported in the literature.[61–64] MV presents as another acute, life-threatening condition whereby the underlying etiopathogenesis remains completely unknown. A retrospective study in MWDs identified breed (ie, GSD), increased age, history of gastrointestinal disease, and history of prophylactic gastropexy or of other abdominal surgery as associated risk factors.[64] Despite observing history of prophylactic gastropexy as an associated risk factor, the prevalence of GDV in MWDs has declined significantly after the military instituted their prophylactic gastropexy policy; therefore, the military continues to support and performs the prophylactic gastropexy in all MWDs.[64]

Law Enforcement

Occupational hazards specific to LE include exposure to hazardous materials (opioids, cocaine, methamphetamines, explosives, accelerants, others), penetrating injuries from GSWs or knife wounds, and blast injuries subsequent to detonation of explosives or explosive devices.[29,65,66] Penetrating trauma (GSW) and heat-related illnesses represent the 2 leading causes of LOD deaths consistently reported in LE K9s.[11,29] Patrol canines possess a higher risk for orthodontic-related injuries, close-quarter traumatic injuries (eg, GSWs, stabbings, other) and musculoskeletal injuries subsequent to the extreme forces placed on a patrol canine's body during bite work training (**Fig. 1**).

Detection canines can experience intoxication from accidental exposures to various illicit or hazardous materials.[65,67–74] Accidental ingestion of an explosive (eg, cyclonite) training aid is commonly reported for explosive detection canines.[67–69] Threat of exposure to potent opioids (fentanyl, carfentanil) and deadly synthetic cannabinoids poses a major threat for narcotic detection canines.[70–73] Clandestine chemical laboratories place all disciplines of LE K9s at risk for exposure to illicit drugs, home-made explosives and the various chemical precursors used in manufacturing these compounds.[74]

Search and Rescue (Wilderness and Urban)

Past natural disasters (Hurricane Katrina; mudslides in Oso, WA; Haiti, others) and mass casualty events (9-11/World Trade Center; Oklahoma City) provides lessons-learned about occupational hazards common to SAR canines.[24–28] Predominant trauma-induced injuries include paw pad and other soft tissue–related injuries, mainly minor lacerations and abrasions to the lower limbs. Nontraumatic illnesses consist of

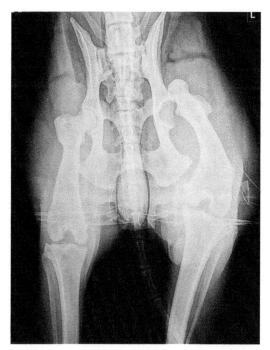

Fig. 1. A 9-year-old male, neutered Belgian Malinois experienced coxofemoral luxation while engaged in bite work training. (Photo courtesy of Dr. Nell Dalton.)

dehydration, fatigue, decreased appetite, ocular irritation, and gastrointestinal issues. Fortunately, these injuries are typically minor and amenable to basic first aid with minimal veterinary medical attention. Terrain features (eg, uneven ground, hot sand or pavement) and scattered ground debris (eg, broken glass, jagged pieces of steel and concrete) contribute to the high risk for paw pad, soft tissue, and musculoskeletal injuries. Wilderness operations experience wild animal interactions (eg, porcupines, wild boars, cougars), venomous encounters (bees, wasps, scorpions, snakes), and infectious vectors such as ticks. Canines working wildfires encounter inhalational exposures to carcinogenic woodland smoke, aerosolized dry ash, and poison oak fumes, as well as contact with hazardous materials hidden under layers of ash (eg, burning ground or roots).[27]

Urban disaster responses commonly operate unprotected in environments contaminated with various liquid, solid, and particulate toxicologic hazards.[75–77] Often, the hazardous material encountered remains completely unknown. A general awareness for potential hazards and common routes of exposure allows personnel to implement preventive strategies and initiate field decontamination procedures to prevent major exposures. Personal protection remains paramount during any suspect or known toxicologic exposure. All personnel must take appropriate personal protection and self-aid measures, such as instituting individual decontamination procedures and donning appropriate personal protection equipment. Awareness and preplanning are critical steps for preventing and managing a potential toxicologic exposure.

CONSIDERATIONS FOR PROVIDING VETERINARY SUPPORT TO AN OPERATIONAL K9 TEAM

The Handler–OpK9 Bond

Veterinary personnel should understand the strong bond between a handler and canine. Handlers rely on their canine partner not only for personal safety but also for companionship.[13] Because of their strong relationship, the handler can identify subtle changes in their canine's routine behavior that may indicate a problem, before the problem becomes apparent to others. During a veterinary visit, handlers serve as an advocate for their canine. In addition, through providing obedience commands, low-stress restraint, and muzzling, handlers protect veterinary personnel from a potential a bite risk; therefore, handler involvement throughout the entirety of the veterinary visit is paramount. In situations in which the primary handler is not available, another handler or person with experience handling OpK9s should be sought to assist in handling.

The handler and OpK9 work as a team. It is imperative that handlers remain aware of the impact any illness, injury, procedure, or medication may have on their canine's working performance. Data regarding pharmaceutical-induced hyposmia in canines remains lacking[78] (See Olfactory Chapter). To date, only high-dose metronidazole (25 mg/kg, by mouth, every 12 hours for 10 days) and high-dose dexamethasone and hydrocortisone combined with deoxycorticosterone were shown to transiently affect a canine's olfactory acuity.[79,80] Intravenous fentanyl followed by reversal with intranasal or intramuscular naloxone does not seem to impair canine olfactory acuity.[81]

General Approach to Handling and Restraint

Special considerations for safety are necessary when examining, handling, and restraining an OpK9. The temperament of each individual canine varies; some are very tolerant during an examination, whereas others present more of a challenge. A canine's behavior can become erratic and unpredictable when exposed to a traumatic, stressful, and/or painful event; they may become overly aggressive even with benign interventions. In general, patrol canines have a different set of drive, focus, and alertness for surrounding events and approaching threats; typically, they are not trained to give into restraint or submission.

Bite wounds present an occupational hazard and debilitating injury for any personnel who work around OpK9s.[82] Adherence to appropriate safety precautions serves as an effective first-line intervention for reducing bite risks. Most animals feed off a person's behavior that, during times of fear, stress, or pain, may add to potential aggression. Harsh restraint may heighten the canine's response of fear aggression and cause a bite event, therefore supporting the need to implement low-stress handling techniques.[83] Overly fractious canines warrant pharmaceutical intervention using a neuroleptanalgesia approach to ensure safety to personnel and the canine (see Anesthesia in Working Dogs Chapter). Awareness of a canine's behavior and associated body language in response to pain, stress or trauma as well as their perception and reaction to a person's body language and actions can help ensure personnel and staff safety when working around an OpK9.

Prevention, Preparedness, and Prehospital Care

Prevention serves as the main focus of treating any injury or illness. Areas of preventive measures should focus on heat-related illness, paw pad and eye protection, physical conditioning, field decontamination, and prophylactic gastropexy for at-risk breeds. All OpK9s should partake in a comprehensive preventive health care program, including appropriate vaccinations and prophylactic treatment against heartworms, fleas, ticks, intestinal parasites, and other common vectors (Marcella Ridgway's article, "Preventative Health Care for Working Dogs," in this issue).

Although OpK9s remain at high risk for experiencing traumatic, potentially life-threatening LOD injuries, access to prehospital care remains limited.[84–86] Point-of-injury first responder field care often falls to the OpK9 handler and/or human prehospital care or emergency medical services provider (EMSP), such as a paramedic or other first responder.[87–89] Although nearly all MWD handlers receive basic emergency canine first aid training, many civilian OpK9 handlers receive little to no training (S. Hansen, DVM, and L. Palmer, DVM, unpublished data, 2018).[88,89] Because handlers and human EMSPs represent the first line of defense in preventing and treating illness and injury in their canine partner, veterinary professionals supporting OpK9 teams should consider taking an active role in educating these personnel in preventive care and basic first aid.[84]

With the lack of veterinary-based emergency medical services (EMS) systems, several states have enacted or are in the process of enacting *preveterinary care legislation* that grants limited authority to EMSPs for rendering emergency life-saving out-of-hospital care to injured animals.[85,90] The legislation provides immunity for EMSPs to render emergency prehospital care to an OpK9s without the direct or indirect supervision of a licensed veterinarian. In some states, it also provides immunity for veterinary personnel that train EMSPs in veterinary prehospital care interventions. The extent of veterinary care allowed by a first responder varies from state to state; however, most allow provision of care to the scope or level of practice the first responder possesses for human patients. To help ensure the quality of care provided, some state's statutes also recommends that nonveterinary first responders receive training in veterinary prehospital care. Preveterinary care legislation affords an injured OpK9 the opportunity to receive the highest level of resuscitative care at the point-of-injury, or as far forward as possible, where the presence of licensed veterinary

Box 3
Prehospital, preveterinary care publications

K9 Tactical Emergency Casualty Care Initiative (K9 TECC, www.k9tecc.org)[3,4]
  The K9 TECC working group formed in 2014 with the primary intent of developing best practice prehospital care guidelines for civilian OpK9s injured under high-threat situations.[3,4] Modeled after the same principles established in human guidelines and lessons-learned from MWDs on the battlefield, the K9 TECC guidelines focus on simple, evidence-based, field-proven medical interventions to eliminate preventable deaths and to improve OpK9 survival.

American College of Veterinary Emergency & Critical Care (ACVECC), Veterinary Committee on Trauma (VetCOT), Prehospital Subcommittee (http://vetcot.org/)
  VetCOT's Prehospital Subcommittee formed in 2014 to address the void in prehospital veterinary care. Two years later in 2016, the subcommittee published their *Best Practice Recommendations of Veterinary Prehospital Care of Dogs and Cats*.[86] These best practices discuss 18 core prehospital care topics with the intent of educating and training veterinary and nonveterinary allied paramedical (physicians, nurses, EMS providers, other) and nonmedical (eg, canine handlers) personnel.

Operation Canine Lifeline: Recommendations for Enhancing Prehospital Care for Government Working Dogs.[84]
  In 2017, graduate students and faculty from Boston University School of Medicine's Healthcare Emergency Management conducted a table-top exercise to discuss recommendations for addressing the needs of prehospital veterinary care for government WDs. The discussion, which focused mainly on exposure to toxins in the field, led to the creation of the following recommendations:
  • Establishing a government-run veterinary toxicology hotline for the sole use of the government.
  • Issuing handlers deployment kits.
  • Preprogrammed smartphones that contain information on the care practices for dogs.
  • Increased effort for civilian integration, through local EMS, in the emergency care of government canines.

Air Medical Transportation of Injured Operational Canines.[91]
  The study assessed the prevalence of air medical transports as well as the existence and content of protocols to conduct air medical transports for injured OpK9s. The investigators' concluding recommendations for Air Medical Programs include the following:
  • Flight programs should determine whether they will honor a request to transport an injured OpK9 before being called on to make an emergent decision.
  • For those flight programs that are willing to transport an injured OpK9 they should
    ○ Work with agencies within their area of operations to develop policy and procedures.
    ○ Obtain expert consultation from a knowledgeable veterinary medical professional regarding the legality of provision of care, care protocols, and specialized equipment that they may wish to obtain if called on to transport an injured OpK9.

The Carle-Illinois (Urbana, Illinois) transport protocol for LEK9s: guidelines for Emergency Medical Service providers.[92,93]
  The authors of this report convened a Joint Task Force on Working Dog Care composed of veterinarians, EMS directors, EMS physicians, and LEK9 handlers to develop a protocol for LEK9s being transported to a veterinary facility. The protocol and manuscript provide the following information based on the legislation and resources:
  • Logistics of getting the LEK9 into the ambulance with or without the handler.
  • Appropriate restraint.
  • The importance of prior arrangements with a veterinary emergency facility.
  • An LEK9 hand-off form.
  • Transport Policy Form (downloadable from www.workingdogHQ.com, and customizable for each EMS provider).

Abbreviations: EMS, emergency medical services; LE, law enforcement; OpK9, operational canine.

personnel is lacking. A successful preveterinary care initiative requires a collaborative working relationship between the veterinary and human EMS communities. **Box 3** lists initiatives and case-based protocols published relevant to prehospital veterinary care for OpK9s.

SUMMARY

Operational K9s are used with increasing demand in the United States and abroad as force multipliers for protecting national security and assisting society in disaster and humanitarian efforts. The nature of their duties comes with inherent occupational hazards that place them at higher risk for LOD injuries and deaths. Veterinary and other medical personnel play a vital role in an OpK9's health and welfare, ensuring their operational performance and longevity. To provide the utmost care to these elite canines, veterinary personnel must take into account numerous considerations. Understanding the handler–canine bond, common occupational hazards, and unique behaviors pertinent to an OpK9 allows veterinarians to provide the highest quality medical care, in the safest way possible. Handlers should receive education and training in preventive care and basic canine first aid. With the gap in veterinary-based EMS systems, providing both handlers and other paraprofessionals (eg, EMSPs) training in canine first aid may decrease the morbidity and mortality of OpK9s.

CLINICS CARE POINTS

- OpK9s deployed in a tactical or high-threat environment remain at high risk for suffering preventable deaths; however, prehospital care for OpK9s injured in the LOD remains lacking. Veterinary and human prehospital medical communities should collaborate together to ensure OpK9s receive the highest level of resuscitative care at the point of injury, or as far forward as possible, where the presence of trained and licensed veterinary personnel is lacking.
- Veterinarians should familiarize themselves with current legislation for prehospital treatment and transport in their state to facilitate appropriate training of first responders for emergent conditions most likely to be encountered in these patients.

DISCLAIMER

The information and views expressed in this article are those of the authors based on cited resources and currently available evidence; they do not reflect the official policy or position of any local, state, or federal governmental or nongovernmental entity.

DISCLOSURE

The author has no financial or other conflicts of interest to disclose.

REFERENCES

1. Olson PN. The modern working dog–a call for interdisciplinary collaboration. J Am Vet Med Assoc 2002;221(3):352–5.
2. Worth AJ, Cave NJ. A veterinary perspective on preventing injuries and other problems that shorten the life of working dogs. Rev Sci Tech 2018;37(1):161–9.
3. Palmer LE, Maricle R, Brenner JA. The Operational Canine and K9 Tactical emergency casualty care initiative. J Spec Oper Med 2015;15(3):32–8.
4. Palmer LE, Yee A. TacMed Updates: K9 tactical emergency casualty care direct threat care guidelines. J Spec Oper Med 2017;17(2):174–87.

5. Parr JR, Otto CM. Emergency visits and occupational hazards in German shepherd police dogs (2008-2010). J Vet Emer Crit 2013;23:591–7.
6. Lazarowski L, Haney PS, Brock J, et al. Investigation of the behavioral characteristics of dogs purpose-bred and prepared to perform vapor Wake® detection of person-borne explosives. Front Vet Sci 2018;5:50.
7. Seck HH. Working dogs are Marines' new 'force multiplier' on ships 2014. Available at: https://www.marinecorpstimes.com/news/your-marine-corps/2014/12/30/working-dogs-are-marines-new-force-multiplier-on-ships/. Accessed July 15, 2020.
8. Mey W, Schuh-Renner A, Anderson MK, et al. Risk factors for injury among military working dogs deployed to Iraq. Prev Vet Med 2020;176:104911.
9. Otto CM. Dogs of DHS: how canine programs contribute to homeland security. Hearing before the Committee on Homeland Security and Governmental Affairs, United States Senate 114th Congress Mar 3, S. Hrg 114-673. 2016. Available at: https://www.hsgac.senate.gov/hearings/dogs-of-dhs-how-canine-programs-contribute-to-homeland-security. Accessed July 15, 2020.
10. Leighton EA, Hare E, Thomas S, et al. A solution for the shortage of detection dogs: a detector dog center of excellence and a cooperative breeding program. Front Vet Sci 2018;5:284.
11. Ingraham C. The surprising reason more police dogs are dying in the line of duty. 20 Nov 2015. Available at: https://www.washingtonpost.com/news/wonk/wp/2015/11/20/the-surprising-reason-more-police-dogs-are-dying-in-the-line-of-duty/. Accessed July 21, 2020.
12. AKC Detection Dog Task Force FAQs. American Kennel Club. Available at: https://www.akc.org/akc-detection-dog-task-force/faqs/. Accessed July 21, 2020.
13. Hart LA, Zasloff RL, Bryson S, et al. The role of police dogs as companions and working partners. Psychol Rep 2000;86(1):190–202.
14. Wyllie D. A K-9 unit has benefits for police departments and communities alike. 2019. Available at: https://www.policemag.com/509962/a-k-9-unit-has-benefits-for-police-departments-the-communities-alike. Accessed July 21, 2020.
15. Hutchison K, Montes D. Dogs of DHS: how canine programs contribute to homeland security. Hearing before the Committee on Homeland Security and Governmental Affairs, United States Senate 114th Congress Mar 3, S. Hrg 114-673. 2016. Available at: https://www.hsgac.senate.gov/hearings/dogs-of-dhs-how-canine-programs-contribute-to-homeland-security. Accessed July 21, 2020.
16. Kmiecik M. Sample report narrative: tracking/trailing people based on last known position. Sheepdog Guardian Consulting, LLC; 2020. Available at: https://www.sheepdogguardian.com/. Accessed July 21, 2020.
17. Kurz ME, Billard M, Rettig M, et al. Evaluation of canines for accelerant detection at fire scenes. J Forensic Sci 1994;39(6):1528–36.
18. Wright RJ. The use of police service dogs in crime scene location and related evidence gathering. Available at: https://www.policek9.com/html/k9_evidence_search.html. Accessed July 21, 2020.
19. Dorriety JK. Police service dogs in the use-of-force continuum. Criminal Justice Policy Rev 2005;16(1):88–98.
20. Fleck T, Kmiecik M. Patrol dog summary. Sheepdog Guardian Consulting, LLC; 2020. Available at: https://www.sheepdogguardian.com/. Accessed July 21, 2020.
21. Merrick BJ. The Bill Blackwood Law Enforcement Management Institute of Texas, . Justification for the creation and implementation of police canine units. TX: Frisco Police Department Frisco; 2014. Available at: https://www.sheepdogguardian.com/. Accessed July 1, 2020.

22. Gilbertson L. How to start and fund a police K-9 unit. Police1; 2019. Available at: https://www.policeone.com/k-9/articles/how-to-start-and-fund-a-police-k-9-unit-94keHTkGMPY5eHkA/. Accessed July 21, 2020.
23. Angle C, Waggoner LP, Ferrando A, et al. Canine detection of the volatilome: a review of implications for pathogen and disease detection. Front Vet Sci 2016; 3:47.
24. Gordon LE. Injuries and illnesses among urban search-and-rescue dogs deployed to Haiti following the January 12, 2010, earthquake. J Am Vet Med Assoc 2012;240(4):396–403.
25. Gordon LE. Injuries and illnesses among Federal Emergency Management Agency-certified search-and-recovery and search-and-rescue dogs deployed to Oso, Washington, following the March 22, 2014, State Route 530 landslide. J Am Vet Med Assoc 2015;247(8):901–8.
26. Otto CM, Franz MA, Kellogg B, et al. Field treatment of search dogs: lessons learned from the World Trade Center disaster. J Vet Emerg Crit Care 2002; 12(1):33–41.
27. Gordon LE, Ho B. Injuries and illnesses among human remains detection-certified search-and-recovery dogs deployed to northern California in response to the Camp Fire wildfire of November 2018. J Am Vet Med Assoc 2020;256(3):322–32.
28. Slensky KA, Drobatz KJ, Downend AB, et al. Deployment morbidity among search-and-rescue dogs used after the September 11, 2001, terrorist attacks. J Am Vet Med Assoc 2004;225(6):868–73.
29. Stojsih SE, Baker JL, Les CM, et al. Review of canine deaths while in service in US civilian law enforcement (2002-2012). J Spec Oper Med 2014;14(4):86–91.
30. Moore GE, Burkman KD, Carter MN, et al. Causes of death or reasons for euthanasia in military working dogs: 927 cases (1993-1996). J Am Vet Med Assoc 2001;219:209–14.
31. Miller L, Pacheco GJ, Janak JC, et al. Causes of death in military working dogs during Operation Iraqi Freedom and Operation Enduring Freedom, 2001-2013. Mil Med 2018;183(9–10):e467–74.
32. Baker JL, Havas KA, Miller LA, et al. Gunshot wounds in military working dogs in Operation Enduring Freedom and Operation Iraqi Freedom: 29 cases (2003-2009). J Vet Emerg Crit Care (San Antonio) 2013;23(1):47–52.
33. Takara MS, Harrell K. Noncombat-related injuries or illnesses incurred by military working dogs in a combat zone. J Am Vet Med Assoc 2014;245(10):1124–8.
34. Baltzer WI, Owen R, Bridges J. Survey of handlers of 158 police dogs in New Zealand: functional assessment and canine orthopedic index. Front Vet Sci 2019;6:85.
35. Otto CM, Cobb ML, Wilsson E. Editorial: Working dogs: form and function [published correction appears in Front Vet Sci. 2020 Feb 26;7:93]. Front Vet Sci 2019; 6:351.
36. Hart BL, Hart LA, Thigpen AP, et al. Neutering of German shepherd dogs: associated joint disorders, cancers and urinary incontinence. Vet Med Sci 2016;2(3): 191–9.
37. Stojish S. A biomechanical assessment of canine body armor. Wayne State University Dissertations; 2015. Available at: https://digitalcommons.wayne.edu/cgi/viewcontent.cgi?article=2295&context=oa_dissertations. Accessed July 21, 220.
38. Pauli AM, Bentley E, Diehl KA, et al. Effects of the application of neck pressure by a collar or harness on intraocular pressure in dogs. J Am Anim Hosp Assoc 2006; 42(3):207–11.

39. Carter A, McNally D, Roshier A. Canine collars: an investigation of collar type and the forces applied to a simulated neck model. Vet Rec 2020 Oct 3;187(7):e52.
40. Nottingham Trent University. Collars risk causing neck injuries in dogs, study shows. 2020. Available at: https://phys.org/news/2020-05-collars-neck-injuries-dogs.html. Accessed July 21, 2020.
41. Baker JL, Hollier PJ, Miller L, et al. Rethinking heat injury in the SOF multipurpose canine: a critical review. J Spec Oper Med 2012;12(2):8–15.
42. Davis MS, Marcellin-Little DJ, O'Connor E. Comparison of postexercise cooling methods in working dogs. J Spec Oper Med 2019;19(1):56–60.
43. Niedermeyer GM, Hare E, Brunker LK, et al. A randomized cross-over field study of pre-hydration strategies in dogs tracking in hot environments. Front Vet Sci 2020;7:292.
44. Otto CM, Hare E, Nord JL, et al. Evaluation of three hydration strategies in detection dogs working in a hot environment. Front Vet Sci 2017;4:174.
45. Robbins PJ, Ramos MT, Zanghi BM, et al. Environmental and physiological factors associated with stamina in dogs exercising in high ambient temperatures. Front Vet Sci 2017;4:144.
46. Angle TC, Gillette RL. Telemetric measurement of body core temperature in exercising unconditioned Labrador retrievers. Can J Vet Res 2011;75:157–9.
47. Bruchim Y, Aroch I, Eliav A, et al. Two years of combined high-intensity physical training and heat acclimatization affect lymphocyte and serum HSP70 in purebred military working dogs. J Appl Physiol (1985) 2014;117(2):112–8.
48. Baker J, DeChant M, Jenkins E, et al. Body temperature responses during phases of work in human remains detection dogs undergoing a simulated deployment. Animals (Basel) 2020;10(4):673.
49. O'Brien C, Karis AJ, Tharion WJ, et al. Core temperature responses of military working dogs during training activities and exercise walks. US Army Med Dep J 2017;(3–17):71–8.
50. Brockman DJ, Holt DE, Washabau RJ. Pathogenesis of acute gastric dilatation-volvulus syndrome: is there a unifying hypothesis? Comp Cont Ed Pract Vet 2000;22:1108–14.
51. Ward MP, Patronek GJ, Glickman LT. Benefits of prophylactic gastropexy for dogs at risk of gastric dilatation-volvulus. Prev Vet Med 2003;60(4):319–29.
52. Glickman LT, Glickman NW, Schellenberg DB, et al. Incidence of and breed-related risk factors for gastric dilatation-volvulus in dogs. J Am Vet Med Assoc 2000;216(1):40–5.
53. Glickman LT, Glickman NW, Schellenberg DB, et al. Non-dietary risk factors for gastric dilatation-volvulus in large and giant breed dogs. J Am Vet Med Assoc 2000;217(10):1492–9.
54. Schellenberg DB, Yi Q, Glickman NW, et al. Influence of thoracic conformation and genetics on the risk of gastric dilatation-volvulus in Irish Setters. J Am Anim Hosp Assoc 1998;34(1):64–73.
55. Buckley LA. Are dogs fed a kibble-based diet more likely to experience an episode of gastric dilatation volvulus than dogs fed an alternative diet? Vet Evid 2017;2(2):1–21.
56. Jennings PB Jr, Butzin CA. Epidemiology of gastric dilatation-volvulus in the military working dog program. Mil Med 1992;157(7):369–71.
57. Pipan M, Brown DC, Battaglia CL, et al. An Internet-based survey of risk factors for surgical gastric dilatation-volvulus in dogs. J Am Vet Med Assoc 2012;240(12):1456–62.

58. Allen P, Paul A. Gastropexy for prevention of gastric dilatation-volvulus in dogs: history and techniques. Top Companion Anim Med 2014;29(3):77–80.
59. Przywara JF, Abel SB, Peacock JT, et al. Occurrence and recurrence of gastric dilatation with or without volvulus after incisional gastropexy. The Can Vet J 2014;55(10):981–4.
60. Hammel SP, Novo RE. Recurrence of gastric dilatation-volvulus after incisional gastropexy in a Rottweiler. J Am Anim Hosp Assoc 2006;42(2):147–50.
61. Andrews SJ, Thomas TM, Hauptman JG, et al. Investigation of potential risk factors for mesenteric volvulus in military working dogs. J Am Vet Med Assoc 2018; 253(7):877–85.
62. Halfacree ZJ, Beck AL, Lee KC, et al. Torsion and volvulus of the transverse and descending colon in a German shepherd dog. J Small Anim Pract 2006;47(8): 468–70.
63. Javard R, Specchi S, Benamou J, et al. Ileocecocolic volvulus in a German shepherd dog. Can Vet J 2014;55(11):1096–9.
64. Gagnon D, Brisson B. Predisposing factors for colonic torsion/volvulus in dogs: a retrospective study of six cases (1992-2010). J Am Anim Hosp Assoc 2013;49(3): 169–74.
65. Llera RM, Volmer PA. Toxicologic hazards for police dogs involved in drug detection. J Am Vet Med Assoc 2006;228(7):1028–32.
66. Barberi D, Jennifer C, Gibbs JC, et al. K9s killed in the line of duty. Contemp Justice Rev 2019;22(1):86–100.
67. Bruchim Y, Saragusty J, Weisman A, et al. Cyclonite (RDX) intoxication in a police working dog. Vet Rec 2005;157(12):354–6.
68. Fishkin RA, Stanley SW, Langston CE. Toxic effects of cyclonite (C-4) plastic explosive ingestion in a dog. J Vet Emerg Crit Care 2008;18(5):537–40.
69. De Cramer KG, Short RP. Plastic explosive poisoning in dogs. J S Afr Vet Assoc 1992;63(1):30–1.
70. Palmer LE, Gautier A. Clinical update: the risk of opioid toxicity and naloxone use in operational K9s. J Spec Oper Med 2017;17(4):86–92.
71. Williams K, Wells RJ, McLean MK. Suspected synthetic cannabinoid toxicosis in a dog. J Vet Emerg Crit Care 2015;25(6):739–44.
72. Brutlag A, Hommerding H. Toxicology of marijuana, synthetic cannabinoids, and cannabidiol in dogs and cats. Vet Clin North Am Small Anim Pract 2018;48(6): 1087–102.
73. Culler CA, Vigani A. Successful treatment of a severe cannabinoid toxicity using extracorporeal therapy in a dog. J Vet Emerg Crit Care (San Antonio) 2019;29(6): 674–9.
74. Department of Homeland Security, Intelligence and Fusion centers. 201. (U// FOUO) DHS Identifying and Differentiating among Clandestine Biological, Chemical, Explosives, and Methamphetamine Laboratories. Available at: https:// publicintelligence.net/ufouo-dhs-identifying-clandestine-biological-chemical-explosives-and-methamphetamine-laboratories/. Accessed July 21, 2020.
75. Gwaltney-Brant SM, Murphy LA, Wismer TA, et al. General toxicologic hazards and risks for search-and-rescue dogs responding to urban disasters. J Am Vet Med Assoc 2003;222(3):292–5.
76. Murphy LA, Gwaltney-Brant SM, Albretsen JC, et al. Toxicologic agents of concern for search-and-rescue dogs responding to urban disasters. J Am Vet Med Assoc 2003;222(3):296–304.

77. Wismer TA, Murphy LA, Gwaltney-Brant SM, et al. Management and prevention of toxicoses in search-and-rescue dogs responding to urban disasters. J Am Vet Med Assoc 2003;222(3):305–10.

78. Jenkins EK, DeChant MT, Perry EB. When the nose doesn't know: canine olfactory function associated with health, management, and potential links to microbiota. Front Vet Sci 2018;5:56.

79. Jenkins EK, Lee-Fowler TM, Angle TC, et al. Effects of oral administration of metronidazole and doxycycline on olfactory capabilities of explosives detection dogs. Am J Vet Res 2016;77(8):906–12.

80. Ezeh PI, Myers LJ, Hanrahan LA, et al. Effects of steroids on the olfactory function of the dog. Physiol Behav 1992;51(6):1183–7.

81. Essler JL, Smith PG, Berger D, et al. A randomized cross-over trial comparing the effect of intramuscular versus intranasal naloxone reversal of intravenous fentanyl on odor detection in working dogs. Animals (Basel) 2019;9(6):385.

82. Schermann H, Eiges N, Sabag A, et al. Estimation of dog-bite risk and related morbidity among personnel working with military dogs. J Spec Oper Med 2017;17(3):51–4.

83. Yin S. Low stress handling® restraint and behavior modification of dogs & cats. Davis, CA: Cattledog Publishing; 2009.

84. Corse T, Firth C, Burke J, et al. Operation canine lifeline: recommendations for enhancing prehospital care for government working dogs. Disaster Med Public Health Prep 2017;11(1):15–20.

85. Wright KM. Equal Treatment for Man's Bets Friends, . White Paper on police canine legislation. Boston: Suffolk University; 2020.

86. Hanel RM, Palmer L, Baker J, et al. Best practice recommendations for prehospital veterinary care of dogs and cats. J Vet Emerg Crit Care 2016;26(2):166–233.

87. Reeves LK, Mora AG, Field A, et al. Interventions performed on multipurpose military working dogs in the prehospital combat setting: a comprehensive case series report. J Spec Oper Med 2019;19(3):90–3.

88. Edwards TH, Scott LL, Gonyeau KE, et al. Comparison of military and civilian canine traumas. Abstracts from the ACVECC VetCOT Veterinary Trauma and Critical Care Conference 2019. J Vet Emerg Crit Care 2019;29:S2–50.

89. Vegas Comitre MD, Palmer LE, et al. Assessment of prehospital care in canine trauma patients presented to veterinary trauma centers (VTC). J Vet Emerg Crit Care, in press.

90. Palmer L. Language in current state EMS practice acts and statutes allowing for prehospital medical care to animals by EMS personnel without direct or indirect veterinary oversight. 2019. Available at: http://users.neo.registeredsite.com/1/2/1/13151121/assets/Prehospital_PreveterinaryCare_Legislation_Information_2020__Updated_Feb_2020.pdf. Accessed July 21, 2020.

91. Hogan CS, Nesbit CE. Air medical transportation of injured operational canines. Air Med J 2019;38(1):36–8.

92. Weir WB, Mitek AE, Smith M, et al. The Carle-Illinois (Urbana, Illinois USA) transport protocol for LEK9s: guidelines for emergency medical service providers. Prehosp Disaster Med 2019;34(4):422–7.

93. Mitek A, McMichael M, Weir W, et al. The Carle-Illinois (Urbana, Illinois USA) treatment protocol for law enforcement K9s: guidelines for emergency medical services. Prehosp Disaster Med 2019;34(4):428–37.

Assistance, Service, Emotional Support, and Therapy Dogs

Maureen A. McMichael, DVM, MEd[a,b,*],
Melissa Singletary, DVM, PhD[c]

KEYWORDS

• Guide dogs • PTSD dogs • Service canine • Assistance animal • K9

KEY POINTS

- Definitions regarding assistance, service, emotional support, and therapy dogs differ, and veterinarians should be familiar with the current definitions.
- Laws regarding assistance, service, emotional support, and therapy dogs differ and allow various levels of access depending on the dog, the location, and the current version of the law.
- Veterinarians need to understand and respect the important bond that occurs between the handler and the canine.
- Temporary or permanent loss of the canine will have a significant impact on the handler's life and may lead to financial losses due to lost work time.

INTRODUCTION

Estimates are that approximately 61 million adults in the United States (1 in 4) report some form of a disability.[1] The value of dogs and animals to assist persons with a disability is increasing in recognition and exploration. This is a broad area of working dogs subdivided into many specialties, not all of which are covered in this article. There are several definitions across organizations describing assistance dogs, service dogs, emotional support animals (ESA), and therapy dogs. Based on sources, these may vary slightly in their definitions and associated limitations. Some of the access or limitations will be defined separately by the Americans with Disabilities Act (ADA), the US Department of Housing and Urban Development (HUD) Fair Housing Act

[a] Emergency & Critical Care, Department of Clinical Sciences, College of Veterinary Medicine, Auburn University, Auburn, AL 36849, USA; [b] Carle-Illinois College of Medicine, University of Illinois; [c] Canine Performance Sciences Program, Department of Anatomy, Physiology, and Pharmacology, Auburn College of Veterinary Medicine, Auburn University, Auburn University College of Veterinary Medicine, 109 Greene Hall, Auburn, AL 36849, USA
* Corresponding author. Department of Clinical Sciences, College of Veterinary Medicine, Auburn University, Auburn, AL 36849.
E-mail address: mam0280@auburn.edu

Vet Clin Small Anim 51 (2021) 961–973
https://doi.org/10.1016/j.cvsm.2021.04.012
0195-5616/21/© 2021 Elsevier Inc. All rights reserved.
vetsmall.theclinics.com

(FHA), or the Department of Transportation (DOT) Air Carriers Access Act (ACAA). This collective category of working dogs is clouded in confusion regarding terminology and levels of public access and rights to access. Readers are encouraged to review Maureen A. McMichael and Martha Smith-Blackmore's article, "Current Rules and Regulations for Dogs Working in Assistance, Service and Support Roles," in this issue where the logistical and legal framework surrounding working dogs are discussed.

Collectively the category that these specialized animals fall under is rapidly expanding for application toward new areas of service. The focus extends beyond individuals with physical disabilities and impairments into medical, psychiatric, and emotional conditions. Although this article discusses dogs, there are a host of other species and inanimate objects that are also being used and explored.[2] This rapidly growing field increases the likelihood of general practitioners becoming engaged in support for medical care, which results in a need for veterinarians to generally understand the terminology, breeding, training, selection, and specific jobs and tasks of these animals. This understanding will improve client communication and outcomes for the patient.

TRAINING AND CERTIFICATION

Currently, there are no legal requirements for training or certification of assistance dogs, and the ADA does not specify any training standards for any category of service animal or ESA. However, independent organizations have set forth minimum standards on training and certification (through them) to help guide this growing field. These organizations aid in providing certification, registration, or establishing minimum training and behavior standards to assistance dogs to support access to public areas. The Assistance Dogs International (ADI), the International Association of Assistance Dog Partners (IAADP), and the International Guide Dog Federation (IGDF) have high standards for certification through their organizations and provide valuable assistance across the guide dog industry in quality control and standards. ADI is a volunteer membership organization that accredits service dog teams across North America. Multiple organizations are registered through ADI to provide certifications, including Canine Companions for Independence (CCI), Guide Dogs for the Blind, Guiding Eyes for The Blind, The Seeing Eye Inc., and Service Dogs for America.[3] In the 2019 ADI fact sheet, they reported 16,868 active service dogs accredited within North America representing 43% guide dogs, 5% hearing, and 52% service.[3] For Animal Assisted Intervention (AAI), there are organizations engaged in setting standards for animal selection and requirements, although these vary by organization.

DEFINITIONS
Assistance Animals

This is the broadest category as defined by various legislative bodies. It refers *to any animal that provides assistance or emotional support or performs tasks or work for a person with a disability*. It encompasses the categories of service animal and ESA and is not limited by species. Although both service dogs and ESA are included under assistance animal, there are clear distinctions. Service dogs are specifically trained to accomplish a task, whereas an ESA does not have a specific task or job, and their support is solely through their presence. Therapy dogs are similar to assistance dogs but distinct as well.

Service Animal

This category, as defined by title II and III of the ADA, was originally restricted to dogs but has been updated to include miniature horses.[4] These are the only 2 species currently covered under the ADA guidelines. This definition of a service animal requires that *the dog or miniature horse be trained to perform specific tasks or do specific work for the benefit of an individual with a recognized disability and the tasks or work must be directly related to the disability.* This definition includes disabilities of the physical (eg, seizures, wheelchair), sensory (eg, blindness, deafness), psychiatric (eg, posttraumatic stress disorder [PTSD]), and intellectual, or other mental health categories.[4] Under this definition, other species are not considered service animals.

Types of work or tasks that may be provided for by the service animal include, but are not limited to, navigation (eg, guide dog for visually impaired persons), interrupting a pattern of behavior (eg, placing paw on thigh to bring the person back into the present moment and interrupt a panic attack), alerting a person to sounds (eg, for hearing impaired persons), retrieving items (eg, medications, communication devices, etc.), and alert dogs (eg, alerting a person that blood sugar is low, allowing them to eat). A Psychiatric Service Dog (PSD) has been trained to perform tasks to assist individuals with disabilities to detect the onset of and lessen the effect of various psychiatric episodes. These tasks may include medication reminders, providing room searches or safety checks, turning on lights, interrupting patterns of self-mutilation by persons with dissociative identity disorders, and keeping disoriented individuals from danger. As the popularity of these dogs grows, the areas where they could be helpful expand.

Emotional Support Animal

An ESA is defined by various legislation (see Maureen A. McMichael and Martha Smith-Blackmores' article, "Current Rules and Regulations for Dogs Working in Assistance, Service and Support Roles," in this issue) as *"any species that provides physical, psychological and/or emotional support through companionship"*. Although the guidelines are not specific as to the species, this article focuses on canines that function as ESAs. The key differentiating factor that separates ESAs from other categories is that these dogs are not specifically trained to perform any task or work related to the disability. Dogs in this category provide their benefits mainly through companionship. An important distinction is that ESAs are not PSDs, which are trained to perform a specific task to mitigate psychiatric symptoms. For example, a PSD may detect the beginning stages of a panic attack in a person with PTSD and then attempt to interrupt the pattern, bringing the person back to the present (more on PTSD in the later section). PSDs are afforded protection under the ADA, whereas ESAs are not.

The benefits of having a companion dog approved as an ESA are mainly for housing. The Department of Housing and Urban Development (HUD) provides landlord guidelines under the Fair Housing Act (FHA) and allows landlords to require documentation from a qualified physician, psychiatrist, or other mental health practitioner for the person's specific disability and need for that species. A health professional must determine that the presence of the dog will be beneficial in some way (eg, easing anxiety, giving structure to the day, feeling a sense of connection, etc.). Previously, ESA dogs were allowed to fly, in cabin, free of charge under the Air Carrier Access Act (ACAA) but this is no longer the case.

ESAs have been shown to help mitigate symptoms associated with anxiety and depression and to improve general psychosocial health. Quantitative reports document benefits beyond those that an assistance dog is thought to provide, specifically benefits not associated with the specific task they are trained for, such as the aforementioned psychosocial benefits.[5–9] Studies report improvement shortly after receiving an assistance dog, in some cases by 3 months, on human quality of life.[10–12] ESAs along with PSDs have been shown to have an effect on their handler's use of health services.[13] In most cases the person had decreased use of services, and this was mainly seen in reduced suicide attempts and lowering of hospitalization needs and medication requirements. In some cases, use of health services went up, and this was due to increased ability to attend medical appointments.[13]

ESAs provide companionship, a sense of purpose, structure, comfort, and unconditional love. They make people feel less vulnerable, help them connect with others, and encourage them to exercise. Use of ESAs is increasing, as more people discover the incredible benefits afforded by these relationships.

Therapy Animal

A therapy animal (any species) is *controlled by the handler but working for the benefit of others*, as opposed to the service animals or ESAs that are for the benefit of the handler. There are umbrella terms animal-assisted activities (AAA), animal-assisted therapy, and AAI that are all somewhat interchangeable, and the definitions are not clearly distinct from each other. AAA may occur in a variety of settings including public schools, assisted living facilities, hospitals, airports, courts of law, and many others. The AAA can be for an individual (eg, as a companion for a child in court) or for groups (eg, to calm travelers at an airport). Therapy animals can enter the buildings where they "work" due to private arrangements, but they are not explicitly covered under the ADA for access to public buildings. A search for this category did not yield any other federal or state legislation that specifically allows therapy dogs access to the public places where they work.

Therapy animals are thought to provide numerous benefits including improvement in muscle strength and balance in older adults with activities that increase movement.[14] Decreases in fear and anxiety, improving mood and improving systemic health by lowering blood pressure and heart rate are also reported.[15] The benefits may be in part due to increased levels of oxytocin that have been shown to occur after physical touch with a friendly animal.[15,16] A systematic review of 7 studies looking at AAIs on wellness reported that all showed beneficial effects for depression, anxiety, addiction, trauma symptoms, behavior, communication, and social skills, particularly for autism spectrum disorders (ASD).[17–25] Improvement in sleep patterns and pain levels occur after AAI but sleep quality degenerated after the evaluation period ended in one study.[26–28]

Addition of a canine to the therapeutic regimen leads to improvements in a wide range of populations. Various beneficial effects were seen in children with ASD, children with attention-deficit hyperactivity disorder (ADHD), children with trauma, adults with trauma, adults with schizophrenia, adults with substance abuse, and women with breast cancer.[29–37] Some institutions allow AAI during end-of-life care, which can be calming for people during this transition.[38] A study in minimally responsive patients reported near-infrared spectroscopy results during 3 sessions with a live animal and 3 sessions with a mechanical toy.[39] All participants (including the healthy control group) showed elevated neural activity in the frontal cortex, which was stronger with the live animal than the mechanical toy. Most of the studies of AAI report positive outcomes that are either superior or equivalent to current treatment outcomes.[40–45]

The type of dog along with the nature of the engagement may have an impact on outcomes, although these are rarely considered. A mismatched team (eg, young puppy with elderly population) may affect the outcome. Using a gentle Collie was not as effective for depressed college students as using a puppy.[46] Future research should explore the implications of canine temperament and behavior in different populations.

It is essential to take the health and welfare of the dog into consideration, and it has been suggested that researchers follow guidelines for animal welfare.[47] In one study, researchers evaluated salivary cortisol every 2 weeks in shelter dogs that were transported to a prison for AAI.[48] Samples were collected in the kennel, after transportation and after the visits. There was a significant decrease in cortisol at the end of the AAI, suggesting a beneficial effect on the dogs. Cortisol increased after transportation in these dogs, and this deserves further consideration.

Feasibility, including financial, practical, physical, and cultural limitations of AAI is important to consider when designing these programs. Logistical (eg, who greets the handler-dog team, familiarize them with location, grant access, etc.) and training requirements for the handler-dog team as well as the humans at the institution place constraints on implementation of these programs. Veterinarians should be familiar with the Centers for Disease Control and Prevention (CDC) Guidelines for Environmental Infection Control for Animals in Health Care Facilities, which suggests that animals may serve as a reservoir for antibiotic-resistant organisms. They recommend service animals be screened for parasites, in good health and up to date on required vaccinations.[49]

Therapy dogs provide comfort and a calming presence that is much needed for the many groups seeking these visits. Dogs are in courtrooms (eg, to assist children testifying against a perpetrator), at hospice centers (eg, to comfort those in their last moments of life) and assisted living facilities. The desire and need for these special animals is increasing, and veterinarians play a crucial role in keeping these pets healthy to allow continued access to the facilities where they provide such valuable services.

SPECIFIC CONDITIONS
Posttraumatic Stress Disorder

PTSD is defined as avoidance, reexperiencing, negative alterations in cognition and mood, and hyperarousal.[50] The syndrome is becoming more prevalent with estimates of up to 23% of military personnel returning with a diagnosis since 9/11.[51] PTSD classically occurs after a traumatic event and is a growing concern in society at large, and in the military community especially. PTSD significantly diminishes quality of life, as the victim starts out avoiding specific and direct signals that are a reminder of the traumatic event. For instance, if an explosion was the triggering event the victim will start out by avoiding loud sounds that are similar (eg, fireworks show, war movies, etc.). Over time as the victim is exposed to more unexpected sounds that are similar (eg, car backfiring) they begin to avoid more exposures. The avoidance, as it widens, serves to shrink the world of the victim, and they may elect to remain indoors with very little social contact.

There are several treatment options to help mitigate the symptoms, but the dropout rates are high and none are thought to be curative. Demand for specially trained PSD for PTSD has skyrocketed partially due to low perceived stigma compared with other mental health treatments, and the waitlist can be years.[52,53] Although, there is no single regulating body, proposed standards suggest these dogs must be trained to perform tasks.[3] The specific tasks the dogs are trained on vary among providers.[54] Tasks that are often covered include alerting to and interrupting patterns of anxiety, waking the victim to interrupt nightmares, and standing behind the person to "watch their back." Use of a canine for PTSD could fall under service dog (covered by ADA) or ESA, depending on what assistance the dog is providing. For example, if a dog is trained to wake the victim up from nightmares and to interrupt the onset of a panic attack (eg, places a paw on the thigh as the victim is rubbing their leg and starting the cycle of panic), then it is considered a service dog and is covered under the ADA. On the other hand, if the dog is providing companionship and is not trained to do tasks it would be considered an ESA and not be afforded the protections associated with the ADA.

Several cross-sectional studies comparing PTSD symptoms in veterans with service dogs demonstrate a higher quality of life, better social functioning, lower PTSD symptoms, and better regulation of cortisol compared with veterans on the wait-list.[21,55,56] A study of post-9/11 veterans either with a service dog or waiting for one evaluated sourcing, requirements, and training. All dogs were provided by K9s for Warriors, an ADI-accredited nonprofit service dog provider[57] (K9s for Warriors, Ponte Vedra Beach, FL, USA). Dogs were acquired primarily from shelters and rescues and selected based on age, temperament, and size. K9s for Warriors requires that dogs be at least 50 pounds and 24 inches tall in order to serve as potential bracing for the veteran. Dogs were mostly Labrador Retrievers or Lab crosses and trained for 120 hours on basic obedience and specific PTSD-related tasks before placement.[57] The veteran and the K9 participate in a 3-week onsite training program just before placement and must pass certification tests to demonstrate appropriate control and behavior. Interestingly, this study found that the most important aspect for helping PTSD symptoms in veterans was having something to love and to feel loved in return, and this was considered more important than the trained tasks the dogs performed.[57]

Training methods, although not standardized, do have an impact on canine welfare.[58–60] Generally, providers use one or more of the following: positive reinforcement (reward), positive punishment (active punishment when behavior occurs such as tugging the leash), negative reinforcement (removal of an aversive stimulus such as releasing pressure on the collar), and negative punishment (removing rewards such as removing attention by ignoring the dog).[61] The methods chosen are critical in setting up the human-animal bond that will occur between the veteran and the dog. In addition, the handler's psychological status has been shown to have an impact on the canine. One study of handlers that were depressed or had PTSD reported the development of separation anxiety, aggression, and attention seeking in the dogs.[62] Men with moderate depression were 5 times more likely to use aversive training methods in their dogs compared with men without depression.[63] A study of post-9/11 veterans with service dogs found that more frequent use of punishment (positive punishment) was associated with higher levels of fear and less eye contact in the dogs.[61] In this study greater than 40% of vets reported their service dogs showed apparent anxiety or fear and 46% were anxious when alone. As dogs for PTSD become more popular, research into the welfare of dogs after placement and optimization of training methods to strengthen the human-animal bond will become essential.

Seizure Alert Dogs

Dogs can be trained to detect when a seizure is occurring and to provide various levels of protection (seizure response dog). The tasks a dog is specially trained to perform depend on the person's needs and can include standing guard over the person during a seizure or getting help.[64] Some dogs seem to be able to predict when a seizure is about to occur (seizure detection dog) and can then warn the person in advance to sit down or move to a safe place. This does not, however, seem to be a trainable task at this time and is not included in the training for seizure response.[64]

Autism Spectrum Disorder Dogs

Dogs trained to assist persons with ASD are called SSigDOG (sensory signal dogs or social signal dog), and they can alert the handler to distracting repetitive movements common among those with ASD and prevent the person from wandering into danger. Decreases in anxiety and outbursts are reported with use of dogs for children with ASD.[65]

Diabetic Alert Dogs

Diabetic alert dogs are trained on sweat samples from people with diabetes during either hyperglycemia or hypoglycemia. These samples are then used to train the dogs to alert the handler if one of these alterations in blood glucose occurs. Tasks include reminding the person to check their blood sugar or getting help if the person is unresponsive.[66]

There are numerous applications either in use or being studied that use the dog's inherent senses, intelligence, and their demeanor to assist humans with disabilities.

PROCUREMENT AND CLINICAL MANAGEMENT

The difference between service dogs and ESAs or therapy dogs highlight differences in methods of procurement. When specific training is not required, temperament and behavior will place a role in selection, but these dogs are pets much of the time and come from many breeds and sources. Typically, these are highly sociable dogs (https://petpartners.org). More skilled training demands drive the need for more specialized dogs and established breeding colonies. Breeding and production considerations are covered under Pamela S. Haney and Robyn R. Wilborn's article, "Breeding Program Management"; and Robyn R. Wilborn and Pamela S. Haney's article, "Production and Reproductive Management," in this issue. Maximizing reproductive techniques and managing behavioral and medical outcomes in selection to improve the success of the overall litter is essential. The selection process for phenotypic characteristics that a production colony will focus on for breeding and successful field placement will vary from those considered most ideal for other work dog groups, and behavioral variations between working dog categories are discussed in Lucia Lazarowski and colleagues' article, "Development and Training for Working Dogs," in this issue. Behavior and temperament are important considerations for this highly public category of working dogs, as many are provided additional levels of access to public spaces not commonly available to pet dogs. For the handler/owner and the public, these dogs should not be selected if they exhibit disruptive or disturbing behaviors such as aggression or excessive barking.

Medical management starts with preventative care, and veterinarians working with therapy dogs or ESAs should familiarize themselves with the CDC guidelines for animals in health care facilities.[49] The foundational considerations for preventative health care can be found in more detail in Marcella Ridgway's article, "Preventative Health Care for Working Dogs," in this issue. The public access provided requires careful consideration to address diseases of zoonotic concern with both prophylactic measures and when diagnosis and treatment require important handler education. The importance of the dog's sensory capabilities for their ability to work and perform is discussed in Melissa Singletary and Lucia Lazarowski's article, "Canine Special Senses: Considerations in Olfaction, Vision and Audition," in this issue. General cognition is also of key importance in assistance dogs and recognition of medications that may cause temporary impairment require consideration for limited use, a well-communicated limitation of use with handler, and a return-to-work plan. Examples of medications may include analgesics, some antihistamines, seizure medications, and antianxiety medications. The critical nature of the role these animals may play for an individual highlights the need to minimize any impacts on performance and minimize the time out of work and educate the handler on adverse signs and symptoms that may require an adjustment to a treatment plan.

Communication with the client/handler may require an accommodation such as additional methods or use of technology. Taking the time to establish a clear method of communication is important for both the handler and the at-home care and welfare of the assistance dog. Guide and service dog clients may use additional methods to communicate and respectful inquiry as to what communication method they would prefer is helpful. Using language that is "people first" and explaining any personal limitations with communication options as well as asking the client for tips can be useful. Examples can be found through a resource designed for health care, Communicating with People with Disabilities.[67]

It is common for service and guide dogs to be trained to respond to cues for when to be "on-duty" and when "off-duty," such as putting on or taking off their vest or harness. When the equipment is on, the animals should be respected as on duty, and distractions (eg, petting, feeding, or providing attention) should be limited so they can focus on their task. Active engagement with the handler throughout the examination and completion of procedures should be offered. Treats are commonly used as motivation in training, and the handler may have preference to provide the reward for good behaviors in the clinic themselves rather than the clinic staff. If cleared by the handler for staff to reward, the treats themselves may need to be from the handler's supply. Appreciation for common conditions in pet dogs that can be significant disruptors for the role service and guide dogs play in daily routines are important. Ear infections for example, common to pet dogs, can serve as a distraction and impair hearing. Many training programs provide assistance and instruction to the handler during initial training on ear care and regular cleanings along with body condition assessment techniques for routine health monitoring that can be useful information to communicate with the veterinary team (https://www.guidedogs.com/explore-resources/alumni-resources/). Service and guide dogs may present with a head collar used for training. These do not impede normal function of jaw movement as opposed to muzzles commonly used in other working dog specialties such as operational canines.

Animal on animal attacks are not uncommon in pet populations. However, there are additional considerations when these occur on a dog guide or service dog (https://www.guidedogs.com/explore-resources/general-information/dog-attacks-on-guide-dogs).

Dog guides may be considered an extension of the handler, as their senses are being used to augment the person's. The close relationship that is established between a handler and their dog guide makes these incidents challenging to navigate, and the immediate loss of that animal to assist the individual along with the emotional distress must be considered. Training facilities and guide dog programs are working to address dog attacks in their foundational training and providing support through financial assistance and counseling programs (https://www.guidedogs.com/explore-resources/general-information/, https://www.gdb-official.com). Some programs encourage establishing veterinary partners, and many states have enacted dog guide protection laws, although this is not uniform and what is covered varies by state. It is recommended to be familiar with state laws and local programs/training facilities in the area that may have resources for the handler. The Animal Legal and Historical Center, Michigan State University College of Law (https://www.animallaw.info/topic/table-state-assistance-animal-laws) maintains an up-to-date Website on all aspects of animal law and is a vital resource for veterinarian.

When presented with a traumatic injury involving a dog guide or service animal, such as a dog attack, consideration of the additional needs the handler may have, along with frequent communication, is essential, as the temporary (or permanent) loss of their dog may place the handler at higher risk for experiencing significant levels of grief.[68]

Having an appreciation for the resource that dogs play in assistance and service promotes respect for the unique bond between the handler and dog, resulting in a pro-active approach to preventative care and medical management and minimizing time out of service or impacts on performance when treatments are necessary. Taking a dog out of service has significant implications for many working dogs, which can impede independence and mobility, and result in disruption of daily routines and lost wages of the handler.[69] Numerous studies have physiologically and behaviorally evaluated the relationship between handlers and their dog guides demonstrating a unique bond.[70–72] Specialty areas for service and assistance dogs are continuing to grow, as their capabilities and applications are adapted to fill needs in the everyday lives of individuals. The impact, both physically and psychologically, that these ani-mals have on the quality of life for millions of people is incredible and the role that vet-erinarians can play in supporting their work is critical.

CLINICS CARE POINTS

- Familiarization with the crucial bond between a service dog and their handler is an essential component of excellent care for the canine.
- A knowledge of the equipment and the essential tasks that a service dog provides will help veterinarians care for these dogs.
- Veterinarians should be familiar with national, state, and local laws regarding service dogs as well as the CDC guidelines for therapy dogs.

DISCLOSURE

The authors report no conflicts of interest. This document represents current rules and regulations as of the time of this writing. Local, state, and national legislation changes frequently, and veterinarians are advised to remain up to date on the changes by accessing real-time data via individual or collective Websites mentioned in this article.

REFERENCES

1. Okoro CA, Hollis ND, Cyrus AC, et al. Prevalence of disabilities and health care access by disability status and type among adults— United States, 2016. MMWR Morb Mortal Wkly Rep 2018;67:882–7.
2. Liang A, Piroth I, Robinson H, et al. A pilot randomized trial of a companion robot for people with dementia living in the community. J Am Med Dir Assoc 2017; 18(10):871–8.
3. Assistance Dogs International. ADI Fact Sheet 2019. Available at: https://assistancedogsinternational.org. Which one to follow? Service animal policy in the United States; Emily R.ZierMPA, PhD. Accessed December 1, 2020.
4. Code of Federal Regulations 28 C.F.R. §§ 35.104; 36.104 "Americans with Disabil-ities Act Title III Regulations" Department of Justice, Sep 15 2010, p33. Accessed December 1, 2020.
5. Barker SB, Wolen AR. The benefits of human-companion animal interaction: A re-view. J Vet Med Educ 2008;35(4):487–95.
6. Matuyszek S. Animal facilitated therapy in various patient populations: System-atic literature review. Holist Nurs Pract 2010;24(4):187–203.

7. Modlin SJ. Service dogs as interventions: State of the science. Rehabil Nurs 2000;25(6):212–9.

8. Sachs-Ericsson N, Hansen NK, Fitzgerald S. Benefits of assistance dogs: a review. Rehabil Psycology 2002;47(3):251.

9. Winkle M, Crowe TK, Hendrix I. Service dogs and people with physical disabilities partnerships: A systematic review. Occup Ther Int 2012;19(1):54–66.

10. Guest CM, Collis GM, McNicholas J. Hearing dogs: a longitudinal study of social and psychological effects on deaf and hard of hearing recipients. J Deaf Stud Educ 2006;11(2):252–61.

11. Allen K, Blascovich J. the value of service dogs for people with severe ambulatory disabilities. A randomized controlled trial. JAMA 1996;275(13):1001–6.

12. Vincent C, Gagnon DH, Dumont F. Pain, fatigue, function and participation among long term manual wheelchair users partnered with a mobility service dog. Disabil Rehabil Assistive Technol 2017;1–10. https://doi.org/10.1080/17483107.2017.1401127.

13. Lloyd J, Johnston L, Lewis J. Psychiatric Assistance Dog use for people living with mental health disorders. Front Vet Sci 2019;6:166.

14. Grubbs B, Artese A, Schmitt K, et al. A pilot study to assess the feasibility of group exercise and animal assisted therapy in older adults. J Aging Phys activity 2016;24(2):322–31.

15. Beetz A, Uvnas-Moberg K, Julius H, et al. Psychosocial and psychophysiological effects of human animal interactions: the possible role of oxygocin. Front Psychol 2012;3:234.

16. Jones MG, Rice SM, Cotton SM. Incorporating animal assisted therapy inmental health treatments for adolescents: a systematic review of canine assisted psychotherapy. PLoS One 2019;14(1):e0210761.

17. Julius H, Beetz A, Kotrschal K, et al. Attachment to Pets: An integrative review of human-animal relationships with implications for therapeutic practice. Cambridge (MA): Hogrefe; 2013.

18. Kamioka H, Okada S, Tsutani P, et al. Effectiveness of animal assisted therapy: a systematic review of randomized controlled trials. Complement Ther Med 2014;22☺2:371–90.

19. Maujean A, Pepping CA, Kendall E. A systematic review of randomized controlled trials of animal assisted therapy on psychosocial outcomes. Antrozoos 2015;28(1):23–36.

20. Nimer J, Lundahl B. Animal Assisted therapy: a meta-analysis. Antrozoos 2007;20(3):225–38.

21. O'Haire ME, Guerin NA, KirkHam AC. Animal assisted intervention for trauma: a systematic literature review. Front Psychol 2015;6:1121.

22. Germain SM, Wilkie KD, Milcourne VMK, et al. Animal Assisted psychotherapy and trauma: a meta-analysis. Anthrozoos 2018;31(2):141–64.

23. Hoagwood KE, Acri M, Morrissey M, et al. Animal assisted for youth with or at risk of mental health problems: a systematic review. Appl Dev Sci 2017;21(1):1–13.

24. Souter MA, Miller MD. Do animal assisted activities effectively treat depression? A Meta-analysis. Anthrozoos 2007;20(2):167–80.

25. Cherniack EP, Cherniack AR. The benefit of pets and animal assisted therapy to the health of older individuals. Curr Gerontol Geriatr Res 2014. https://doi.org/10.1155/2014/623203.

26. Chitic V, Rusu AS, Szamoskozi S. the effects of animal assisted therapy on communication and social skills; a meta-analysis. Transylvanian J Psychol 2012;13(1):1–17.

27. Zaw CC, Ahmad NB, Hohd MM. the effect and benefits of pet facilitated therapy in the elderly. Scholars J Appl Med Sci 2017;5(12C):4954–60.
28. Thodburg K, Sorensen LU, Videbech PB, et al. Behavioral responses of nursing home residnets to visit from a person with a dog, a robot seal or a toy cat. Anthrozoos 2016;29(1):107–21.
29. Becker JL, Rogers EC, Burrows B. animal assisted social skills training for children with autism spectrum disorders. Anthrozoos 2017;30(2):307–26.
30. Schuck SE, Emmerson NA, Fine AH, et al. Canine assited therapy for children with ADHD; preliminary findings from the positive assertive cooperative kids study. J Atten Disord 2015;19(2):125–37.
31. Signal T, Taylor N, Prentice K, et al. Going to the dogs; a quasi experimental assessment of animal assisted therapy for children who have experienced abuse. Appl Dev schience 2016;21(2):81–93.
32. Hunt M, Chizkov R. Are therapy dogs like Xanax? Does animal assisted therapy impact processes relevant to cognitive behavioral psychotherapy. Anthrozoos 2014;27(3):457–69.
33. Nathans-Barel I, Feldman P, Berger B, et al. Animal Assisted therapy ameliorates anhedonia in schizophrenia patients. Psychotherapy and psychosomatics 2005; 74:31–5.
34. Calvo P, Foruny JR, Guzman S, et al. Animal Assisted therapy program as a useful adjusnct to conventional psychosocial rehabilitation for patients with schizophrenia. Front Psycol 2016;7:631.
35. Wesley MC, Minatrea NB, Watson JC. Animal Assisted therapy in the treatment of substance dependence. Anthrozoos 2009;22(2):137–48.
36. Marr CA, French L, Thomson D, et al. Animal Assisted therapy in psychiatric rehabilitation. Anthrozoos 2000;13(1):43–7.
37. White JH, Quinn M, Garland S, et al. Animal assited therapy and counseling support for women with breast cancer; an exploration of patient's perceptions. Integr Cancer Ther 2015;14(5):460–7.
38. Kumasaka T, Masu H, Kataoka M, et al. Changes in patient mood through animal assisted activities in a palliative care unit. Int Med J 2012;19(4):373–7.
39. Arnskotter W, Marcar VL, Wolf M, et al. Animal presence modulates frontal brain activity in patients in a minimally conscious state: A pilot study. Neuropsychol Rehabil 2021;18:1–13.
40. Lubbe C, Scholtz S. The application of animal assisted therapy in the South African context. A case study. South Afr J Psychol 2013;43(1):116–29.
41. Stefanini MC, Martino A, Allori P, et al. The use of animal assisted therapy in adolescents with acute mental disorders: a randomized controlled clinical study. Complement therapies Clin Pract 2016;21(1):42–6.
42. Stefanini MC, Martino A, Bacci B, et al. The effect of animal assisted therapy on emotional and behavioral symptoms in children and adolescents hospitalized for acute mental disorders. Eur J Integr Med 2016;8(2):81–8.
43. Hartwig EK. Buidling solutions in youth: evaluation of the human animal resilience therapy intervention. J Creativity Ment Health 2017;12(4):468–81.
44. Hamama L, Hamama-Raz Y, Dagan K, et al. A preliminary study of group intervention along with basic canine training among traumatized teenagers: a 3 month longitudinal study. Child Youth Serv Rev 2011;33(10):1975–80.
45. Lange AM, Cox JA, Bernert DJ, et al. Is Counseling Going to the Dogs? An exploratory study related to the inclusion of an animal in group counseling with adolescents. J Creativity Ment Health 2007;2(2):17–31.

46. Fine AH, Beck AM, Ng Z. The state of animal assisted interventions: addressing the contemporary issues that will shape the future. Int J Environ Res Public Health 2019;16(2):3997.
47. Folse E, Minder C, Aycock M, et al. Animal assisted therapy and depression in adult college students. Anthrozoos 1994;7(3):188–94.
48. D'Angelo D, d'Ingeo S, Ciani Fm, et al. Cortisol levels of shelter dogs in animal assisted interventions in a prison: an exploratory study. Animals 2021;11(2):345.
49. Centers for Disease Control and Prevention. Guidelines for environmental infection control in health care facilities. 2019. Available at: https://cdc.gov/infectioncontrol/pdf/guidelines/environmental-guidelines-P.pdf. Accessed December 1, 2020.
50. American Psychiatric Association. Diagnostic and statistical manual of mental disorders: DSM-V. 5th edition. Washington, DC: American Psychiatric Association; 2013. https://doi.org/10.1176/appi.books.9780890425596. Accessed December 1, 2020.
51. Fulton JJ, Calhoun PS, Wagner HR, et al. The prevalence of PTSD in Operation Enduring Freedom/Operation Iraqi Freedom (OEF/OIF) veterans; a meta-analysis. J Anxiety Disord 2015;31:98–107.
52. Walther S, Yamamoto M, Thigpen AP, et al. Asistance dogs: historic pattern androles ofdogs placed by aDI or igDF accredited facilities and by non-accredited US facilities. Front Vet Sci 2017;4:1.
53. Walther S, Yamamoto M, Thigpen AP, et al. Geographic availability of assistance dogs; dogs placed in 2013-14 by ADI or IGDF-accredited or candidate facilities in the United States and Canada and non-accredited US facilities. Front Vet Sci 2019;6:349.
54. Vincent C, Gagnon DH, Dumont F, et al. Service dog schools for PTSD as a tertiary prevention modality; assessment based on assistance dogs international criteria and theoretical domains framework. Neurophysiol Rehabil 2019;2:29–41.
55. Yarborough BJH, Ashli A, Owen sMith SP, et al. An observational study of service dogs for veterans with post traumatic stress disorder. Psychiatr Serv 2017;68:730–4.
56. Rodriguez KE, Bryce Cl, Granger DA, et al. The effect of a service dog on salivary cortisol awakening response in a military population with post traumatic stress disorder. Psychoneuroendocrinology 2018;98:202–10.
57. Rodriguez KE, Greer J, Yatchilla JK, et al. The effects of assistance dogs on psychosocial health and wellbeing; a systematic literature review. PLoS One 2020;15(12):e0243302.
58. Blackwell EJ, Twells C, Seawright A, et al. The relationship between training methods and the occurrence of behavior problems, as reported by owners, in a population of domestic dogs. J Vet Behav 2008;3:207–17.
59. Fernandez JG, Olsson IAS, Vieira de Castro AC. Do aversive based training methods actually compromise dog welfare? A literature review. Appl Anima Behv Sci 2017;196:1–12.
60. Hiby EF, Rooney NJ, Bradshaw JWS. Dog training methods; their use, effectiveness and interactions with behavior and welfare. Anim Welf 2004;13:63–70.
61. Lafollette MR, Rodriguez KE, Ogata N, et al. Military veterans and their PTSD service dogs: associations between training methods, PTSD severity, dog behavior, and the human animal bond. Frontiers in Veterinary Science 2019;6(23). https://doi.org/10.3389/fvets.2019.00023.
62. Hunt M, Otto CM, Serpell JA, et al. Interactions between handler well being and canine health and behavior in search and rescue teams. Antrozoos 2012;25:323–35.

63. Dodman NH, Brown DC, Serpell JA. Associations between owner personality and psychological status and the prevalence of canine behavior problems. PLoS One 2018;13:e0192846.
64. Brown SW, Godlstein LH. Can seizure alert dogs predict seizures? Epilepsy Res 2011;97:236–42.
65. Stace LB. Welcoming Max; increasing pediatric provider knowledge of service. Complement therapies Clin Pract 2016;24:57–66.
66. Hardin DS, Anderson W, Cater J. Does can be successfully trained to alert to hypoglycemia samples from patients with type I diabetes. Diabetes Ther 2015; 6(509):509–17.
67. Smeltzer SC, Mariani B, Meakim C. Villanova University College of Nursing teaching resources. 2017. Available at: http://www.nln.org/professional-development-programs/teaching-resources/ace-d/additional-resources/communicating-with-people-with-diabilities. Accessed December 1, 2020.
68. Olson P, Samco K, Brown-Leist E. Neurophysiological correlates of affiliative behavior between humans and dogs. Vet J 2002;165:296–301.
69. Bennett G. American Psychiatric Association. Diagnostic and statistical manual of mental disorders. 4th edition. Washington, DC: Author. Bennett, G.; 2001.
70. Fallani G, Prato PE, Valsecchi P. Guide dog attacked, not "just a dog fight. Casper J 2007;1:10.
71. Naderi S, Miklosi A, Doka A, et al. Co-operative interactions between blind persons and their dogs. Appl Anim Behav Sci 2001;74(1):59–80.
72. Odendaal J, Meintjes R. Neurophysiolical correlates of affiliative behavior between humans and dogs. Vet J 2003;165:296–301.

Herding Dogs

Marcella Ridgway, VMD, MS

KEYWORDS

- Sheepdog • Border collie • Canine • K9 • Agility

KEY POINTS

- Herding dogs control the movement of other animals, usually groups of domesticated farm animals.
- Selective breeding to enhance and stabilize traits has resulted in herding breeds possessing the skills and versatility to make them the preferred breeds across most dog occupations, including law enforcement, detection work, service/assistance, obedience, agility, and other performance sports.
- Handler monitoring and intervention is critical to keep dogs from literally working themselves to death, and veterinarians should take an active role in training handlers on the skills of detection.

INTRODUCTION

Herding dogs are used to control the movement of other animals, usually groups of domesticated farm animals. Herding and hunting, unlike other canine occupations, are done predominantly by dogs of breeds developed over centuries to millennia specifically for that purpose. Selective breeding to enhance and stabilize traits[1–3] such as athleticism, endurance, work ethic, problem solving, cooperative behaviors, handler responsiveness, and ability to work at distance has resulted in herding breeds highly developed to perform their specialized tasks (eg, border collies and sheepherding) but also possessing the skills and versatility to make them the preferred breeds across most dog occupations, including law enforcement, detection work, service/assistance, obedience, agility, and other performance sports (eg, border collies and agility) (**Fig. 1**). Working-level herding breed dogs are intense, high-drive dogs that will work despite severe illness or pain, thereby masking clues that they are ailing or the nature of their problem. It is therefore incumbent on the handler to be knowledgeable about each individual dog and to recognize subtle changes that might signal ill health. Handler monitoring and intervention is critical to keep dogs from literally working themselves to death, and veterinarians should take an active role in training handlers on the skills of detection. That said, these dogs spend substantial periods of time working at a distance and out of eyesight

College of Veterinary Medicine, University of Illinois, Urbana, IL 61802, USA
E-mail address: ridgway@illinois.edu

Vet Clin Small Anim 51 (2021) 975–984
https://doi.org/10.1016/j.cvsm.2021.04.013
0195-5616/21/© 2021 Elsevier Inc. All rights reserved.

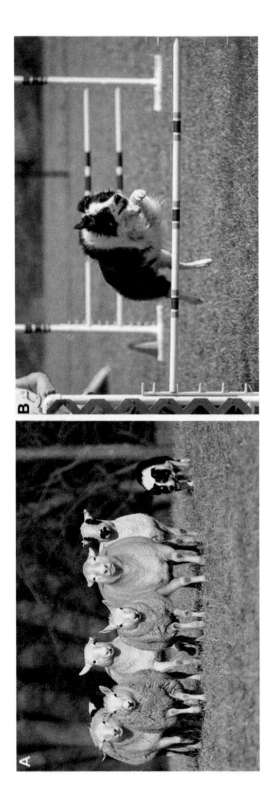

Fig. 1. A) Smooth-coated border collie working sheep. The border collie breed was developed specifically for herding and dominates in herding competitions as well as routine herding purposes (Photo by Dave Stone. Used by permission.); B) Border collie competing in agility. Although purpose-bred for herding, the breed traits of athleticism, speed, and ability to work at distance yet still respond quickly to cues from the handler make border collies an ideal breed for agility as well (Photo courtesy of Laurie Lobdell).

of their handler, so they may incur substantial exposure or injury that is not witnessed, further complicating health monitoring and accurate history acquisition.

Herding dogs typically work entirely outdoors in rural to wilderness environments with continuous exposure to other domestic animals and wildlife, infectious disease reservoirs and vectors, rugged terrain, and weather extremes. Many dogs live outdoors even when not working, further increasing exposure. Through sustained or repeated contact with other animal species and their habitats, these dogs may be affected by infectious diseases, including parasitic infections, not commonly seen in dogs. General principles for preventative care and health considerations for working dogs presented in Marcella Ridgway's article, "Preventative Health Care for Working Dogs," in this issue apply to herding dogs. Specific health concerns of herding dogs are addressed here.

HERDING DOGS

Herding dogs specialize in gathering and controlling the movement, direction, and speed of other animals and in sorting and partitioning particular individuals within a larger animal group in cooperative response to the guidance of their handler. The most commonly herded animals are sheep, goats, and cattle. When humans transitioned from hunting to farming cultures and domesticated farm species (11,000-7000 BC), their use of dogs transitioned in parallel.[4] Herding dogs likely developed from hunting dogs and retained many hunting dog characteristics. Some characteristics, such as prey drive, were modified through selective breeding to develop dogs ideal for managing domesticated stock rather than pursuing wild animals. In early references (pre-2900 BC) to shepherd's dogs, it is unclear if the reference is to guardian-type dogs (likely) or dogs that functioned as herders but use of dogs for herding was clearly already well established by the early 1570s. The most popular breeds for herding livestock are border collies, Australian cattle dogs, Australian kelpies, and Australian shepherds. Herded animals are usually much larger than the herding dog and are often hooved, sometimes horned. Dogs are used to maneuver stock into chutes or trailers, through confined spaces and paddocks, larger fields, and open spaces or a combination, with somewhat different skill sets necessary for each context. Depending on the size of the flock/herd and the expanse or complexity of the working context, dogs may work singly or collectively. Stock dogs have been estimated to provide their owners with a 5.2-fold return on investment over their working life with median age of 10 years at retirement.[5]

SPECIAL HEALTH CONSIDERATIONS IN HERDING DOGS

Canine health conditions associated with the occupation of herding have received limited investigation. Musculoskeletal problems, cutaneous injury, and dental trauma were the most common abnormalities in a study of 641 working New Zealand farm dogs[6]: only 6% of these dogs were spayed/neutered, 69% had been vaccinated, and 33% were insured. Husbandry and feeding practices can contribute to disease risk in herding dogs. In addition to working outdoors in close proximity to livestock and wildlife and over variable and difficult terrain, they usually spend nonworking hours outside in individual or group pens or tethered (only a small proportion of farm dogs live in the house with the handler),[7] further increasing exposure to environmental and vector-mediated diseases.

General: Breed-related differences in normal hematological and biochemical values should be considered when interpreting laboratory work.[8–11] Breed variations in drug metabolism and response arise from differences in genes encoding drug transporters and receptors. A well-characterized example is the ABCB1-1Δ (MDR-1) gene mutation, which is most prevalent in the herding breeds: Australian shepherds, collies, Shetland sheepdogs, and border collies are most commonly affected.[12-15] This gene encodes P-glycoprotein, a cell membrane pump that acts as a drug transporter for several pharmacologic agents used in veterinary medicine. P-glycoprotein is expressed in various tissues, including the intestine and brain capillary endothelium, and functions to limit drug absorption from the intestine, restrict drug entry into the central nervous system, and generally reduce accumulation of substrate drugs. Dogs heterozygous or homozygous for the mutation are more susceptible to toxicosis from substrate drugs, including ivermectin, milbemycin, selamectin, moxidectin, loperamide, acepromazine, vincristine, doxorubicin, and cyclosporine, and show suppression of the hypothalamic-pituitary-adrenal axis, making them potentially more susceptible to relative adrenal insufficiency under periods of stress.[16] This enhanced risk for adverse reactions to drugs should be considered when planning pharmacologic therapy, including heartworm prophylaxis, in herding breeds, although the low concentrations of drugs in commercial preventatives is safe.[17,18] Dogs can be tested for the ABCB1-1Δ mutation using a blood or cheek-swab sample.[a] Routine infectious disease screening appropriate for all regions in which the dogs live and work is vital in light of the heightened year-round exposure to outdoor environments and animal reservoirs. Comprehensive parasite control is important to counter increased exposure associated with working in areas where animals are concentrated as well as feeding practices in which dogs are fed raw animal products.

Hydration and Nutrition: nutritional needs of herding dogs have not been specifically evaluated, but energy and water requirements are expected to increase proportionally with total work and further increase with work in hot or, especially, cold conditions.[19] Working farm dogs are usually an appropriate or low Body Condition Scoring (see Debra L. Zoran's article, "Nutrition of Working Dogs: Feeding for Optimal Performance and Health," in this issue). Of 126 working farm dog owners in New Zealand,[6] 90% fed commercial dog foods, 83% fed some proportion of meat sourced on the farm (mostly livestock but also game), and 21% fed fresh meat. Cooking or freezing meat before feeding should be recommended to reduce transmission of parasites and other infectious organisms, which infected dogs may then transmit to other dogs, livestock, or humans.

Disease Considerations

Trauma: Musculoskeletal and skin injuries are the most common illnesses in working farm dogs.[6] Herding dogs work to control animals, usually in groups, that are much larger than the dog, may resist the dog's influence, perceive the dog as a threat, or may be protecting their young (**Fig. 2**). Dogs may sustain blunt, crush, or penetrating injury from being stomped, kicked, trampled, butted, or gored. Additional risks include injury from working through heavy brush; barbed and other wire, farm equipment and debris, encounters with wild animals, and musculoskeletal injury from exertion, uneven terrain, and quick turns. Handlers use topical products such as Tuf-Foot, Pad-Tough, or Musher's Secret to prevent and treat foot pad tears, which are common in dogs working rocky terrain. Gastrocnemius musculotendinopathy attributed to myotendinous strain was reported in a group of herding dogs; border collies made up 8 of the 9 affected dogs, possibly related to their naturally crouched working posture.[20] Outcomes for these dogs and for return to work in herding dogs treated

---

[a] MDR-1 testing at Washington State University WSU Veterinary Clinical Pharmacology Laboratory.

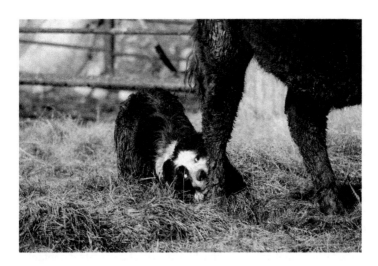

Fig. 2. Border collie working cattle. Herding dogs work animals that are 3-30 times larger than the dog and work in very close proximity to the animals, typically working groups of animals at a time, with obvious potential for injury to the dog (Photo courtesy of CKF Stock Dogs, Manitoba Canada. Used by permission)

surgically for humeral condylar fractures[21] and with pancarpal arthrodesis for carpal injuries[22] were good. Plant foreign bodies, particularly foxtail grass awns, are a concern across many regions.

Toxins: Working farm dogs are exposed to agricultural chemicals, drugs, and feed additives given to livestock including residues passed in urine and feces as well as rodenticides and other intentionally placed poisons aimed at control of pest animals. Herding dogs working in open ranges may encounter poison baits placed by landowners other than their own handlers. Secondary poisonings are possible through feeding of farm-origin meats containing toxic feed additives.[23]

Infectious disease: Herding dogs experience close, sustained exposure to the domestic animals they herd as well as other domestic species present on the same property and potentially sharing the same areas of confinement. Congregating groups of animals together in defined, frequented to permanent areas or enclosures, where feces, urine, and birthing tissues may be randomly deposited, allows high concentrations of infectious organisms to accrue with unrestricted opportunity for resident animals to be exposed. Although herding dogs may not interface with wildlife as much as hunting dogs, they encounter wildlife species such as coyotes, deer, and raccoons that share land used by domestic livestock. Infected dogs may be a source of transmission of disease to humans, other dogs, or other resident animals by shedding infectious disease agents, acting as fomites (feet, haircoat) or carrying insect vectors into proximity of others. Inconsistent preventative care (vaccination, parasite prophylaxis) for farm dogs and the common practice of feeding them raw meat exacerbates risk of infection and spread.[6,24] *Neospora caninum* is a significant protozoal pathogen in dogs (neurologic disease) and cattle (abortion, neurologic disease in calves) and occasionally sheep, goats, and camelids. Deer and moose are important intermediate hosts in sustaining a sylvatic cycle of infection.[25] Dogs and wild canids (coyotes, wolves, Australian dingoes) are the only known definitive hosts. Cattle become infected by ingestion of sporulated oocysts shed in feces of an infected definitive host (horizontal transmission) or by vertical (transplacental) transmission (most common). Dogs become infected initially by ingestion of tissues of an infected intermediate host (most common) or fecal transmission. Infection is then maintained in the dog population principally by transplacental transmission. Seropositivity to *Neospora* is higher in farm and hunting dogs than pet dogs[26–28]: dogs are exposed through feeding fresh meat from infected cattle or deer; eating or licking placentas, uterine discharge, or aborted fetuses from infected cattle; or interfacing with other intermediate hosts in the domestic or sylvatic cycles.[26,29,30] Dogs or incompletely cooked meats can be a source of transmission to humans: humans seroconvert to *N caninum* but its potential to cause zoonotic disease is unclear. *Brucella abortus* (another agent of bovine abortion), *Brucella melitensis*, and *Brucella ovis* can infect dogs in contact with cattle and small ruminants. Infected dogs are then a source of transmission to uninfected livestock and humans.[31–33] Farm dogs are at increased risk for leptospirosis and often show seropositivity to the *Leptospira interrogans* serovar for which the primary reservoir host is the farm animal species with which the dog has greatest contact.[34–36] Farm dogs associating with cattle, sheep, or goats may become infected with *Coxiella burnetii* (bacterial agent of Q fever), especially if exposed to the placenta, aborted fetus, or other birth fluids or tissues from infected livestock: parturition triggers shedding of high numbers of organisms.[37–39] Transmission also occurs via feces, urine, milk, or tissues of an infected animal; contaminated fomites; aerosolization of infected material; and transmission by ticks, fleas, and lice. Coxiellosis, a zoonotic disease, may be subclinical, cause reproductive abnormalities, or may present as acute febrile illness with lethargy, anorexia, and neurologic signs in dogs. Farm dogs are at increased risk not only from contact with livestock but also through increased exposure to ticks and other reservoir species and through the practice of being fed raw meat.[40] Dogs may transmit infection to humans directly or by carrying infected ticks into proximity to humans. Farm dogs have an increased exposure to other vector-borne diseases, including ehrlichiosis, anaplasmosis, borreliosis, babesiosis, hepatozoonosis, bartonellosis, and coinfections with multiple vector-borne agents,[41,42] due to prolonged periods spent outdoors compounded by inconsistent use of preventative medications.[6] Herding breed dogs were more than twice as likely to be seropositive for *Bartonella* spp. antibodies than other breed groups in northern California,[43] possibly because of increased exposure to disease vectors. Ticks were found on 108/113 sheep herding dogs in a German study.[44] Endoparasitism is common in farm/herding dogs with 26% to 46% of studied dogs testing positive for one or more parasites including zoonotic parasite species.[44–49] Canine echinococcosis is of tremendous significance in herding dogs because of the zoonotic potential of *Echinococcus* spp., which cause severe disease (cystic echinococcosis/hydatid disease and alveolar echinococcosis) in infected humans, and the important role that farm dogs play in transmission. *Echinococcus granulosus*, the cause of cystic echinococcosis, occurs worldwide, especially in grazing areas. *Echinococcus multilocularis,* the cause of alveolar echinococcosis, is also widely dispersed in regions north of the equator. Adult tapeworms live in the intestine of the definitive host (canids: *E granulosus*, *E multilocularis*, *Echinococcus vogelii*; cats: *E multilocularis*), which are usually asymptomatic although diarrhea and, rarely, cystic or alveolar echinococcosis may occur. Eggs shed in feces of the definitive host are ingested by intermediate hosts (sheep, cattle, horses, rodents), and hatch and penetrate the intestine wall and then distribute to various tissues, especially liver and lung, where they form thick-walled hydatid cysts. Dogs become infected by ingesting cyst-containing tissues of infected intermediate hosts. Humans are aberrant intermediate hosts exposed by ingestion of eggs, usually from dog feces. The occupation of herding brings dogs, humans, and intermediate hosts into close proximity and is a significant risk factor for human echinococcosis.[50–54] Prevention in dogs includes routine fecal testing, appropriate anthelmintic use, and discontinuing feeding raw meat. *Echinococcus* vaccines are available for sheep and cattle. Proper hygiene and care when handling dogs or dog feces are critical for preventing transmission to humans. *Heterobilharzia americanum*, a trematode "blood fluke" and causative agent of canine schistosomiasis, is widespread across the southern and east central United States, especially prevalent along the Gulf Coast: in a study of 238 affected Texas dogs, herding dogs (breed group, not occupational group) made up the largest number of cases referable to a specific breed type.[55] Canids and raccoons are the definitive hosts for the parasite, which have an indirect life cycle with an aquatic snail intermediate host. Dogs are infected by water-borne cercaria, released from infected snails, which penetrate the dog's skin while the dog is swimming or otherwise in contact with contaminated water. Cercaria migrate through the lungs to the liver where they mature, then migrate through portal veins to mesenteric veins where they reproduce and deposit ova. Ova penetrate mesenteric vessels and the intestinal mucosa, inducing an intense granulomatous inflammatory response, to enter the intestinal lumen and pass in the feces: if exposed to fresh water, these ova hatch to release miracidia, which can infect the snail intermediate. Some ova may lodge in the dog's liver, pancreas, or lymph nodes, inciting severe inflammation in those tissues. Clinical presentation is generally that of gastrointestinal (GI) disease (diarrhea, vomiting, anorexia, weight loss, and hematochezia) that may progress to protein-losing enteropathy; hypercalcemia, hepatic disease, pancreatic insufficiency, and collapse may also occur. Infection can be treated with praziquantel or fenbendazole but, in many cases, *Heterobilharzia* infection is not considered as a differential, so infections go undiagnosed.

Other disease considerations: Dogs that herd fiber-producing animals may ingest enough wool from gripping the animals during herding activities or from picking up shorn or shed fibers to cause GI obstruction. Herding competitions and training seminars introduce additional health concerns in bringing together dogs from multiple different farms, risking spread of infectious diseases present in one home farm environment to other dogs and subsequently other farms. At these events, water tubs are usually available that are shared by all dogs for whole-body cooling: this can facilitate transmission of disease organisms that survive in water or wet areas around the tub (leptospirosis, giardiasis). Disease transmission through these events is fortunately uncommon. Participating dogs may travel and compete in environments to which they may not be acclimated (elevation, heat) and develop related health problems, especially because competition herding requires periods of intense activity. Herding dogs that eat manure may be exposed to medications and feed additives administered to livestock species as well as infectious organisms.

CLINICS CARE POINTS

- Herding dog breeds have the skills and versatility to make them the preferred breeds across most dog occupations, including law enforcement, detection work, service/assistance, obedience, agility, and other performance sports
- Because of their high drive and strong work ethic, handler monitoring and intervention are critical to keep dogs from overwork and exhaustion.
- Veterinarians should take an active role in training handler's physical examination skills to be able to detect problems before they become critical.

- Because of work environment (eg, entirely outdoors in rural to wilderness environments) and exposure (exposure to other domestic animals and wildlife) they may be exposed to musculoskeletal trauma, cutaneous injuries, and dental trauma as well as toxin exposure, infectious diseases, and parasitic infections.

DISCLOSURE

The author declares no conflicts of interest.

REFERENCES

1. Spady TC, Ostrander EA. Canine behavioral genetics: pointing out the phenotypes and herding up the genes. Am J Hum Genet 2008;82:10–8.
2. Konno A, Romero T, Inoue-Murayama M, et al. Dog breed differences in visual communication with humans. PLoS One 2016. https://doi.org/10.1371/journal.pone.0164760.
3. Arons CA, Shoemaker WJ. The distribution of catecholamines and β-endorphin in the brains of three behaviorally distinct breeds of dogs and their F1 hybrids. Brain Res 1992;594:31–9.
4. Clutton-Brock J. Man-made dogs. Science 1977;197(4311):1340–2.
5. Arnott ER, Early JB, Wade CM, et al. Estimating the economic value of Australian stock herding dogs. Anim Welf 2014;23:189–97.
6. Isaksen KE, Linney L, Williamson H, et al. TeamMate: a longitudinal study of New Zealand working farm dogs. I. Methods, population characteristics and health on enrolment. BMC Vet Res 2020;16:59–76.
7. Arnott ER, Early JB, Wade CM, et al. Environmental factors associated with success rates of Australian stock herding dogs. PLoS One 2014;9(8):e104447.
8. Greenfield CL, Messick JB, Solter PF, et al. Results of hematologic analyses and prevalence of physiologic leukopenia in Belgian Tervuren. J Am Vet Med Assoc 2000;216(6):866–71.
9. Ruggerone B, Giraldi M, Paltrinieri S, et al. Hematologic and biochemical reference intervals in Shetland Sheepdogs. Vet Clin Pathol 2018;47(4):617–24.
10. Chang YM, Hadox E, Szladovits B, et al. Serum biochemical phenotypes in the domestic dog. PLoS One 2016;11(2):e0149650.
11. Lawrence J, Chang YM, Szladovits B, et al. Breed-specific hematological phenotypes in the dog: a natural resource for the genetic dissection of hematological parameters in a mammalian species. PLoS One 2013;8(11):e81288.
12. Mealey KL, Munyard KA, Bentjen SA. Frequency of the mutant MDR1 allele associated with multidrug sensitivity in a sample of herding breed dogs living in Australia. Vet Parasitol 2005;131(3–4):193–6.
13. Mealey KL, Meurs KM. Breed distribution of the ABCB1-1Δ (multidrug sensitivity) polymorphism among dogs undergoing ABCB1 genotyping. JAVMA 2008;233:921–4.
14. Gramer I, Leidolf R, Doring B, et al. Breed distribution of the nt230(del4) MDR1 mutation in dogs. Vet J 2011;189:67–71.
15. Soussa RW, Woodward A, Marty M, et al. Breed is associated with the ABCB1-1Δ mutation in Australian dogs. Vet J 2020;98(3):79–83.
16. Mealey KL, Gay JM, Martin LG, et al. Comparison of the hypothalamic-pituitary-adrenal axis in MDR-1-1Δ and MDR1 wildtype dogs. J Vet Emerg Crit Care 2007;17:61–6.

17. Mealey KL. Canine ABCB1 and macrocyclic lactones: heartworm prevention and pharmacogenetics. Vet Parasitol 2008;158:215–22.
18. Geyer J, Janko C. Treatment of MDR1 mutant dogs with macrocyclic lactones. Curr Pharm Biotechnol 2012;13(6):969–86.
19. Stephens Brown L, Davis M. Water requirements of canine athletes during multi-day exercise. J Vet Intern Med 2018;32:1149–54.
20. Stahl C, Wacker C, Weber U, et al. MRI features of gastrocnemius musculotendinopathy in herding dogs. Vet Radiol Ultrasound 2010;51(4):380–5.
21. Nortje J, Bruce WJ, Worth AJ. Surgical repair of humeral condylar fracture in New Zealand working farm dogs – long-term outcome and owner satisfaction. N Z Vet J 2015;63(2):110–6.
22. Jerram RM, Walker AM, Worth AJ, et al. Prospective evaluation of pancarpal arthrodesis for carpl injuries in working dogs in New Zealand, using dorsal hybrid plating. N Z Vet J 2009;57(6):331–7.
23. Espino L, Suarez ML, Mino N, et al. Suspected lasalocid poisoning in three dogs. Vet Hum Toxicol 2003;45(5):241–2.
24. Kardjadj M, Yahiaoui F, Ben-Mahdi M-H. Incidence of human dog-mediated zoonoses and demographic characteristics/vaccination coverage of the domestic dog population in Algeria. Rev Sci Tech 2019;38(3):809–21.
25. Gondim LFP, McAllister MM, Mateus-Pinella NE, et al. Transmission of Neospora caninum between wild and domestic animals. J Parasitol 2004;90(6):1361–5.
26. Hornok S, Edelkofer R, Fok E, et al. Canine neosporosis in Hungary: screening for seroconversion of household, herding and stray dogs. Vet Parasitol 2006;137:197–201.
27. Collantes-Fernandez E, Gomez-Bautista M, Miro G, et al. Seroprevalence and risk factors associated with Neospora caninum infection in different dog populations in Spain. Vet Parasitol 2008;152:148–51.
28. Arunvipas P, Inpankaew T, Jittapalapong S. Risk factors of Neospora caninum infection in dogs and cats in dairy farms in Western Thailand. Trop Anim Health Prod 2012;44(5):1117–21.
29. Dijkstra T, Barkema HW, Eysker M, et al. Natural transmission routes of Neospora caninum between farm dogs and cattle. Vet Parasitol 2002;105:99–104.
30. Gharekhani J, Yakhchali M. Neospora caninum infection in dairy farms with history of abortion in West of Iran. Vet Anim Sci 2019;8:100071.
31. Baek BK, Lim CW, Rahman MS, et al. Brucella abortus infection in indigenous Korean dogs. Can J Vet Res 2003;67(4):312–4.
32. Mortola E, Miceli GS, Meyer LP. Brucella abortus in dog population: an underestimated zoonotic disease. BJSTR 2019;15:11266–8.
33. Forbes LB. Brucella abortus infection in 14 farm dogs. J Am Vet Med Assoc 1990;196(6):911–6.
34. Ward MP, Glickman LT, Guptill LF. Prevalence of and risk factors for leptospirosis among dogs in the United States and Canada: 677 cases (1970-1998). J Am Vet Med Assoc 2002;220(1):53–8.
35. Lee HS, Guptill L, Johnson AJ, et al. Signalment changes in canine leptospirosis between 1970 and 2009. J Vet Intern Med 2014;28:294–9.
36. Adesiyun AA, Hull-Jackson C, Mootoo N, et al. Sero-epidemiology of canine leptospirosis in Trinidad: serovars, implications for vaccination and public health. J Vet Med 2006;53:91–9.
37. Capuano F, Parisi A, Cafiero MA, et al. Coxiella burnetii: what is the reality? Parassitologia 2004;46(1–2):131–4.

38. Ma GC, Norris JM, Mathews KO, et al. New insights on the epidemiology of *Coxiella burnetii* in pet dogs and cats from New South Wales, Australia. Acta Trop 2020;205:105416.

39. Shapiro AJ, Norris JM, Heller J, et al. Seroprevalence of *Coxiella burnetii* in Australian dogs. Zoonoses Public Health 2016;63(6):458–66.

40. Shapiro A, Bosward K, Mathews K, et al. Molecular detection of *Coxiella burnetii* in raw meat intended for pet consumption. Zoonoses Public Health 2020;67(4): 443–52.

41. Gizzarelli M, Manzillo VF, Ciuca L, et al. Simultaneous detection of parasitic vector borne diseases: a robust cross-sectional survey in hunting, stray and sheep dogs in a Mediterranean area. Front Vet Sci 2019. https://doi.org/10.3389/fvets.2019. 00288.

42. Hornok S, Tanczos B, Fernandez de Mera IG, et al. High prevalence of *Hepatozoon*-infection among shepherd dogs in a region considered to be free of *Rhipicephalus sanguineus*. Vet Parasitol 2013;196:189–93.

43. Henn JB, Liu C-H, Kasten RW, et al. Seroprevalence of antibodies against *Bartonella* species and evaluation of risk factors associated with seropositivity in dogs. Am J Vet Res 2005;66(4):688–94.

44. Rehbein S, Kaulfuss K, Vissar M, et al. Parasites of sheep herding dogs in central Germany. Berl Munch Tierartzl Wochenschr 2016;129(1–2):56–64.

45. O'Connell A, Scott I, Cogger N, et al. Parasitic nematode and protozoa status of working sheepdogs on the North Island of New Zealand. Animals 2019;9:94–105.

46. Frey CF, Regotz J, Rosenberg G, et al. Uberblick uber intestinale Parasiten bei Herdenschutzhunden und Hutehunden in der Schweiz. Schweiz Arch Tierheilk 2010;152(12):569–73.

47. Papazahariadou M, Founta A, Papadopoulos E, et al. Gastrointestinal parasites of shepherd and hunting dogs in the Serres Prefecture, Northern Greece. Vet Parasitol 2007;148:170–3.

48. Michalczyk M, Sokol R, Galecki R. Internal parasites infecting dogs in rural areas. Ann Parasitol 2019;65(2):151–8.

49. Edwards GT, Hackett F, Herbert IV. *Taenia hydatigena* and *Taenia multiceps* infections in Snowdonia, U.K. I. Farm dogs as definitive hosts. Br Vet J 1979;135(5): 426–32.

50. Baldock FC, Thompson RC, Kumaratilake LM, et al. *Echinococcus granulosus* in farm dogs and dingoes in south eastern Queensland. Aust Vet J 1985;62(10): 335–7.

51. Yuan R, Wu H, Zeng H, et al. Prevalence of and risk factors for cystic echinococcosis among herding families in five provinces in western China: a cross-sectional study. Oncotarget 2017;8(53):91568–76.

52. Merino V, Westgard CM, Bayer AM, et al. Knowledge, attitudes, and practices regarding cystic echinococcosis and sheep herding in Peru: a mixed-methods approach. BMC Vet Res 2017;13(1):213–22.

53. Conrath FJ, Probst C, Possenti A, et al. Potential risk factors associated with human alveolar echinococcosis: systemic review and meta-analysis. Plos Negl Trop Dis 2017;11(7):e0005801.

54. Hao L, Yang A, Yuan D, et al. Detection of *Echinococcus multilocularis* in domestic dogs of Shiqu County in the summer herding. Parasitol Res 2018;117:1965–8.

55. Rodriguez JY, Lewis BC, Snowden KF. Distribution and characterization of *Heterobilharzia americana* in dogs in Texas. Vet Parasitol 2014;203:35–42.

Moving?

Make sure your subscription moves with you!

To notify us of your new address, find your **Clinics Account Number** (located on your mailing label above your name), and contact customer service at:

Email: journalscustomerservice-usa@elsevier.com

800-654-2452 (subscribers in the U.S. & Canada)
314-447-8871 (subscribers outside of the U.S. & Canada)

Fax number: 314-447-8029

Elsevier Health Sciences Division
Subscription Customer Service
3251 Riverport Lane
Maryland Heights, MO 63043

*To ensure uninterrupted delivery of your subscription, please notify us at least 4 weeks in advance of move.